GOING**HIGHER**

Oxygen, Man, and Mountains

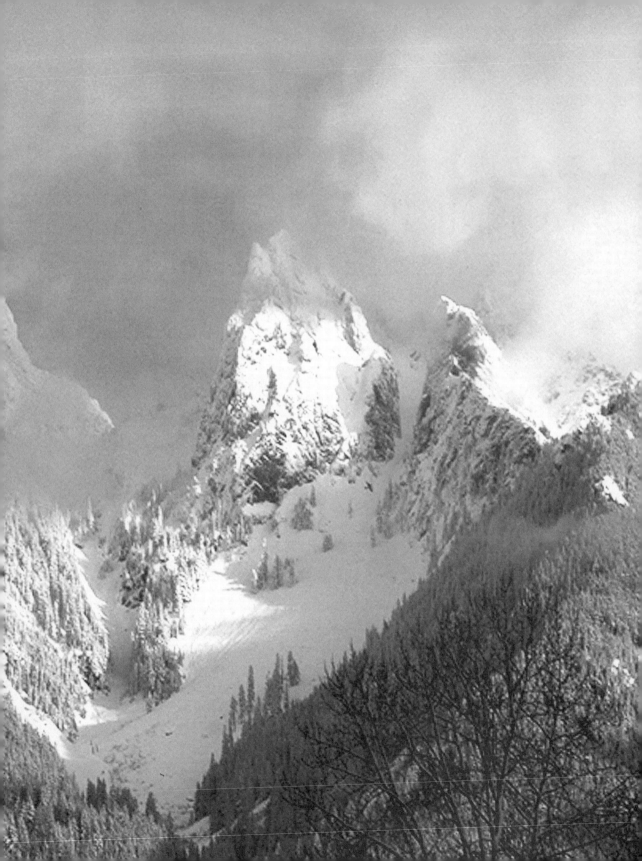

GOING**HIGHER**

Oxygen, Man, and Mountains

Charles S. Houston, M.D.
David E. Harris, Ph.D.
Ellen J. Zeman, Ph.D.

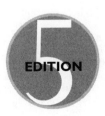

THE MOUNTAINEERS BOOKS

THE MOUNTAINEERS BOOKS
is the nonprofit publishing arm of The Mountaineers Club, an organization founded in 1906 and dedicated to the exploration, preservation, and enjoyment of outdoor and wilderness areas.

1001 SW Klickitat Way, Suite 201, Seattle, WA 98134

© 2005 by Charles S. Houston, M.D., David E. Harris, Ph.D., and Ellen J. Zeman, Ph.D.

Fifth edition, 2005

First published in 1980 as *Going Higher: The Story of Man and Altitude*. Revised 1983, 1987, 1998, 2005.

Published simultaneously in Great Britain by Cordee, 3a DeMontfort Street, Leicester, England, LE1 7HD

Manufactured in the United States of America

Project Editor: Kathleen Cubley
Copy Editor: Uma Kukathas
Cover and Book Design: Kristy Thompson
Layout Artist: Marge Mueller, Gray Mouse Graphics
Illustrations: Gary Nelson, except as noted

Cover photographs: Top: © Gordon Wiltsie; bottom and back cover: © Bill Stevenson/Outdoorpics

THE MOUNTAINEERS, founded in 1906, is a nonprofit outdoor activity and conservation club, whose mission is "to explore, study, preserve, and enjoy the natural beauty of the outdoors . . . ." The club sponsors many classes and year-round outdoor activities in the Pacific Northwest, and supports environmental causes through educational activities, sponsoring legislation and presenting educational programs. The Mountaineers Books supports the club's mission by publishing travel and natural history guides, instructional texts, and works on conservation and history.

Library of Congress Cataloging-in-Publication Data
Houston, Charles S.
 Going higher : oxygen, man, and mountains / Charles S. Houston, David E. Harris, Ellen J. Zeman.— 5th ed.
  p. ; cm.
 Includes bibliographical references and index.
 ISBN 0-89886-631-6 (pb.)
 1. Mountaineering—Physiological aspects. 2. Altitude, Influence of.
 [DNLM: 1. Altitude Sickness—physiopathology. 2. Adaptation, Physiological. 3. Mountaineering—physiology. 4. Oxygen—physiology. WD 715 H842g 2005] I. Harris, David E. II. Zeman, E. J. III. Title.

RC1220.M6H68 2005
616.9'893—dc22

                2005005840

♻ Printed on recycled paper

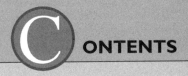
CONTENTS

LIST OF ILLUSTRATIONS

LIST OF TABLES

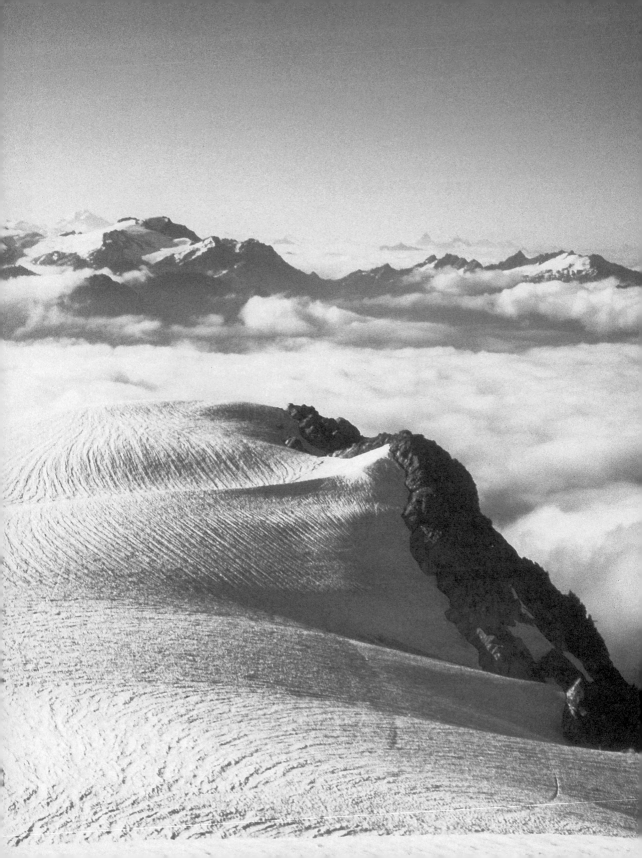

PREFACE

The motivation for the fifth edition of this book is essentially the same as for the first edition, written twenty-five years ago. As a physician, I was interested in decreasing the incidence of illness and death among travelers to the mountains, and as a scientist I was curious about *why* people got sick in the mountains. There was added urgency because, with the beginning of the Golden Age of Himalayan climbing in the mid-twentieth century and the ascent of Annapurna, greater numbers of people were thronging to the high peaks, and more were paying a fearsome price. In addition, modern transportation had begun to penetrate into ever more remote areas, so that travelers also began to travel too high, too fast, and too easily. One hundred and fifty years ago the Alps went through a similar Golden Age when thousands of people went climbing, when increasing numbers of travelers climbed to heights they would not have considered attempting before.

But the unprepared adventurers who go to the high mountains are not alone in being victims of mountain sickness. Skiers, hikers, and trekkers who go from sea level to even the low mountains, where thousands of resorts have sprung up, are also at risk. And modern science has kept alive many people with diseases that cripple their ability to obtain enough life-giving oxygen.

The causes of mountain sickness were fairly well recognized by the beginning of the nineteenth century, but the physiology was yet to be defined. Intriguing questions begged answers. There was the possibility that healthy individuals going to a low-oxygen environment might teach us something to help individuals made sick by disease or injury that prevented adequate respiration at or near sea level.

I began work on the fifth edition of *Going Higher* to clarify many of the new discoveries and ideas that have appeared in the last decade. But as I was partway along the road, my vision began to fail. The revision of this book would have died had it not been for the generous and adept help of Ellen Zeman and David Harris, who became my colleagues and to whom the book owes most of its quality. David—a physiologist, climber, and teacher—wrote new material on genetics, cell biology, and physiology. Ellen—a hiker, science writer, and editor—helped research, reorganize, and rewrite many sections of the book. Her patience and meticulous attention to detail, plus her determination to "get the job done," made this new edition possible. I hope and believe that this collaboration was as happy for my coauthors as it was for me, and that the result is a much better book than if I had tried to finish by myself.

I have had many friends and helpers. In addition to Ellen and David, I want to particularly thank several others: Tom Hornbein, Browney Shaney, Peter Hackett, Ray Huey, Jessica Panko, Lorna Moore, Jennifer Jordan, Norman Alpert, Natalie Powell, and my secretary, Jenny Larrabee. All helped me through some difficult times. It has been a rewarding experience.

We wanted a book that would be highly readable, enjoyable, and informative for the novice, the inquisitive amateur climber, and the physician. Writing for a broad audience is rather tricky, and we have tried to keep the information as simple as possible. However, where it is desirable to be more deeply engaged we have included some quite technical information that might challenge, but nevertheless intrigue, the novice.

It is exciting to watch new techniques being applied to old problems, and to see new ideas developing as these problems are solved. Life really should be a never-ending journey of discovery—of the world around us and of the world within. We inhabit a miraculously intricate external environment, but also an even more exciting environment we call the body. It is my hope that this book will inspire not only those who love mountains, but also those who wish to understand and to cherish the world around us. May such journeys never end.

Charles S. Houston, M.D., M.A.C.P., 2004

ABOUT THIS BOOK

This book contains contributions from three authors. However, the book truly belongs to its original author, Charles Houston. Most of the words are his, and furthermore, it is his experience, insight, and philosophy that provide the heart, soul, and spirit of the entire text. In creating this new edition, the authors have made every effort to retain and follow Dr. Houston's voice. His personal experiences in mountaineering, medicine, and research all are told in the first person, and designated by italic text.

The fifth edition contains more biology than the previous edition and is organized more coherently around high-altitude physiology. As was the case with the previous edition, this book is divided into four parts, each with several chapters. Part I deals with the atmosphere around us and our forebears' gradual realization of its weight and ubiquity. Oxygen is a small but essential component of air, and so these chapters trace how we have come to learn that oxygen is indispensable for life, not only for humans, but for nearly every living organism.

Part II deals with how the human body obtains, moves, and uses oxygen. Chapter 3 describes how we draw in and exhale air and where oxygen goes in our body. Respiration is inseparable from circulation (detailed in Chapter 4), and the two are intertwined in both their histories and functions. Moving air and moving blood serve several purposes, but the most important is to provide food and fuel to the cells. The third chapter of Part II, Chapter 5, summarizes how the living cell—the secret of life itself—works.

Part III addresses the main topic of this book: mountain sickness. Here too the history (Chapter 6) is fascinating and important. Primarily, however, we discuss mountain sickness in relation to our understanding of normal respiration and circulation. First we describe the most frequent forms of mountain sickness and what we know about their pathophysiology. Then we look at some of the less common but important problems due to lack of oxygen at altitude. The last—but in some ways most interesting—part of this section is a brief look at how we might become short of oxygen in our everyday lives. This is a large subject related to mountain sickness, and one that leaves much to be explored.

In Part IV we cover the processes by which our bodies "learn" to survive the gradual onset of a lack of oxygen (which, if it occurred rapidly, would be fatal). Acclimatization (Chapter 13) saves us not only on mountains but, wonderfully, during gradually developing lung and heart conditions that threaten our oxygen supply. The lives of those who summit the highest mountains depend on acclimatization. Yet to be explored are the ways in which genetics might confer advantage in one becoming acclimatized to the high-altitude environment (Chapter 14). We include here the latest understanding of the prevention and treatment of mountain sicknesses (Chapter 15) as well as the limits to human performance at high altitude (Chapter 17, which includes the unresolved issues of training for athletic competition and differences—where they exist—between gender and age groups). Chapter 18 deals with the question of who can, and who should not, go to high altitude and the important subject of environmental hazards other than hypoxia that threaten mountaineers at great altitude.

A glossary of medical and scientific terms is found at the back of the book, to make the denser, more technical material easier to grasp. For those with a special interest in the past, we include an appendix that contains brief biographies of some of the most important—and sometimes least known—people who brought us the knowledge we have today.

Some readers may want to explore the medical facts and theories more deeply, so we include a list of helpful books and articles for further reading. Some of the works cited in the bibliography are sources for the excerpts found throughout the book. The World Wide Web provides a more complete and ever-growing source of information on high-altitude medicine and physiology. Unfortunately, quite a bit of it is inaccurate, incomplete, or totally misleading. After you've read this book, you will be better able, we hope, to sort out the good from the bad advice about high altitude.

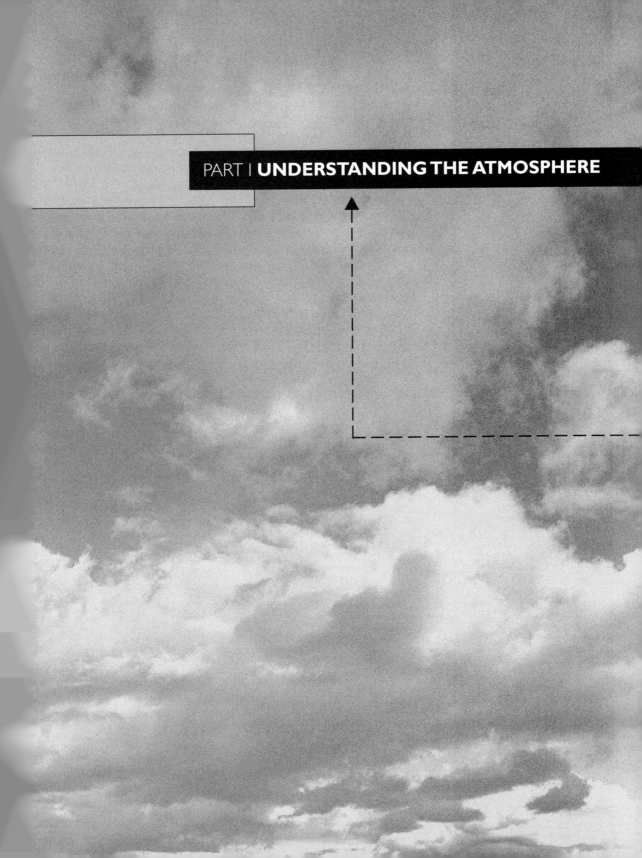

PART I **UNDERSTANDING THE ATMOSPHERE**

CHAPTER 1

THE AIR ABOUT US

In October 1950 Bill Tilman and I stood on Kala Pattar and looked into the West Cwm and up to the dark summit of Everest—the first Westerners to have crossed Nepal from India and to have seen the great southern wall of Lhotse, Nuptse, and Everest. The whole Khumbu Valley and most of the country to the southern border between Nepal and India had not yet been touched by tourism and climbers. That year was the beginning of the Golden Age of Himalayan mountaineering, a century after a similar debut in the European Alps. We wondered then about what the future might bring to this sheltered land; even today the answer to that question is ambiguous.

In May 1996 the tragedy unfolding high on Mount Everest was followed with shocked fascination by millions of people around the world.

During that ten-day period, more than eighty-eight men and women from several countries and their Sherpas were somewhere on the mountain. Of these, forty were caught in a furious storm near the top of Mount Everest, on the "ordinary" route. Eight had reached the summit and were on their way down, a few were still pushing toward the top but were tired and moving slowly, while others had halted, delayed by the slowly moving crowd at the crux of the final climb, or too exhausted to go on. Around midnight on May 10, most had reached safety in their high camp, but some were missing. During the night, two rescuers (one a doctor) made desperate rescue sorties and found two of the missing; both were unconscious and covered with ice; both were barely breathing. In the black, stormy night the exhausted rescuers decided that the two were too near death to be saved, and they did not have strength to carry them down. Six hours later one of them, a male pathologist, staggered into camp; next day they found the other, a small woman, dead where the rescuers had found her. Four others had also died higher up. Twelve died during the first part of May, eight in the furious storm.

This was not the first, nor is it likely to be the last, high-mountain tragedy. In fact Everest 1996 was eerily like an equally bad disaster ten years before on K2, the second-highest mountain in the world.

In the summer of 1986, eighty men and women from twelve countries attempted K2 on different routes. By August 10, twenty-seven had reached the summit and thirteen had died, many while descending the "ordinary" route, the Abruzzi Ridge. The worst of the awfulness played out between August 2 and 10 when, despite worsening weather, some had pushed on toward the summit and were lost near the top when a severe storm struck. Other parties had changed their plans, leading them to use the tents and supplies of others. When those descending climbers, already exhausted, tried to find refuge in their own already overcrowded tents, some were refused. At this point, language barriers led to major misunderstandings, and differences in philosophy or ethics arose. It was bitterly cold, shelter was inadequate, food and drink were scarce, and what little togetherness there had been in a crowd of mostly strangers disappeared. Some started down and survived, but others fell. Most of those who decided to wait for better weather died. In the end, five of the seven who had occupied the ill-fated camp were dead.

In 1986 there were no satellites sending instant news and live photographs from K2 around the world. No celebrities or journalists phoned or faxed news while other climbers struggled for their lives. The full story of K2 1986 was slow to reach the public, and the shock was muted.

As one reads the often conflicting reports about K2, it seems incredible that the same terrible mistakes of 1986 would be repeated on Everest only a decade later. Even given the competitive force that drives climbers and the overwhelming impact of the high-mountain environment, perhaps these tragedies need not be inevitable. But history shows they will be repeated too many times by those who climb for motives other than the love of mountains.

At an earlier time, when big-time Himalayan mountaineering was in its infancy, nine men died when national pride led an expedition to ignore the basics.

In 1934 a party of ten elite German climbers and thirty Sherpas were high on Nanga Parbat (26,100 feet). Their supply line was overextended when a major storm came on them, dumping 8 feet of snow in six days. As their supplies and strength dwindled, climbers tried to get down to safety as best each one could. They struggled through the immense snow alone or in pairs. When the storm finally ended, three German climbers and six Sherpas had died of exhaustion. Two Sherpas, who might have made it to safety, had opted to stay with their sahibs and died with them. Far from acknowledging the awful disaster, the returning climbers were greeted in Germany as national heroes.

The causes of these and other lesser-known tragedies, although complex, were mainly the lack of oxygen in the atmosphere at high altitudes. We call this *hypoxia*, or, less accurately, *anoxia* or *anoxemia*. Its subtle impact has caused many deaths not only on mountains but near sea level, too. We have learned about oxygen and its absence slowly over centuries.

Looking to the sky on a clear day, it is easy to understand why our distant ancestors were puzzled by what could be out there. At night they saw tiny lights and a large one that moved and changed; in daylight the sun also moved and changed. But what and where were these objects, and what, if anything, surrounded them?

Sometimes clouds and fog, rain or snow, and wind could be seen and felt, but how did these natural phenomena relate to the invisible, impalpable, tasteless stuff they breathed and without which they could not live? On clear days they could see forever into the void—and wonder. Today science can tell us a thousand things about the atmosphere in which we live, but our forebears could only look and speculate.

Two thousand years ago, the Chinese recognized that an uninterrupted supply of "good" air was necessary to support most life. During the age of the Pharaohs, Egyptian physicians described the pathways through which air entered and left the chest. The Greco–Roman philosopher–scientists, building on these beliefs, taught that the purpose of breathing was to cool the "innate heat" of the heart.

In the fifth century B.C., Anaximenes of Miletus proposed that *aer* was an invisible spirit that was sometimes manifested when it condensed into water vapor or mist. He saw this as a divine and universal living spirit. As the ancients had, he suggested that this invisible stuff sustains the soul that animates life, and introduced the name *pneuma* for it. Erasistratus later expanded this concept to found the Pneumatic school. A few centuries later the word *pneuma* was being used for the mixture of air and blood that sustained life and was found in both arteries and veins.

The term *klepsydra* is commonly used to describe an ancient "waterclock," but it was also the name of a device for collecting a small amount of liquid from a large container. The great experimentalist Empedocles in the fifth century B.C. apparently saw something more in a *klepsydra* (see Figure 1). Inadvertently or not, he showed that a vacuum could exist—a concept that was, and would be for centuries, contrary to accepted beliefs. His little experiment led him to state that air had weight and therefore substance. Thus he laid the groundwork for understanding the atmosphere.

Aristotle, who lived and taught in the fourth century B.C., and was one of the greatest of the philosopher–scientists, used observation and experience rather than theory to define what he saw about him. Looking toward the heavens, he could not conceive that space could be empty, because then it would have no dimensions. Light could not penetrate a space that did not exist and therefore could not be visible through a vacuum—but he could see the distant stars and therefore space was not a vacuum. Thus he differed with Empedocles about the nature of air even while agreeing that "In its

The Klepsydra

History does not tell us just what mathematician, explorer, and inventor Empedocles had in mind when he used this curious jar almost 500 years before the Christian era. But whatever his purpose, he did in fact show that the atmosphere had weight. He showed that when the vessel, with one small hole in the top (the view on the right in Figure 1) and several small holes in the bottom (the view on the left), was held under water with the hole in the top closed, water could not enter until the top was opened. Conversely, once the vessel was filled and the top closed, when he held it in air, water would not flow out—because, as we now recognize, the weight of the air prevented a vacuum from being formed in the jar. This did not persuade doubters until a more impressive demonstration was done 2,000 years later by Gaspar Berti.

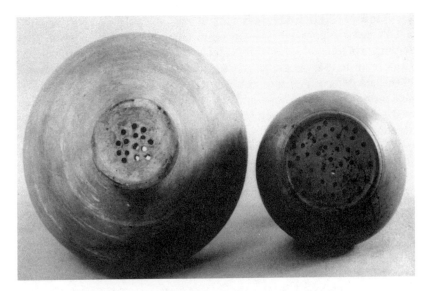

Figure 1. *The* klepsydra: *bottom of vessel* (left); *top of vessel* (right)

own place, every body has weight except fire, even air.... It is proof of this that an inflated bladder weighs more than an empty one."

A century later, Strato(n) of Lampsacus theorized that everything—solids, liquids, gases, even light rays—consisted of particles separated by "void," and the heavier the substance, the less "void" it contained. He showed that a "void" could be produced by sucking air out of a closed container, and thus took another step toward the concept of a vacuum.

During the next few centuries, philosophers of the Pneumatic school advanced more theories, but with little or no experimental evidence.

Another school, the "Atomists," came very close to describing the atomic theory we know today.

To us, swept along in the frantic expansion of knowledge, it seems strange that it took our ancestors so many centuries to understand such basics. But remember, only a few score scholars were involved, and their resources were limited. In fact it is really a marvel that they laid such a broad base for what we do know today.

Aristotle's writings pervaded European thought for 1,500 years. Many of his principles were accepted without question and slowly became fundamental to the religious doctrine of the time, which held that the universe was static and perfect. Aristotle had been vague about the possibility of a vacuum, but much later the Roman Catholic Church denied the existence of a vacuum, and all that this implied, even while conceding that if God wanted to create a vacuum, He could certainly do so. Those who differed were heretics.

THE NATURE OF AIR

These views prevailed for many centuries. In this worldview the universe was made of four elements—fire, water, earth, and air. Although the importance of air to life was recognized, its nature was unknown and debatable. In the late sixteenth century, as the Age of Enlightenment began, a remarkable series of new ideas blossomed like spring flowers after the long winter of the Dark Ages. A few short years opened the way for exciting studies of air and altitude.

A big step came when the vague idea suggested by Aristotle and Empedocles—that air had substance—was brilliantly restated in 1618 by a young student, Isaac Beeckman, who wrote in his doctoral thesis: "It happens that air, in the manner of water, presses upon things and compresses them according to the depth of the super-incumbent air." Beeckman and others opened new windows on the natural world. From his bold pronouncement it followed that air must be flexible and could be expanded, even far enough to create a vacuum.

This hypothesis put Beeckman in direct conflict with the Catholic Church and also with the distinguished Galileo Galilei, who accepted Aristotle's somewhat ambiguous position that air had weight, even while arguing that a vacuum could not exist. Beeckman persisted: Air did weigh something, and it was also elastic and compressible. His career suffered from this heresy, but he was twenty years ahead of a monumental experiment that would show his intuitive statement to be correct. Soon after Beeckman, others began to challenge the Church and Aristotle with direct experiments.

CREATION OF A VACUUM

One of the early challenges came from Giovanni Baliani, who made an experiment with a long flexible pipe or hose. When this hose was filled with

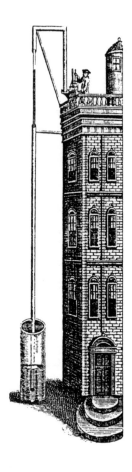

Figure 2A. *Gaspar Berti's barometer, ca. 1642*

water and extended from a tub of water over a small elevation, it created a siphon, drawing water from the higher end, sending it over the rise, and discharging it at the lower. But if the elevation was too high, the siphon failed and water simply ran out of each end. Baliani described this in a long letter to Galileo in 1630, implying that the weight of the air pushed the column of water up over the elevation in the hose, but could not do so if the slight elevation were too high. Galileo did not accept Baliani's explanation, which rested on the creation of a vacuum, because he still would not accept the idea that a vacuum could exist. Three months later, Baliani wrote again, clearly stating his agreement with Beeckman, and added, "The higher you go in the air, the lighter it is." He concluded that the siphon failure was due to the formation of a vacuum in the hose.

The first firm proof that air had weight came from a young Italian mathematician and astronomer, Gaspar Berti. Berti was modest and left little record of what he did or why, so we rely on his philosopher friend Emmanuel Maignan, who described the great experiment that Berti did in Rome between 1640 and 1642 (see Figure 2A), in the presence of a handful of friends, all scientists, all churchmen. They too wrote accounts, differing only slightly in details.

From his experiment (see sidebar, below), Berti concluded that there

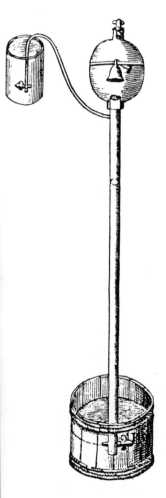

Figure 2B. *Robert Boyle's barometer, 1665*

The First Barometer

Gaspar Berti wanted to prove to Galileo that a vacuum could exist. He probably knew about Giovanni Baliani's demonstration (ca. 1630) of the limitations of a siphon, and planned his own experiment a decade later to prove Baliani right. He erected a long leaden pipe against the wall of his house and filled it with water. The pipe was closed by a stopcock at the bottom end, which was then immersed in a tub of water. The upper end was filled with water and closed with a stopcock, and the lower stopcock opened (see Figure 2A). Supported by the atmospheric pressure on the water in the tub, water in the pipe fell in the tube to a level some 34 feet above the level in the lower reservoir, leaving a vacuum at the top, which Berti demonstrated by closing the lower stopcock and opening the upper stopcock.

W. E. K. Middleton wrote a scholarly book, *The History of the Barometer*, about this first experiment, showing how Galileo's student Evangelista Torricelli recognized its importance and went on to make the barometer we know today, using mercury instead of water. Berti had made his point and went back to his mathematics, leaving credit for this great accomplishment to Torricelli. Robert Boyle, of London's newly formed Royal Society, quickly made a number of different models using glassware (see Figure 2B), and foresaw how useful the device might be in predicting weather.

must be a vacuum between the water and the upper sealed end of the tube, which was exactly what he hoped to show was present in order to convince Galileo of the existence of a vacuum. But, more importantly, Berti had made the first barometer!

Little publicity attended this epoch-making demonstration, but word soon reached physicist Evangelista Torricelli, a devoted student of Galileo's. He immediately recognized its importance and took the next great step: He substituted mercury for water, which reduced the necessary length of the tube from 34 feet to 40 inches. Mathematician René Descartes later added a scale—which converted the device into a measuring instrument.

THE BAROMETER

In a famous letter dated June 11, 1644, Torricelli took another step toward understanding altitude, referring to Berti's experiment:

> I have already hinted to you that some sort of philosophical experiment was being done concerning the vacuum; not simply to produce a vacuum, but to make an instrument which might show the changes in the air, now heavier and coarser, now lighter and more subtle... above the peaks of very high mountains air begins to be very pure, and of very much less weight... [than at sea level].

Torricelli went further in an experiment designed to determine the nature of the vacuum at the upper end of the tube: He placed a mouse in the lower reservoir of his barometer and allowed it to swim up through the mercury to the empty space. The mouse died, but it was not clear whether from struggling through the mercury or because of the vacuum at the top. He tried fish and butterflies and other animals, with little success. Others quickly made different models of his barometer and conducted many ingenious experiments.

Once he accepted the firm evidence of atmospheric pressure, Torricelli suggested that he might be able to observe (and perhaps predict) changes in weather, as Robert Boyle would do a few years later. He described the atmosphere, which he estimated might be 50 miles thick, in words almost identical to Beeckman's:

> We live submerged at the bottom of an ocean of elementary air which is known by incontestable experiments to have weight, and so much weight, that the heaviest part near the surface of the earth weighs about one four hundredth as much as water....

Torricelli's prestige along with his rapid-fire experiments and publications attracted notice among scientists, and very quickly an unseemly competition for recognition began. New players appeared, claiming to have had the idea first, or to have told Berti what to do. One, Viviani Magni, demonstrated the barometer in Poland, claiming it had been his idea in the first place.

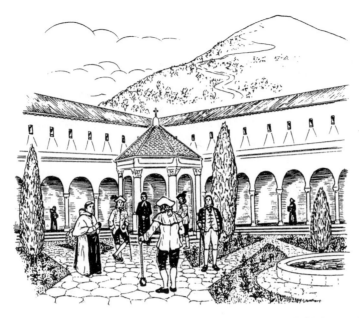

Figure 3. *Perier uses a Torricellian barometer*

National pride was at stake, and French scientists claimed the honor for the city of Rouen. The squabble spread to other countries; charges of forgery and falsification of documents flew back and forth. It was all unfortunately similar to the competition among some scientists today.

Still more evidence for understanding the effect of altitude was needed, solid proof that air was really thinner and weighed less on mountains, as Giovanni Baliani had hypothesized. Just who pressed for the definitive experiment remains unclear; it may have sprung from a demonstration of the barometer that was staged by physicists Pierre Petit and Blaise Pascal (who had a flair for the dramatic). Among the audience was Pascal's brother-in-law, Florin Perier.

A few years after Berti's experiment, Perier carried a Torricellian barometer up a small mountain, the Puy de Dôme, and, after carefully preparing his control observations at the foot of the mountain, showed that the mercury was lower on the summit (see Figure 3). The importance of this neat little project immediately prompted other claimants for priority, one of whom, already widely known, may have suggested the idea—but Perier did the necessary work before the others. Perhaps Perier realized that this was a great moment in the history of science, and his astonishment suggests that he really did not expect it—and his nicely designed experiment was quite unbiased! But whose idea was it?

Young Blaise Pascal, already a distinguished mathematician, claimed credit for the idea in a letter to Perier, the date of which has been challenged. Descartes might also have done so, and certainly the idea had been around for some time. Anonymous pamphlets were published, dates of documents

---

Air Weighs Less the Higher One Goes

On September 18, 1648, Florin Perier filled two Torricellian barometers with re-distilled mercury (to remove all air) and meticulously compared the readings in the courtyard of a monastery at the foot of a small mountain, the Puy de Dôme (3,500 feet). With him were several distinguished local citizens to attest to the experiment. Leaving a monk, Father Chastin, to record the readings at the monastery, the party carried one barometer up the path, pausing halfway up and again at the top to measure the height of the mercury. Between the readings at the bottom and the top of the mountain, Perier later wrote that "there was a difference of 3 inches and one and a half lines which ravished us all with admiration and astonishment and surprised us so much that for our own satisfaction we wished to repeat it"—which of course they did.

When they returned to the monastery, Father Chastin assured them that the level of the mercury had not changed, and indeed it showed the same as in the instrument brought back from the summit.

---

were altered; it was all quite nasty for several years, and the brouhaha has resurfaced now and then ever since. Only one fact is unquestioned: Florin Perier did the work.

Priority in science is a will-o'-the-wisp; few great ideas have sprung fully hatched from a single person, and all of us learn from the work of those who have gone before. As Lucan wrote at the start of the Christian era: "Even pygmies, placed on the shoulders of giants, can see further than the giants can." The exact sequence of events that occurred from 1640 to 1645, who did what when, and whose ideas inspired successive steps, are debatable and not terribly important. Torricelli gave us the mercury barometer by using Berti's demonstration, and his device, with many refinements, is the basic instrument we use today. It is quite fitting that his name should be remembered in the unit of pressure measurement—torr. But at the same time, let us honor and respect Gaspar Berti for his imaginative and almost forgotten experiment, and honor Florin Perier as well.

There it is in the span of one short decade—proof that a vacuum could exist, recognition of the weight of the atmosphere, and invention of a sensitive instrument with which to measure atmospheric pressure. Word of these experiments spread rapidly through Europe with amazing speed considering the famine, epidemics, and wars that plagued so much of the region.

THE ROYAL SOCIETY

In 1645 a small group of men soon to become imperishably famous, calling themselves "The Invisible College," met in London to discuss scientific subjects. Soon they were meeting regularly, and by 1660 the college was chartered as The Royal Society. They began studies of the atmosphere, recognizing that the experimental proof by Berti and Torricelli had established that air had weight and, equally important, that a vacuum could be produced with a new kind of pump.

Otto von Guericke, mayor of Magdeburg in Bavaria (later made baron), had built a pump with which he sucked water out of wine barrels, and found that the weight of the atmosphere caused these to collapse. In 1654, in a dramatic demonstration of atmospheric pressure, he fitted together two copper hemispheres, carefully made to be airtight, and then pumped the air out of the sphere. Then he showed that two teams of horses could not pull the hemispheres apart until the vacuum inside the sphere was released—because of the weight of the atmosphere.

Robert Boyle, a prime mover in the new Royal Society, asked his assistant Robert Hooke to improve on von Guericke's pump. Hooke was curator of the Society and charged with bringing to the meetings several new experiments each week.

The *Proceedings of the Royal Society of London* during an incredibly productive five years present a fascinating record of ingenious and imaginative experiments of many kinds. The Society heard tales from travelers and examined strange minerals, plants, and animals. They were an extraordinary group of scholars. Many of their experiments used the "New Pneumatical Engine" to examine all sorts of animals, snakes, insects, fish, and materials like wood and cork and rock in a vacuum.

One of the most significant glimpses into the future came when a mouse and a lighted candle were placed under a bell jar, which was then evacuated. Over and over again Hooke and Boyle found that the candle went out a short time before the mouse died. This led to the mistaken belief that life and combustion were fueled differently.

After many experiments on animals, plants, and nonliving materials, in December 1670 Hooke proposed to make a vessel large enough to hold a man, from which air could be extracted with his pump. There was some delay, but on February 2, 1671, Hooke reported in the *Proceedings of the Royal Society of London*:

> ...that the air-vessel for a man to fit in was ready. . . . Being asked how it was contrived, he said that it consisted of two tubs, one included in the other; the one to hold a man, the other filled with water thereby to keep it staunch; with tops to put on with cement, or to take off; one of them having a gage to see to what degree the air is rarefied; as also a cock to be turned by the person who sits in the vessel.

Finally Hooke entertained the members of the Society in his rooms to demonstrate the device. He entered the inner barrel, the outer one sealing it with water, and one-tenth of the air was extracted by his pump. This "took

The First Decompression Chamber

In 1654 Otto von Guericke's vacuum pump attracted immediate attention, and Fellows of the young Royal Society commissioned the curator, Robert Hooke, to build an improved model. After many years of experiments in the vacuum made possible by the pump, Hooke was asked to make a vessel large enough to hold a man (Figure 4). After some time, he described this to the Society, and in 1671 demonstrated its use in his home. Watched by several other members, he entered the barrel, an assistant operated the pump, and Hooke was "taken up" about 4,000 feet. Considering what had happened to animals under an evacuated bell jar, this was rather brave, and so far as we have found, the barrel was not used again.

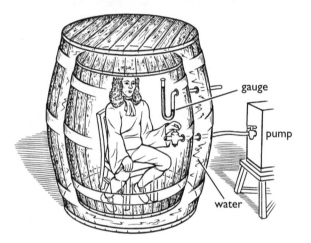

Figure 4. *Hooke's barrel*

him up" to about 4,000 feet, and he noticed no discomfort save for slight pressure in his ears when the experiment was ended. The first human study in a decompression chamber had been completed. It was a courageous experiment, in view of what had been learned from mice and other forms of life, and perhaps it is not surprising that there seems to be no record of its being repeated for a hundred years.

COMPOSITION OF AIR

By 1660 Boyle had repeated Berti's experiment and had made many types of Torricellian barometers. He knew all about the Perier/Torricelli experiment and probably had read descriptions of the symptoms suffered by Jesuit missionaries Father Alonzo Ovalde and Father Jose Acosta while crossing the high Andes (see Chapter 8, "The Spectrum of High-Altitude Illness: AMS/HACE"). He corresponded with many other travelers who had been on high mountains. All this confirmed Perier's observation that air was thinner the higher one went, but did little to answer the question of what substance in air was necessary for life or combustion. Boyle tried to explain:

> ... the atmospherical air consists of three different kinds of corpuscles ... first these numberless particles ... in the form of vapors ... the second more subtle consists of those exceedingly minute atoms, the magnetic effluvia of earth ... the third sort is its characteristic and essential property, I mean permanently elastic parts.

Boyle did not continue these studies, which might have led him to discover oxygen, but John Mayow, a lawyer-turned-physician and a prominent member of the Royal Society, picked up Boyle's theory and suggested that the atmosphere consisted of two kinds of gases, one of which he called "nitro-aerial particles," which were necessary for the support of life and combustion. The other would not support either life or combustion. He showed this by burning a candle under a bell jar sealed with water, and watched the water level rise in the bell jar as the candle slowly went out. Then he showed that a mouse confined in a small bell jar consumed the air in the jar, and soon died.

In 1674 Mayow reached a short and wonderfully perceptive conclusion, recorded in the *Proceedings of the Royal Society of London*: "From what has been said it is quite certain that animals in breathing draw from air certain vital spirits that by means of respiration are transmitted into the mass of the blood, and the fermentation and heating of the blood are produced by it."

Some believe that Mayow deserves credit for so clearly showing the necessity for life and

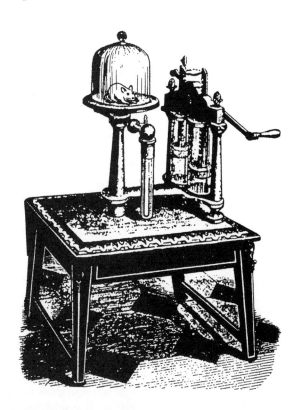

Figure 5. *Bell jar and mouse*

Life Cannot Exist in a Vacuum

The vacuum pump was used to examine anything that caught the fancy of the Fellows of the Royal Society: stones, fish, wood, minerals, liquids, and a great variety of living animals. In the mid-1600s, John Mayow found that a mouse could not live very long in the evacuated bell jar, concluding that something in air was essential to life (Figure 5). But proof would not come for a hundred years.

combustion of a "vital substance" (which would be christened "oxygene" 150 years later). Alas, to history he remains in the background—but an important player.

Despite the many difficulties that made travel slow and uncertain, word of new ideas and discoveries spread throughout Europe surprisingly fast. In Denmark Olaus Borrichius (aka Ole Borch) also theorized that air contained a special life-giving substance and in 1678 actually isolated oxygen from the decomposition of potassium nitrate—but he did not appreciate the importance of what he had done and remains largely unrecognized.

Carbon Dioxide

Much earlier in the seventeenth century a restless, unorthodox Belgian scholar, Johann Baptista Van Helmont, had coined a new word, *gas,* to describe a substance different from solids and liquids. He made carbon dioxide by dripping acid over limestone, and showed that this was the same gas which, heavier than air, pooled in the bottom of a famous cave (La Grotte de Cane) in Italy, where dogs who entered perished but their taller masters survived. Modern cavers often face such pools of bad air through which they can only pass by breathing artificial air with special equipment. He went on to show that his new gas would extinguish fire and would not support life. It was still too early to relate this to combustion.

A century later Joseph Black found that what he christened "fixed aire" was formed by burning charcoal. Furthermore, in an ingenious experiment, he arranged for the air exhaled by 1,500 people during ten hours inside a church at a religious gathering to pass through a ceiling vent and over rags saturated with limewater. By weighing the calcium carbonates thus formed, he showed that the expired gases contained what he called "fixed aire"; it was carbon dioxide. Thus, even before oxygen was isolated, the gas exhaled during respiration and generated by combustion, and presumably by bodily functions too, had been identified.

The next step would be to determine what this "aerial spirit" or "vital essence" really was, and to connect it clearly with combustion of inert materials, and with the metabolism of living animals.

OXYGEN: THE VITAL ESSENCE

My introduction to oxygen—or rather the lack of it—occurred in 1936 when I was preparing for my first expedition to the high Himalayas. Someone introduced me to Dr. Ross McFarland, one of the leading authorities in aviation medicine. He was interested in our plans to climb a 26,000-foot mountain and offered to check my tolerance for altitude. Ross had a special room in which the percentage of oxygen could be reduced to simulate ascent. I knew little or nothing about altitude, but I had read about the British attempts on the Tibetan side of Everest, in which they used bottled oxygen, but the equipment was heavy and unreliable. I had also read that Edward Norton had climbed to 27,000 feet, and Noel Odell almost as high, without oxygen.

So Ross "took me up" to over 26,000 feet, an experience about which I have only a vague memory, and tried to educate me. The team and I climbed the Nanda Devi, and that meeting with Ross has influenced much of my life ever since.

When I talk about and show pictures of my climbs among the highest mountains, people invariably ask whether we used oxygen. Although most have never heard of Berti or Torricelli, almost everybody knows we need oxygen to live and has heard that there is less oxygen on "high mountains," even though they may not know why.

Once the existence of a vacuum and the fact that air had weight had been demonstrated by Berti, Torricelli, and Perier in the seventeenth century, the composition of the atmosphere began to attract more attention. By the middle of the eighteenth century it was clear that air, or some part of it, was essential for life. In fact, that essential part had been isolated several times during the previous 200 years (and even earlier)—although its importance was not recognized. Finally came the climactic experiments, one of them by a British clergyman, Joseph Priestley, who wrote in his laboratory notes on November 21, 1774:

> I procured a mouse and put it into a glass vessel containing two ounce measures of the air obtained from mercuris calcinatus. Had it been common air, a full grown mouse such as this was would have

lived in it about a quarter of an hour. In this air, however, my mouse lived a full half hour.

I did not certainly conclude that this air was any better because, though one mouse would live only a quarter of an hour in a given quantity of air, I knew it was not impossible but that another mouse might have lived in it for half an hour. [So I] procured another mouse and putting it into less than two ounce measures of air extracted from mercuris calcinatus. . . I found it lived three quarters of an hour. Being now fully satisfied of the goodness of this kind of superior air I proceeded to measure that degree of purity with as much accuracy as I could.

This is the first clear and unequivocal description of how essential for life is the unique substance we now know as oxygen.

Long before this, however, in A.D. 756, a Chinese scientist, Nao Hoa, had generated a "purified" air by heating potassium nitrate to produce oxygen, but history does not tell us whether he did anything with it. Pliny the Elder wrote in his *Natural History* that Roman well diggers would lower a lighted lamp into the well, deciding that if the lamp went out, the air was dangerous for them to breathe. Anticipating Robert Boyle by 150 years, Leonardo da Vinci recognized that "air" in which fire would not burn would not support life either.

Alchemists in the sixteenth and seventeenth centuries, trying to change base metals into gold, had released oxygen by heating mercuric oxide, potassium nitrate, or lead oxide, but although they saw that this "gas" supported fire and life, few seem to have asked why: Their interests lay in other directions. The "philosopher's stone" they sought would not only miraculously cure disease but also make them wealthy; the "gas" was only a distraction.

PHLOGISTON

While the brilliant members of the fledgling Royal Society were exploring the relationship of air to fire and life, Danish chemist Georg Stahl proposed a theory that all combustible materials contained an impalpable substance, which his followers called *phlogiston*, or "fire substance," that enabled them to burn. But this idea was hard to sell, because some substances weighed more *after* they were burned. So his followers decided that phlogiston must have a new property the opposite of weight—levity—which was what made the substance heavier when phlogiston was consumed or escaped during combustion. This seems rather absurd today, but it captured the minds of many scientists for a century.

Sixty years earlier, Jean Rey was puzzled by his own finding that some matter (he used tin) heated in air gained weight. He proposed that this was due to air, which somehow became "adhesive" and clung to the substance as it burned. Like the ancient Chinese and many alchemists, Ole Borch also had isolated oxygen, but he too has been forgotten.

Finally, between 1770 and 1773, Swedish pharmacist Carl Scheele, in an extraordinary and systematic series of experiments, not only generated

How to Make Oxygen

Over the centuries many alchemists had extracted a gas from different substances, but none realized that the gas was far more important than the precious metals they were trying to make. Among those who did, Swede Carl Scheele in the 1770s began studying the properties of a gas he extracted from silver carbonate. He soon showed that this gas would support life and fire in a confined space, and he sought help from prominent French chemist Antoine-Laurent Lavoisier, who had a very powerful magnifying glass with which he could concentrate the sun's rays to create a higher temperature than in a conventional furnace (Figure 6). Scheele asked Lavoisier to use this lens to make the new gas, to confirm Scheele's own observations.

Figure 6. *Lavoisier's compound lens. (From Oeuvres de Lavoisier, Tome III [Mémoires de chimie et de physique]. Paris: Imprimerie Impériale, 1865, planche 9. Reproduced with permission.)*

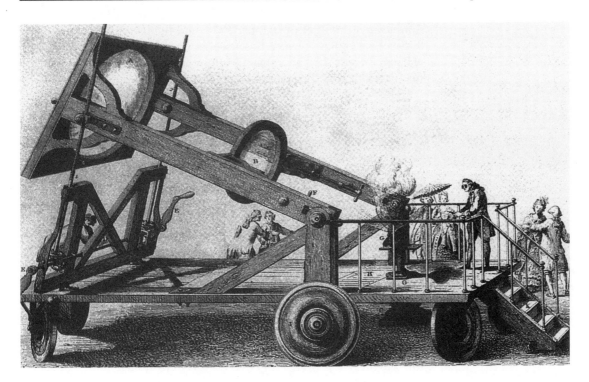

a special gas but had the boldness to challenge the popular "phlogiston" theory, which did not endear him to his elders. He noted that his new gas supported life as well as combustion, and at first called this gas "vitriol air" but soon changed the name to "fire air."

During the same period in Paris, Antoine-Laurent Lavoisier, a young chemist from a well-to-do family, had been looking at oxidation of inorganic substances, and perhaps was interested in phlogiston. In 1772 he sent a letter to the French Academy describing this work, asking that the letter be sealed until he was ready to publish.

On September 30, 1774, Scheele wrote Lavoisier thanking him for a book and added a description of his experiment. Scheele asked Lavoisier to repeat it, using his much larger burning glass to "reduce" silver carbonate in a bell jar sealed with water containing quicklime to combine with the "fixed air" (carbon dioxide), some of which he expected would be generated. Scheele did not tell Lavoisier what he had learned about this new gas, but explained that he sent him the information "… so that you will see how much air is produced by this reduction and whether a lighted candle can carry on its flame, and animals live in it," as Scheele already had found.

OXYGEN RECOGNIZED

Joseph Priestley, who had been studying a gas formed from fermentation, visited Lavoisier in October 1774, and the two probably discussed Scheele's letter. Both seemed to sense that something important was close at hand, because right after their meeting, each hurried home to isolate the new gas using slightly different methods.

On Saturday, November 19, 1774, Priestley set up the crucial experiment, but on Sunday he was occupied at church, and not until Monday did he actually generate oxygen, as described in the preceding section. Excited by what he had done with the mouse, he took another step, as a good scientist would, and in his lab notes added an appealing personal note:

> My reader will not wonder that, after having ascertained the superior goodness of dephlogisticated air by mice living in it and the other tests mentioned, I should have the curiosity to taste it myself. I have gratified that curiosity, by breathing it, drawing it through a glass siphon, and, by this means I reduced a large jar full of it to the standard or common air. The feeling of it to my lungs was not sensibly different from that of common air but I fancied my breast felt peculiarly light and easy for some time afterwards. Who can tell but that in time this air may become a fashionable article in luxury. Hitherto only two mice and myself have had the privilege of breathing it.

It didn't take long for his prediction to come true: Within two years, others throughout Europe were using the new gas to treat many different conditions, but with mixed results.

Priestley described his work to the Royal Society in a letter dated March 15, 1775, which was accepted and formally read to the Society on March 23. This was the first formal announcement of the isolation of oxygen.

Five weeks later, on April 26, 1775, Lavoisier read to the French Academy his own paper describing oxygen. The existence of oxygen had been confirmed. There followed years of controversy, but debating who was first to "discover" oxygen is irrelevant. There is ample honor for both of these men, and neither should their unsung predecessors be forgotten.

Then Lavoisier went further; he placed guinea pigs in pure oxygen and found that they died from a "burning fever and an inflammatory illness." He soon concluded that "healthy air is therefore composed of a good proportion between vital air (oxygen) and atmospheric moffete (nitrogen);... when there is an excess of vital air the animal undergoes a severe illness; when it is lacking, death is almost instantaneous." Others quickly confirmed the toxicity of pure oxygen.

Scheele also continued his studies, and at about this same time recognized the importance of his new gas, writing:

> ...our atmosphere consists of two very different kinds of air: the one is called corrupted air, because it is dangerous and fatal as well to living animals as to vegetables; it constitutes the greatest part of our atmosphere. The other is called pure air, fire air. This kind of air is salutary, supports respiration, and consequently the circulation; without it we could form no distinct idea, either of fire, or how it is kindled. It constitutes but the smallest part of the whole atmosphere. Now as we know this air is of the most immediate necessity for the support of our health.

Unfortunately his book was delayed for two years by a dilatory publisher and appeared after Priestley and Lavoisier had published their papers, so Scheele has not shared in their fame. But he continued his work, and a few years later stated that air always consisted of the same percentage (27 percent) of "fire air." This puzzled him; because both combustion and respiration consumed oxygen and formed "corrupted air," he had expected that the composition of air would vary from place to place, but he reached no conclusion about why it did not.

OXYGEN FROM PLANTS

Even before he isolated his "dephlogisticated air," Priestley had started some pioneering studies with plants, the great importance of which would soon be recognized. (See Figure 7.) His was the first demonstration that plants can convert carbon dioxide into oxygen.

In Paris, Benjamin Franklin, envoy from the rebellious American colonies, hearing about these experiments with plants, wrote several letters to friends calling Priestley's experiment very important, and adding:

I hope this will give some check to the rage of destroying trees that grow near houses, which has accompanied our late improvements in gardening. . . We Americans have everywhere our country habitations in the midst of woods, and no people on earth enjoy better health or are more prolific.

Plants Can Convert Bad Air to Good Air

Joseph Priestley was a careful researcher who understood the importance of controls in his experiments. Three years before he isolated oxygen, he did a well-planned experiment that was almost as important in the broad scheme of life. In his laboratory notebook he wrote: "On the 17th of August, 1771, I put a sprig of mint into a quantity of air, in which a candle had burned out, and found on the 27th of the same month [that] another candle burned perfectly well in it. . . . I took a quantity of air made thoroughly noxious by mice breathing and dying in it, and divided it into two parts; one of which I put into a phial immersed in water, and into the other . . . I put a sprig of mint . . . and after eight or nine days I found that a mouse lived perfectly well in that part of the air in which the sprig of mint had grown, but died the moment it was put into the other part of the same original quantity of air, and which I had kept in the very same exposure, but without any plant growing in it." The fact that green plants can convert carbon dioxide into oxygen makes life possible for all animals on this earth today.

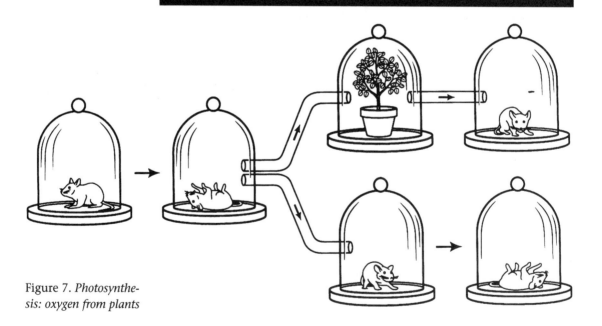

Figure 7. *Photosynthesis: oxygen from plants*

Priestley's experiment of growing mint in "corrupted" air led in a few years to an equally momentous discovery by Jan Ingenhousz, a Dutch physician who showed that green plants can isolate oxygen from "common aire" when exposed to sunlight—the first demonstration of photosynthesis.

Ingenhousz also advocated the use of Priestley's new gas for treatment of various illnesses, as did many other physicians hurrying to demonstrate Priestley's prediction that this pure air would become fashionable. Thomas Beddoes, a leading proponent of therapeutic oxygen, expected considerable benefit from oxygen in a variety of diseases, and founded the Pneumatic Institute in England, with Humphrey Davy as superintendent. Davy soon moved into other major studies for which he was later knighted. Others used the new gas for asthma, tuberculosis, and many other illnesses, with predictably variable success, before the fad subsided.

OXYGEN AS A COMPONENT OF AIR

By the end of the eighteenth century, the phlogiston theory was effectively dead, although a few scientists—among them, surprisingly, Priestley—never completely abandoned it; and the composition of air had been approximated. The next question was whether Scheele was right that air everywhere contained the same amount of "oxygene," or did it vary from place to place? Priestley and others soon devised tests to measure the proportion of oxygen in air, and most found that it was the same everywhere, but in his lab notes Priestley wrote:

Doctor Ingenhousz discovered that the atmosphere at Vienna contains a greater proportion of vital air than in Holland and to this he attributes the remarkable increase in appetite felt by strangers on their arrival in Vienna.

Lavoisier too relied on imperfect analytical methods when he reported that the percentage of oxygen was 18.5 percent at floor level but 25 percent at ceiling level in a hospital ward, and he urged that society be alerted to these health hazards.

Lavoisier would be executed during the Reign of Terror in 1794, along with thirty-two "ex-nobles and former Farmers tried and convicted of conspiracy against the State." Priestley at first defended the principles of the French Revolution, but was disenchanted by the extremism during the Reign of Terror. A mob destroyed his laboratory, and two years later his anti-revolutionary sentiments led him to flee to Philadelphia, where he lived for the next ten years.

These two, building on those who had gone before, established the importance of oxygen. Like others before them, they asked why, if combustion and life were equally dependent on oxygen, the heat generated in living tissues did not consume them as it did other substances when they were ignited. It would be almost another hundred years before this question was answered.

In a short decade, several brilliant men had put one more piece of the puzzle of air, fire, and life on the table, but a few more pieces were needed before the relationship of oxygen to altitude sickness would be understood. How did life-supporting oxygen enter lungs and blood to be carried throughout the body? The next two chapters describe breathing and circulation and the substance that carries the essential gas.

PART II **HOW THE BODY GETS OXYGEN**

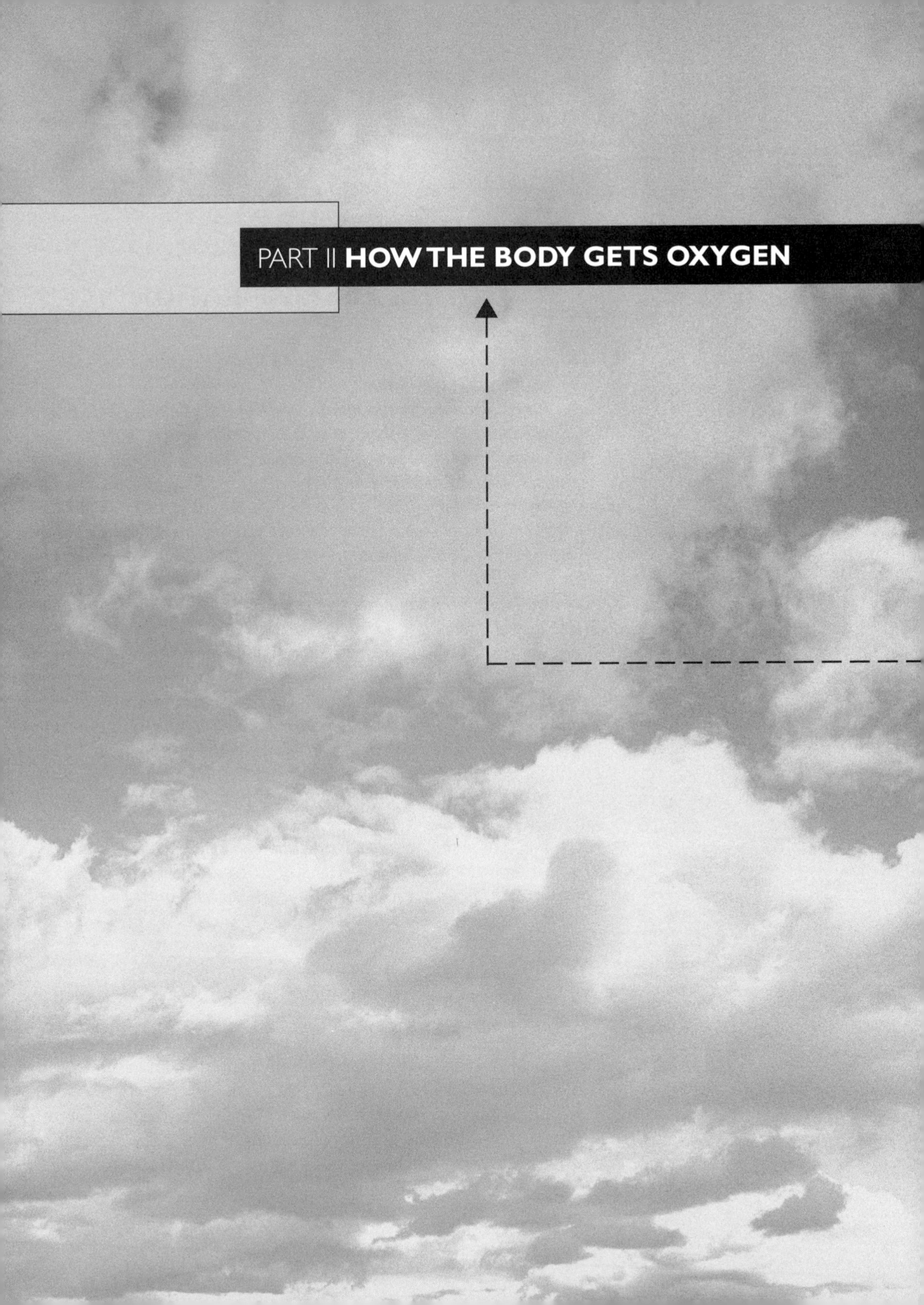

MOVING AIR: RESPIRATION

My own journey into the milieu of atmosphere began with a very small step in 1929, when my father arranged a summer job for me as a lowly apprentice to Dr. Martha Washburn, a patient and motherly biochemist at the Cold Spring Harbor Laboratories, a biological research center on New York's Long Island. I was as ignorant about the air around us as the early philosopher–scientists had been—but just as eager to learn. I began by doing simple chores; my duties were to feed the laboratory cats and rabbits, collect and analyze their excreta, and help with measuring their vital functions. These were recorded with a moving stylus touching a smoked paper drum—which I learned to make and later to paint with shellac for preservation. Dr. Washburn showed me that this was research in the old tradition, and I lapped it up.

Apparently I was adequate, and Dr. Washburn next taught me how to use the Haldane gas analyzer to measure levels of oxygen and carbon dioxide in blood serum. This was basically the same instrument that John Haldane and his contemporaries had used in their pioneering work around the turn of the century, but I didn't have a sense of history then, and all I knew was that it was fussy and rather delicate work. Fortunately Dr. Washburn was patient as I wasted samples and spilled mercury until I finally learned to be reasonably reliable.

This was an unforgettable introduction to the exploration of gases. Dr. Washburn showed me the excitement of research and taught me to be precise, although I never really learned much biochemistry. I had already decided I would be some sort of doctor, and she opened a wondrous vista before me.

Everything we do—thinking or dreaming, running or climbing mountains, eating, getting angry or making love—requires an uninterrupted supply of the "vital spirit"—oxygen. Oxygen allows us to release the energy we need to breathe, pump blood, move muscles, secrete hormones, and excrete wastes. We need oxygen to live.

Lavoisier named it "oxygene." Scheele, Boyle, Priestley, and forgotten others made it clear that all animals required it to live, to "burn" foodstuffs that fuel every activity, much as a candle must have air in order to burn. This idea was not really new: Long before these great men, the Chinese recognized that a continuous supply of "good" air was necessary to support most life.

Our body's supply of oxygen must be replenished almost as rapidly as it is used. This places severe limits on where we go and what we can do. Unlike the turtle, man cannot spend a long, cold winter buried snugly in mud at the bottom of a pond. Nor can we hibernate like bears or ground squirrels, or stay under water for an hour like whales and seals. True, we do have what might be called temporary stores from which to draw, but for practical purposes we must breathe to live—we must take in as much oxygen as we need for whatever task we undertake, as fast as needed. And the intake system must be virtually fail-safe.

During the age of the Pharaohs, 4,000 to 5,000 years ago, Egyptian physicians were forbidden to dissect the human body, but they learned a good deal of anatomy by preparing the dead for mummification. They accurately described the respiratory tract through which air is drawn into the chest. But they also believed that air entered through the ears and other orifices as well as through the skin. Centuries later Greco–Roman philosopher–scientists taught that breathing cooled the "innate heat" of the heart. They developed various theories about how air entered the blood, mixing with it to form *pneuma*, which could be found in both arteries and veins.

Galen, the best-known physician at the start of the Christian era, described the process of breathing. His explanation is sometimes vague because, even though he could not accept the notion of a vacuum, he did believe that air was drawn into the lungs by expansion of the chest, and he supported this concept by showing that the lungs collapsed when the chest was opened. For the next 1,500 years Galen's theory went unchallenged.

In 1640 Gaspar Berti's demonstration of a vacuum, showing that air had weight, revived interest in Galen's theory that during inspiration the thorax actively expanded, which implied, but did not state explicitly, that air was pushed into the lungs by the weight of the atmosphere. When the thoracic muscles and diaphragm relaxed, Galen saw that the expanded thorax returned to its relaxed position, and air flowed out. "Sucked in" or "pushed in"—a fine but important distinction. During his studies in 1674 of the vital spirit in air, John Mayow described the process of breathing, and wrote in the *Proceedings of the Royal Society of London*:

> With respect then to the entrance of air into the lungs, I think it is to be maintained that it is caused . . . by the pressure of the atmosphere. For as the air, on account of the superincumbent atmosphere, . . . rushes into all empty places . . . it follows that air passes through the nostrils and the trachea up to the bronchia. . . . When the inner sides of the thorax . . . are drawn outwards by muscles. . . and the space in the thorax is enlarged, the air which is nearest the bronchio-inlets. . . rushes under the full pressure of the atmosphere into the cavities of the lungs. . . . From this we conclude that the lungs are distended by

air rushing in, and that they do not expand of themselves, as some have supposed.

Sylvius, aka Franciscus de la Boe, had written much the same thing in 1660:

The lungs do not move naturally of their own motion but they follow the motion of the thorax and the diaphragm. . . . The lungs are not expanded because they are filled with air, they are filled with air because they are expanded.

Another pioneer, mathematics professor Giovanni Borelli, friend and disciple of Galileo, applied his imagination and talent to physiology and also recognized that breathing air was essential for life in animals. Borelli made the new and important observation that air dissolved in water could pass through certain membranes, and thus introduced the basic principles of gaseous diffusion, an essential part of respiration.

These theories were beginning steps toward understanding how the essential part of air moves from the surrounding atmosphere into the lungs and onward toward the living cells. Today we call this the oxygen transport system: the process of acquiring, transporting, delivering, and using oxygen.

THE OXYGEN TRANSPORT SYSTEM

Oxygen is acquired by breathing in air. After the lungs are filled, the oxygen diffuses from the lungs into the blood. The diffusion occurs throughout the ventilatory cycle. Oxygen is transported by the flowing blood where it is loosely combined with the red pigment called *hemoglobin*. Oxygen is delivered to all the tissues of the body through large blood vessels, which divide into ever smaller ones and end in *capillaries*, tiny, thin-walled vessels barely large enough for red cells to tumble through. It is in the capillaries that oxygen leaves hemoglobin and diffuses into the fluid-filled tissue around our living cells and into the cells themselves. Utilization of oxygen—for which the whole system is organized—takes place within the cell in a multistep process. Some important steps—the steps that use oxygen—take place in tiny compartments within the cell called *mitochondria*.

The oxygen transport system is beautifully suited to its task. It is flexible, can double its capacity by changes at each stage, and—through an intricate web of feedback loops—can respond swiftly to changes that occur both inside and outside the body. This system is specially designed to carry oxygen, and will do so unless interfered with by a rare alien molecule such as carbon monoxide or cyanide. It has multiple checks and balances and redundant control points that function so smoothly we are seldom aware of them. And this system is capable of performing multiple tasks: Respiration, working together with blood circulation, maintains a constant

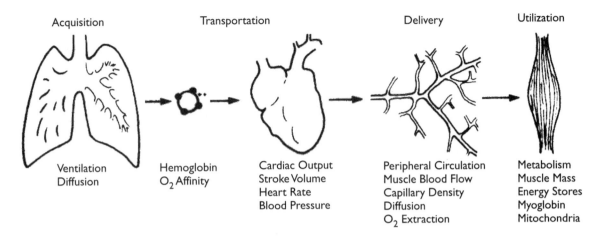

Acquisition	Transportation	Delivery	Utilization
Ventilation Diffusion	Hemoglobin O_2 Affinity	Cardiac Output Stroke Volume Heart Rate Blood Pressure	Peripheral Circulation Muscle Blood Flow Capillary Density Diffusion O_2 Extraction	Metabolism Muscle Mass Energy Stores Myoglobin Mitochondria

Figure 8. *The oxygen transport system*

The Oxygen Transport System

John Sutton used a deceptively simple diagram to show how oxygen is taken in and dispersed throughout the body. (See Figure 8.) Inhaling brings air deep into the air sacs (*alveoli*) of the lungs (*acquisition*), from which oxygen diffuses into the lung capillaries. The rate of diffusion of oxygen from the alveoli to the blood is determined by several factors, including the distance separating the alveoli from the capillaries and the difference in oxygen levels between alveoli and the capillaries. Having entered the blood, oxygen is picked up by red blood cells (*transportation*). The amount of oxygen that each volume of blood can carry is determined by the amount of circulating hemoglobin and its affinity for oxygen. The amount of oxygenated blood pumped by the heart is a function of the heart rate and stroke volume (the volume of blood pumped by the heart with each beat). The product of the heart rate times the stroke volume is known as the *cardiac output* (the volume of blood the heart pumps each minute). The heart rate and stroke volume (and thus the cardiac output) are controlled by nerve impulses and hormones communicated to the heart from elsewhere in the body.

After passing through increasingly smaller and more widely branching blood vessels (*delivery*), blood carries oxygen into the capillary network throughout the body for diffusion into each living cell. The amount of oxygen delivered to each tissue is affected by blood flow in the capillary net supplying that tissue and by the blood oxygen level. Finally, living cells everywhere in the body receive oxygen (*utilization*), more or less according to demand. In muscle, a pigment resembling hemoglobin (*myoglobin*) provides an extra safeguard against hypoxia by holding in reserve some oxygen until it is urgently needed. Other organs must take what they are given, but that, too, is dictated according to demand, as monitored by the nervous system.

body temperature, a stable acidity, and a suitable level of body water. Blood also carries hitchhikers, important molecules such as *hormones* (messenger substances) and *enzymes* (catalysts), as well as essential nutrients and other substances, like alcohol. Blood also carries away the waste products of *metabolism*, the chemical changes of life.

Less appreciated but just as important as the transport of oxygen is carriage of carbon dioxide in the opposite direction—from cells to blood to lungs to outside air. Carbon dioxide is carried by the blood in three ways: dissolved in the liquid portion of blood (*plasma*), chemically combined with water as carbonic acid (which dissociates to form hydrogen ions and bicarbonate), and bonded with hemoglobin. Because carbon dioxide molecules are smaller than oxygen molecules and have different chemical properties, carbon dioxide diffuses through membranes twenty times as rapidly as oxygen. For this reason, carbon dioxide moves readily in the tissues from the cells to the blood of the capillaries, and in the lung from the blood to the alveoli. We breathe out the carbon dioxide when we exhale.

Because carbon dioxide, through its ability to form carbonic acid, is the primary regulator of blood serum acidity, its easy mobility enables rapid adjustment of the acidity of blood and tissues. If blood becomes too acid, we automatically breathe more deeply or faster to eliminate more carbon dioxide. Or, should we err on the alkaline side, our breathing tends to slow, and we hold back this weak acid.

To understand the human body's successful response to the stresses of high altitude, we need to look at each part of the oxygen transport system—acquisition, transportation, delivery, and utilization—as well as the transport and discharge of carbon dioxide. Each component responds individually and to the responses of the others as well.

Acquisition: Mechanics of Breathing

Breathing in and out is the first step in the oxygen transport system. This action, called ventilation, or *respiration*, is, as Mayow pointed out, a purely mechanical function that, absent illness or injury, occurs automatically.

The chest is separated from the abdominal cavity by a great plate-like muscle, the *diaphragm*, that Galen recognized was activated by the *phrenic nerve*, which originates from the cervical spinal cord. When relaxed, the diaphragm is domed upward into the chest cavity; when the diaphragm contracts, it flattens, enlarging the chest cavity. Simultaneously, small muscles positioned diagonally between the ribs (*intercostal muscles*) contract, spreading the ribs and enlarging the chest. Air is then pushed in by atmospheric pressure (*inspiration*). When the intercostal muscles and diaphragm relax, the chest wall (*thorax*), which is quite elastic, relaxes and becomes smaller; this is *expiration*.

As outside air rushes in through the nose or mouth, it is warmed to body temperature and rapidly saturated with water vapor from the moist mucous

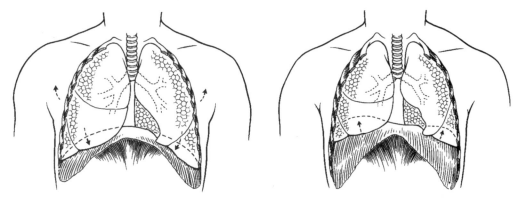

The Mechanics of Breathing

Even though he did not accept that a vacuum could exist, Galen taught that air was *drawn* into the lungs by expansion of the thorax. (See Figure 9.) His somewhat murky explanation was accepted for many centuries. Once a vacuum had been demonstrated, it became clear that air is *pushed* into the lungs when the chest expands, creating a slight vacuum. This expansion is accomplished by contraction of the diaphragm, which is domed upward when relaxed. Flattening of this plate-like muscle, together with contraction of short muscles positioned diagonally between the ribs, enlarges the volume of the chest, making a vacuum that air rushes into to fill the lungs (*inspiration*). Relaxation of these muscles allows the elastic chest wall to contract, driving air out (*expiration*).

Figure 9. *The mechanics of breathing: inspiration (left) and expiration (right)*

lining of these passages. By the time air reaches the windpipe (*trachea*), it is warm and wet; otherwise it would chill and dry the delicate lung tissues.

The trachea splits into the two main *bronchi*, which in turn divide into smaller and smaller *bronchioles* that finally lead into the air sacs (*alveoli*), where gas transfer takes place. In the adult lung there are about 300 million alveoli, whose total membrane lining has a combined area almost the size of a tennis court. Having arrived in the alveoli, oxygen must pass into the lung capillaries—and carbon dioxide must pass out—through the membrane enclosing each alveolus.

From Lungs to Blood: Diffusion of Gases

Borelli demonstrated in the seventeenth century that air could pass through such a membrane, and it could be assumed that oxygen could do so. Eventually it became necessary to ask a new question: If carbon dioxide is carried in the blood, and oxygen inhaled into the lung, could the two gases pass the lung membrane at the same time in opposite directions? Much later, in 1808, John Dalton provided the answer: "When a vessel contains a mixture of such elastic fluids (gases), each acts independently on the vessel...just as if the other were absent.... "

This is the crucial law of partial pressures, which states that the passage of a gas or gases through a membrane is dependent (among other things) on the difference in the pressure of each gas on the opposite sides of the membrane. Of course Dalton's law was not known in the seventeenth century, but those early workers recognized intuitively that it applied to the alveolar walls: Oxygen could pass into blood at the same time that carbon dioxide was passing out of it. Note that the partial pressure of nitrogen is the same on each side of all these membranes because it does not take part in body processes.

Scheele and others had shown that air everywhere on earth is made up of about 21 percent oxygen, and the remainder is mostly nitrogen with traces of other gases. Today, by Dalton's law we easily calculate that the partial pressure of oxygen in air at sea level (barometric pressure 760 torr) is 20.93 percent of 760 torr, or roughly 160 torr. At 18,000 feet, where barometric pressure is half that at sea level, oxygen partial pressure is 20.93 percent of 380 torr, or about 80 torr. Dalton's law enables us to think of the partial pressures of oxygen and carbon dioxide, and to use these values in mathematical equations. We can think of oxygen as having "high" pressure in outside air, lower pressure in the lungs, where it is diluted with carbon dioxide and water vapor, and still lower pressure by the time it has reached the cells. This stepwise drop is called the *oxygen cascade*.

The Oxygen Cascade

Because we do not empty our lungs completely when we exhale, when we breathe in, the entering air mixes with some air left over from previous breaths that has a high carbon dioxide level. The air we breathe in also picks up water vapor, which—like any other gas—has a partial pressure. Once it is warmed to body temperature and fully saturated with water, the partial pressure of water vapor is 47 torr at body temperature. Together, carbon dioxide and water vapor deep in the lungs reduce the partial pressure of oxygen there to about 100 to 110 torr. (See Figure 10.)

At each stage in oxygen's journey from outside air to lungs, into blood and on into cells, its partial pressure decreases. It is by minimizing the loss at each stage of the oxygen cascade that man is able to live and work at altitudes (or in environments) where oxygen pressure is very low. This adjustment is the first part of acclimatization, and without changes in the oxygen cascade we could not survive at high altitude.

Between outside air and the depths of the lungs comes the first "drop" in the oxygen cascade (from atmospheric to alveolar oxygen). We can mitigate this drop by breathing faster or more deeply, bringing more fresh air deep into the lungs. But this accommodation cannot bring alveolar oxygen pressure up to ambient atmospheric levels because carbon dioxide is constantly entering the lungs, and because water vapor pressure is constant.

Once oxygen is in the innermost parts of the lung, it must diffuse from alveolus to lung capillary. First it passes through the lining of the alveolus (the alveolar *epithelium* and *basement membrane*), then through the loose *interstitial space* (spaces between the cells), and finally through the capillary basement membrane and capillary *endothelium* and into the red blood cell. The single layer of cells lining the alveoli,

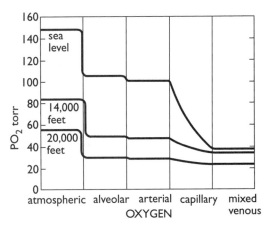

Figure 10. *The oxygen cascade*

The Oxygen Cascade

The partial pressure of oxygen in the air we breathe (*atmospheric oxygen*) decreases markedly when air enters the lungs, where it mixes with water vapor and carbon dioxide. (See Figure 10.) The level of oxygen in the air sacs of the lung (*alveolar oxygen*) falls further during passage from the lungs into the blood (*arterial oxygen*), although normally only slightly. There is a further drop in oxygen as the blood passes through the tissue capillaries (*capillary oxygen*). At this point oxygen is moving from the capillaries into the cells. The oxygen level in the blood that leaves the tissues is known as *mixed venous oxygen*. It is convenient to compare this series of drops in oxygen partial pressure to a waterfall or cascade. The first drop (from atmospheric to alveolar) is the greatest, but is also the most sensitive to change: As ventilation increases, alveolar oxygen more closely approaches that of inhaled air (atmospheric oxygen). Obviously this increase improves oxygenation all the way to the cells. Increased breathing is the first and most important part of adjustment—and later acclimatization—to hypoxia.

Next, under normal conditions, there is only a slight drop in oxygen as it passes from alveolus to blood (arterial oxygen). Finally, as blood courses into ever smaller vessels, the oxygen pressure drops yet again as oxygen leaves the blood and enters the tissues.

At increasing altitudes, reduced oxygen levels in the atmosphere result in lower oxygen pressure at every stage. However, the changes of acclimatization compensate for this reduction to some extent, as shown in Figure 10.

Carbon dioxide moves in the opposite direction, from a high partial pressure in cells, into the capillary blood as it moves toward the venous capillaries, and into larger and larger veins back to the heart and thence to the lungs, where its partial pressure is low.

and those lining the adjacent capillaries, are joined tightly together and are designed to permit diffusion of oxygen, carbon dioxide, and some other gases, but not liquids or large molecular substances.

The Alveolar–arterial Gradient

So large is the alveolar surface area that oxygen diffuses rapidly through the alveolar walls at sea level, where its partial pressure is much higher than in blood arriving in the lungs. Diffusion takes less than a half second at sea level, while a red blood cell takes eight-tenths of a second to traverse the capillary adjoining the alveolus. Transit or exposure time is not normally a limiting factor in loading oxygen into blood at sea level, although it may become so at very high altitude, or during prolonged and extreme exertion.

The oxygen level in lung capillaries is lower than that in alveoli. This small drop in pressure, the second in the oxygen cascade, is called the *Alveolar–arterial*, or *A–a, gradient*. The normal resting A–a gradient in youth is 2 to 5 torr but it increases to 10 to 15 torr in old age. Usually—but not always—the A–a gradient increases during moderate or intense exercise. The few direct measurements of the gradient at extreme altitude show that it decreases to near zero at rest, but increases sharply with exertion.

Obviously the passage of oxygen through the cells and membranes separating alveolus from capillary is a crucial step, leading one to think it possible that there might be a protective capability in case of failure. This notion gave rise to the intriguing theory that alveolar cells can actually *secrete* oxygen into the capillary blood, to overcome low oxygen blood levels. This seemingly reasonable supposition has been very controversial, as will be explained below.

Transportation: Blood Cells

The red blood cell is a selfless and versatile carrier: It has little need for the oxygen it carries, making it a very efficient carrier. There is little drop in the partial pressure of oxygen while it is transported to its destinations. In the arterial stage of the cascade, very little oxygen pressure is lost between the fluid portion of blood and the red blood cell; the cascade is almost flat. (See Chapter 4, "Moving Blood: Circulation," for more about blood cells.)

Delivery and Utilization: Capillaries and Cells

The final stage in the oxygen cascade is arrival in the tissue capillaries, which spread throughout every body tissue to deliver food and oxygen to all cells. From these tiny vessels, oxygen diffuses into the fluid of the interstitial space in which cells live and, from there, through the cell membrane into the cell where the oxygen is utilized. The tissue capillaries do not have a muscular coat but are lined only with a thin endothelium in which the single cells are not tightly joined, but have gaps between them, permitting passage of large molecules.

The major "purpose" of respiration and circulation is to ensure an adequate supply of nutrients and oxygen to, and removal of carbon dioxide and other wastes from, the tissues. Direct measurement of the oxygen within living cells suggests that the cellular oxygen level may be very low. However, this does not indicate that oxygen is unimportant to our cells. Quite the contrary, it shows why disruption of either circulation or respiration has such a devastating impact on our body cells.

FROM LUNGS TO BLOOD, REVISITED

Let us return briefly to the oxygen cascade between lungs and blood—the A–a oxygen gradient. As we measure it, this pressure drop-off reflects the overall difference between alveolar and arterial oxygen pressures—it is an average for all parts of both lungs. We know that in different parts of the lung, the gradient is likely to be different depending on several important influences.

For one thing, the top (*apex*) of the lung is not as well ventilated as the rest of the lung. If there is some local obstruction like pneumonia in a part of the lung, that area may receive less air than normal lung tissue, while its blood flow is normal or even increased. If the alveolar walls are thickened by illness or swelling, oxygen passage from alveolus to blood will be slowed and the A–a gradient increased. On the circulatory side, blood flow may be impeded by any of several causes—by constriction or by small blood clots, for example—while ventilation is normal.

These are examples of imbalance or inequality between alveolar ventilation and circulation, which we call *ventilation–perfusion mismatch*. When mismatch exists, it can only increase the A–a gradient. Mismatch also results when some blood goes through vessels that bypass alveoli. These detours are called *shunts*, because they allow blood to transit the lung without being exposed to oxygen. This blood mixes with blood that did become oxygenated at alveoli, reducing the overall oxygen level in the blood leaving the lung. Small shunts normally occur in many people, and they are usually unimportant. However, a large shunt can significantly reduce the arterial blood oxygen level and seriously hamper oxygen transport.

Early in the twentieth century, the oxygen diffusion theory was challenged by a major question: Does oxygen move through the alveolar–capillary barrier *only by diffusion*, or does the alveolar membrane *actively secrete* oxygen from lung to blood? Wouldn't it seem reasonable that for the acquisition of such an absolutely vital substance as oxygen some additional protection—a fail-safe mechanism—should exist? Might oxygen actually be secreted from lung to blood in special circumstances, making the A–a gradient negative?

After researchers showed low tissue oxygen levels due to decreased barometric pressure to be the cause of mountain sickness, this question became even more compelling: Perhaps the answer would explain why some people become ill at high altitude while others do not. Finding the answer is an interesting story.

Oxygen Secretion Theory

In 1892 Christian Bohr confirmed earlier work by Baptiste Biot showing that the swim bladders of fish contained a very high concentration of oxygen; this appeared to violate Dalton's law and could be explained only by active secretion of oxygen from blood into the swim bladder.

This concept attracted the attention of physiologist John Haldane and his assistant, Lorrain Smith, who were already studying how oxygen moved from lungs to blood. They visited Bohr in 1894 and were intrigued by his suggestion that a similar secretion might occur through mammalian alveolar walls. To test this hypothesis, Haldane and Smith measured the oxygen pressure in their own alveolar air, calculated the arterial oxygen pressure using a carbon monoxide technique, and found that the alveolar oxygen pressure was lower than the arterial. If this were true, it would suggest that oxygen was indeed being secreted from the alveoli into the blood. They were not able to measure oxygen directly in arterial blood.

But by then Bohr's students Auguste and Marie Krogh had devised a more accurate method for measuring blood oxygen by equilibrating a bubble of air with blood and analyzing the oxygen in the bubble. With this technique they could not confirm their respected professor's findings. Reluctantly they published a series of brilliant papers in 1910 and started a famous controversy by their unequivocal statement: "The passage of [oxygen] and the elimination of carbon dioxide in the lungs takes place by diffusion and by diffusion alone."

Haldane and Smith's experiments led them to dispute the Kroghs' diffusion theory. In 1910, at a meeting in Vienna, Haldane met a young American, Yandell Henderson, and told him that he was looking for a "high mountain with a nice hotel on top" where he could do experiments. Henderson immediately suggested the summit of Pikes Peak in Colorado as an ideal location to detect oxygen secretion, if indeed it took place. The following year Haldane and Henderson, with Englishmen Gordon Douglas and Edward Schneider, went to Pikes Peak to study acclimatization, by measuring oxygen pressure in alveolar air and using the carbon monoxide method to estimate oxygen in arterial blood at rest and after exertion.

On Pikes Peak they found that the calculated arterial oxygen pressure was always higher than the alveolar, which convinced Haldane that active oxygen secretion was a specific function of the lung that enabled humans to tolerate altitude. He proposed that differences between individuals in their susceptibility to mountain sickness were due to different degrees of secretion. His later studies did not shake this belief, even when confronted with contrary evidence collected by his former colleague, Joseph Barcroft.

Barcroft had begun his scientific career by studying the metabolism of salivary glands, and in 1901 he, together with Haldane, developed a method for measuring gases in small amounts of liquid. He found that the partial pressure of oxygen in saliva was higher than in the capillary blood in the salivary gland. At first he could explain this observation only by active oxygen secretion. Several years later, however, his study of factors changing the shape of the hemoglobin dissociation curve, and thus the oxygen content of blood, led him to reexamine his data and to renounce oxygen secretion in this instance.

Barcroft was called up in World War I to treat pulmonary edema caused by the military use of chlorine gas, but soon after the Armistice he returned to studies of other causes of hypoxia—such as high altitude. Because of his work with salivary glands, he did not accept oxygen secretion, but challenging the attractive oxygen secretion theory meant opposing his senior, Haldane, and trying to repeat his studies.

To do so, in 1920 Barcroft spent ten days in a sealed glass room where the oxygen was gradually decreased to the partial pressure equivalent of 18,000 feet. Using a method developed a few years earlier by William Christopher Stadie, a physician at the Rockefeller Institute, Barcroft had a large needle (*cannula*) tied into his radial artery (which, as he wrote matter-of-factly, "of course had to be sacrificed"). Through this cannula he drew arterial blood and was able to measure oxygen directly at the same time that he collected his alveolar air sample. His data showed that his alveolar oxygen pressure was higher than the arterial, and thus contradicted the idea of oxygen secretion by the lung.

Haldane countered that Barcroft had studied only himself, and when he was sick (perhaps from altitude?) at that. Haldane repeated and corrected his own studies, and argued that although secretion might not occur during rest or at normal atmospheric pressure, it was one of the means by which man adjusted or acclimatized to altitude. He correlated his data with clinical observations of those who had been sick or well on Pikes Peak but, again, he did not measure arterial oxygen directly.

The argument raged, of course in gentlemanly terms. Barcroft and a strong team went to Cerro de Pasco (14,200 feet) in Peru and, along with much other work, repeated the alveolar–arterial studies on themselves and on well-acclimatized altitude residents. Once again the alveolar air always contained a higher oxygen pressure than the arterial blood, even in the well-adapted natives. Haldane was wrong. This ended the oxygen secretion theory.

There remains, however, the faint possibility that at extreme altitude, the arterial blood may contain a higher oxygen pressure than the alveolar in acclimatized man. After all, there is precedent in the swim bladder of fish...

This tantalizing possibility intrigues me still, because the simultaneous measurements of arterial and alveolar oxygen were done at extreme altitude toward the end of Operation Everest II—and above 25,000 feet for those partially acclimatized men the arterial was often slightly higher than the alveolar oxygen pressure. Critics have said, not unreasonably, that this difference was due to experimental error.

AUTOMATIC CONTROL OF BREATHING

From an examination of the oxygen cascade it is obvious that we can best increase the partial pressure of oxygen in blood by improving alveolar ventilation—that is, by more efficient breathing. We are seldom conscious of our breathing because it is dictated by stimuli we only dimly perceive. The automatic control of breathing is one of the more fascinating chapters in human physiology and of course it is crucial to staying well at altitude and at sea level.

We know that strenuous exertion, sudden excitement, fear, passion, or even stepping under a cold shower makes us breathe faster or deeper, or both, even though there may not be any immediate, obvious demand for more oxygen. We know that during sleep our breathing becomes shallow, often irregular, and consequently our lungs are less well ventilated—an important effect at high altitude (which might help explain why altitude sickness is worse in the mornings). How and where are these changes dictated?

It is obvious that strenuous exertion or fear-induced preparation for fight or flight require more than the customary supply of oxygen. Exertion causes increased breathing because the extra carbon dioxide that is produced and the mechanical activity of the muscles both stimulate the brain. Fear is a more subtle stimulus: Breathing increases even before the demand for oxygen increases. A cold shower stimulates the skin nerve endings that direct blood flow to the skin and, again in anticipation, this calls for more breathing. Passion has both physical and emotional stimuli to greater effort and greater need for oxygen.

We also know that hypoxia per se stimulates breathing—this is an early and effective response to altitude (or other causes of low oxygen levels). It is reasonable to expect that hypoxia would initiate instructions to breathe more deeply. It is also reasonable to expect that when carbon dioxide accumulates, breathing would be increased in order to wash out the excess. In fact, accumulation of carbon dioxide is a more powerful respiratory stimulant than is mild lack of oxygen: When you hold your breath at sea level, it is accumulation of carbon dioxide rather than lack of oxygen that forces you to breathe again.

Oxygen Sensors: The Carotid Bodies

Lack of oxygen in the arterial blood leaving the heart stimulates a small group of cells strategically sited along the carotid arteries on each side of the neck and richly supplied with blood vessels. These two collections of specialized cells are called the *carotid bodies*. When they sense a fall in blood oxygen, they send a signal to the brain, which in turn signals the respiratory muscles (chest and diaphragm) to increase the rate and/or depth of breathing. Because oxygen is so crucial to life, the carotid bodies are a major first line of defense against an early threat of hypoxia.

In the early 1960s there was a fad to treat severe asthma by removal of one—and often both—carotid bodies. Nowhere is the resilience of the body better illustrated than by the continued survival of these patients; most stayed well, but a few were reported to have difficulty above 5,000 feet, possibly because they did not respond to hypoxia with adequate hyperventilation. A long-term follow-up of these unfortunate individuals might be quite interesting.

The Brain's Respiratory Center

Although both lack of oxygen and excess carbon dioxide stimulate breathing, decreased carbon dioxide (but not excess oxygen) slows breathing. These and other stimuli are read by a collection of chemo-sensitive cells in the midbrain called the *respiratory center*, from which appropriate corrective signals are sent by the brain. Like the thermostat in a house, which turns on the furnace when the temperature falls and turns it off when the house is too hot, the respiratory center responds to carbon dioxide and to changes in acidity of blood. The center also stimulates breathing under some conditions of hypoxia; it is an additional fail-safe mechanism that protects those who for some reason have lost the function of their carotid bodies. The entire control system is exquisitely sensitive and versatile, responsive to blood and to spinal fluid (which is influenced, though slowly, by changes in the blood).

In some people, or under special circumstances, the body's ability to respond to low blood oxygen is less sensitive than normal. The reaction to low oxygen is called the *hypoxic ventilatory response,* or HVR. Whether this lowered sensitivity results solely from a flaw in the carotid body or from a defect somewhere else in the neurotransmitter system is not clear. Whatever its cause, this blunting prevents an increase in ventilation appropriate to the degree of oxygen lack and can produce problems at high altitude.

Once scientists demonstrated the importance of oxygen and the influence of barometric pressure, it remained to be shown how oxygen, the vital substance, could be brought to the cells that needed it. The respiratory system is beautifully contrived to bring air repeatedly into the lungs, and to exhale depleted air containing carbon dioxide. As oxygen is transported through a cascade into blood and thence into tissues, the system can change to meet changing needs.

CHAPTER 4

MOVING BLOOD: CIRCULATION

As a teenager growing up in rural America I was captivated by all the living things around me—snakes, frogs, birds, rabbits, and rats. Soon I began opening up dead ones to see what made them tick. Compared to other aspects of anatomy the heart seemed unimpressive, but I also learned quickly that when the heart stopped the animal soon died. Later on, like many first-year medical students, I was awed by my first cadaver, but the dried, shrunken heart seemed to have little relationship to the lively organ whose pounding we could hear with our stethoscopes. Later still, as a flight surgeon in World War II, I measured cardiac function in thousands of aviators and performed experiments on pilots and aircrew at high altitude. I learned more about heart physiology, but it still was not the real thing.

In 1947 I began practice, and faced reality for the first time. Before the days of penicillin, acute rheumatic fever had been prevalent among young people. Caused by hemolytic streptococcus, it produced high fever, severe joint pain, and other symptoms. Ten to twenty percent of young people with acute rheumatic fever developed heart damage. So when I went into practice, it was not uncommon to see older individuals suffering rheumatic heart disease, a consequence of illness decades earlier. One patient of mine was particularly worrisome. Then in his fifties, he had suffered a severe case of rheumatic fever as a child, and one of his heart valves was badly dilated. Every time the heart beat, blood flowed backwards and the heart never emptied completely. The muscle began to fail and soon he developed what we call congestive heart failure. After a few weeks he had made little progress, but I had to fly off to a distant medical meeting and reluctantly left him in the care of another doctor for a few days.

During the long flight I thought a lot about this patient, and slowly—possibly for the first time—recognized that the heart was nothing but a pump that moved blood continuously in one direction. It occurred to me that perhaps the failing heart could be replaced with a mechanical pump. It was an exciting idea, and I immediately began to sketch out various ways it could be made, how it could be attached, and even how it might be powered.

When I returned home my patient went downhill rapidly and soon died. But an idea had been born in my head that would not go away. Soon I was trying to make plastic models of various sizes and shapes, but with little idea of how to do so, I had little success.

Months later I wrote a short letter to the director of the National Heart Institute (NHI) in Bethesda, Maryland (I did not even know his name), in which I tried to summarize my thoughts on the heart as a pump. Some of my excitement must have been communicated in this amateurish letter, because a few days later I received a phone call from him asking for more details. After some discussion, we agreed that $3,000 might be a good start-up, and within a few days a check arrived made out to me personally. Imagine that happening today! By a fortunate coincidence I met Doctor Rozendahl at General Electric, who sent helpful suggestions. I also was able to spend six weeks with Doctor Wilhelm Kolff, a Dutch refugee who during World War II had made the first artificial kidney out of salvaged airplane parts and who had begun building artificial valves at the Cleveland Clinic.

After receiving another surprising grant from the NHI, I took my design forward with much help from others, taking as much time as I could spare from a growing medical practice. About six months later I had a working model constructed from Kolff's design that performed well for artificial circulation. A cardiac surgeon in Denver would replace the living hearts of anesthetized dogs with this device, which pumped successfully for twelve to twenty hours.

More was to happen. Doctor Paul Dudley White, the great cardiologist, visited me, and I told him about the heart. He was impressed, but added, "Very soon we will be replacing the living heart with other living hearts." Of course he was proved right within only a few years. Being a realist about my own abilities, I knew that although I was a good innovator and explorer, I was not a dedicated research worker, and my greater passion was treating patients. I turned my heart pumps over to another person, and moved on to other things. That was the beginning of my lifelong interest in circulation and all that it does for us.

Breathing in and out would not be very useful without some way to carry oxygen from the lungs to hungry cells, and to take carbon dioxide away from them. Wondrous though the whole process of breathing is, the circulatory system seems even more amazing.

Studies of the atmosphere gradually taught us more and more about breathing and the circulation and, consequently, about wellness and illness on the high mountains. The past can be our greatest teacher—if only we will listen.

A Chinese medical text, written early in the first century B.C. and quoted in J. Needham's book of Chinese history, *Science and Civilization in China*, gives a good description of the circulation of the blood, even if the times and distances are a bit off and portions of the text suggest that air was mixed together with blood in the vessels:

> ...the heart regulates all the blood in the body...the blood current flows continuously in a circle and never stops...a circle with no beginning and no end. Blood flows six inches with one respiration making a complete circuit of the body about fifty times in fourteen hours....

Even earlier, in fact five centuries before Christ, the remarkable philosopher–scientist Empedocles compared the circulation of the blood to the ebb and flow of the tides. Aristotle took the next step, observing that there were two types of blood, one "spiritual," which was purified by passing through the lungs, and another "venous," which moved through the rest of the body. He was the first to describe the branching of arteries and veins from large to smaller and smaller, but, like his contemporaries, he thought the veins carried blood, while the arteries were filled with *pneuma*, a mixture of air and blood.

He was almost correct. Had he made the simple observations that Fabricius and William Harvey would make a thousand years later, he might have taken a giant stride and described how blood actually flows from heart to lungs, from lungs to body, and back to the heart and again to the lungs. But he did not, and instead he taught that there were two separate circulations. In the second century Galen hypothesized how these were connected, mixing the two circulations. As an official surgeon for gladiators, whose terrible wounds often exposed the functioning organs, Galen had many opportunities to study anatomy, including the heart, lungs, and blood vessels. He also did many experiments on living animals.

GALEN'S CIRCULATION STUDIES

Galen, the best-known and most influential physician of the Greco–Roman school, made many fundamental studies by animal vivisection. He saw that the heart valves allow passage in only one direction, and he accepted the ancient belief that it was essential to life for air and blood to be distributed to all parts of the body—as of course it is. He thought that during respiration, air flowed from the lungs into the left side of the heart, where it both fueled and cooled the "innate heat," which was life itself. There air mixed with blood to form *pneuma*, which was then pumped through the arteries, which "...in the whole body...communicate with the veins and exchange air and blood with them through extremely fine invisible openings," as Galen is quoted as saying in an article by D. Fleming.

But Galen's dissections had shown that the arteries and veins contained only blood and no air. He escaped this quandary by some complicated speculations about *anastomoses* (connections) of arteries and veins in the lungs as well as elsewhere, and by postulating tiny pores between the two ventricles of the heart. He also believed that air entered arteries through the skin. Even though Galen did not fully understand the circulation in the lungs, his anatomical studies left an enduring and influential legacy to those who would later define the heart and circulation.

In 1553 Michael Servetus challenged Galen's dictum, defied the church, was charged with heresy, and was burned at the stake. His great book of anatomy, only a few copies of which survived, show he was convinced that blood flowed through the lungs to the heart, out to the body, and back through the heart to the lungs. He had no way to see or demonstrate the capillaries in the lung through which venous blood passes, becomes saturated with oxygen, and returns to the heart. Those connections were still to be found. Since most copies of his revolutionary book were burned with him, it is unlikely that William Harvey, whose work came less than a century later, saw one.

In 1543 the Belgian anatomist Andreas Vesalius challenged Galen more subtly: "We are driven to wonder at the handiwork of the Almighty, by means of which blood from the right into the left ventricle sweats through passages which escape human vision." Vesalius also implied that air did not flow in blood vessels, but instead was bound to blood, but he never fully grasped what this meant to respiration and circulation.

In the thirteenth century a Persian physician, Ibn-al-Nafis, described the course of blood that we know today, and stated that the purpose of the lungs was to purify the blood. His theory was remarkably accurate, not only because he was forbidden by his religion to perform dissections, but also because he attributed "purification of the blood" to a process (oxygenation) that would not be discovered for four more centuries.

In the sixteenth century other pioneers like Matteo Realdo Colombo and Renaldo Cesalpino, now largely forgotten, also taught correctly most of the pathways traveled by blood. Plinio Prioreschi has written a magnificent history of medicine. He researched the writings of Cesalpino and offers the following summary of his work:

> Since the publication of *De Motu Cordis* in 1628, William Harvey has generally been considered the discoverer of the circulation. Since then, however, a minority of authors have tried to show that the laurels belong instead to Andrea Cesalpino (c. 1520–1603). Over the years, an endless number of points and opinions on the two sides of the question have been advanced and debated; the consensus to-day, however, is that Harvey deserves the credit and that Cesalpino's contribution was negligible. In the process of writing the history of medicine of the Renaissance, we reviewed the pertinent literature and translated ourselves, from the original Latin, all the passages of Cesalpino concerning the circulation of the blood. The results were surprising on two accounts. First, the conclusion seems inescapable that this author, several decades before Harvey, had a clear general

understanding of the circulation of the blood. Second, the dismissal of Cesalpino's contribution was (and is) based on misunderstandings and misinterpretations resulting, for the most part, from two factors: (1) critics often did not read all the pertinent passages (possibly because his Latin prose is tedious and sometimes unclear); and (2) some passages were inaccurately translated. As for who discovered the circulation, it depends on how we define "discovery."

Almost certainly Harvey did not know of Ibn-al-Nafis's work, which was published in Arabic and not discovered until 1924. Nor is it likely that he saw Servetus's book or Cesalpino's work. Harvey buttressed his argument by calculating that in one hour the heart pumped blood weighing more than three times the weight of the entire body. Like Vesalius, he applied a simple tourniquet to the arm and showed that the veins contained valves that permitted blood to flow in only one direction. As Galen had done, he showed that valves in the heart also allowed only one-way blood flow. His synthesis was so masterful that it seemed no one could challenge him, but old beliefs die hard, and he was harshly attacked at home and abroad. Though stung, he refused to respond. Most of his contemporaries supported him, and he won acceptance from those who mattered most. Harvey was physician to Charles I, and later to James I; in 1628, prefaced with a letter to King Charles, his famous book *De Motu Cordis* was published. In it he wrote:

> Since calculations and visual observations have confirmed all my suspicions, to wit that the blood is passed through the lungs and the heart by the pulsations of the ventricles, is forcibly ejected to all parts of the body, therein steals into the veins and the porosities of the flesh, flows everywhere back through those very veins from the circumference to the center, from small veins into larger ones, and thence comes at last into the vena cava and to the auricle of the heart...I am forced to conclude that...the blood is driven around with an unceasing circular sort of movement.

This is what some of his predecessors had fumbled with, and Harvey sorted through many bits of information to prove it. Four years after Harvey's death, Marcello Malpighi, using the newly developed microscope, was able to add the missing bit when he saw the tiny capillaries (which Harvey called "porosities"), confirming Harvey's speculations. With this demonstration, Harvey's description of the continuity of the vessels that carry blood through the lungs and to all parts of the body was complete and confirmed.

THE HEART

Central to circulation, of course, is the heart, celebrated by poets and lovers. But, as physiologists know, it is nothing but a tireless mechanical pump. If it has emotional or spiritual qualities, these have yet to be found,

The Circulatory System

Shown in Figure 11 is the circulatory system as we know it today, with the branching arteries that carry unoxygenated blood pumped by the right ventricle to the lungs and the veins, which return oxygenated blood to the left auricle and ventricle, which in turn pump this oxygenated blood through arteries to tissues throughout the body. The blood loses oxygen to cells as it passes through body tissues. The unoxygenated blood then returns to the right side of the heart through a network of veins and is once again pumped to the lungs.

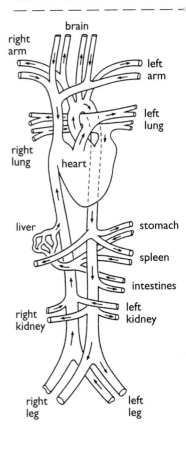

Figure 11. *The circulatory system*

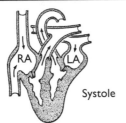
Systole

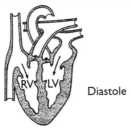
Diastole

though we do know that the heart does produce hormones that stimulate other organs. For example, small granules in some muscle fibers of the heart secrete the hormone *atrial natriuretic peptide* (ANP), which has a powerful effect on salt and water balance. Because ANP increases the output of urine—and, therefore, of sodium—it is believed to play an important role in the spectrum of mountain sicknesses.

In an average person, leading a placid, undisturbed, and inactive life for seventy-five years, the heart will beat some 2,400 million times and pump about 40 million gallons of blood. In our real lives, with excitement, exertion, and stress, these figures are likely to be more than half again as high. That is a lot of work for a small, self-driven, living organ.

After the Royal Society was formed in the seventeenth century, experiments with the heart and blood vessels began to flourish. Stephen Hales, a clergyman better known for his pioneering studies of plant respiration, inserted a thin tube into the carotid artery of a horse and measured blood pressure for the first time; he may have done so in a man as well. He described the capacity of the heart as a pump and, from this and the pulse rate, accurately calculated how much blood was pumped per minute—the first measurement of cardiac output. Hales also made a remarkably accurate count of the size and number of the lung alveoli.

Once again we see how the dreams, the inspiration, and the tedious work of many dedicated people have brought us step by step to the level of understanding we have today. Using the simplest tools, without the fantastic capabilities we now have, well-known scientists—and many more now forgotten—laid the base on which our knowledge rests and developed the hard facts we now take for granted. Sometimes they were wrong, but even their mistakes led others to the correct paths. Honor the forgotten, for they too made science what it is today. Their work showed how respiration and circulation coordinate to create the system that makes life possible for us and all animals.

The heart is absolutely indispensable. Humans can live for weeks, or months, even for years, with little brain activity, and for days or weeks with deficient kidney, digestive, and hormonal functions. But let the heart stop pumping blood for a mere five or six minutes, and first the brain and then other organs are irreversibly damaged and quickly die. An active and effective heart, or a mechanical substitute, must pump blood day in and day out without interruption for us to survive. And when lack of oxygen or lack of blood threatens the supply of nutrients or oxygen to the tissues, the heart increases its output to meet the demand.

Automatic Control of the Heart

The basic rate and rhythm of the heart are dictated by a small strip of tissue called the *sino-atrial* node, located in the wall of the *right atrium*. Amazingly, the S-A node can stimulate the heart to beat at its own intrinsic rate, even if cut off from all outside nerve stimuli, as long as it receives an adequate inflow of blood carrying oxygen and nutrients, and as long as wastes like carbon dioxide are carried away. In fact, the properly nourished and oxygenated heart, removed from the body, may beat for a surprisingly long time, stimulated by the S-A node.

Absent external stimuli, this phenomenal little electric generator, the S-A node, steadily sends tiny electrical impulses that make the heart muscle contract or allow it to relax, unless other "instructions" arrive via the nervous system or in the blood.

External Control of the Heart

The *autonomic nervous system* comprises those parts of the brain and peripheral nerves that automatically control the functions we do not willfully control—among them the heart, the muscles lining the arteries, and the muscles that control breathing. Signals are transmitted from the brain through two subdivisions, the *sympathetic* and *parasympathetic* nervous systems. Broadly speaking, the two are antagonists; the sympathetic system transmits alarm impulses, while the parasympathetic sends relaxing signals. Messages appropriate to the circumstances come from centers deep in the brain to the heart and blood vessels along both systems. Thus the sympathetic system directs the heart to speed up and pump more blood, and the blood vessels to constrict so that arterial pressure rises. The parasympathetic system sends the opposite signals. Both circulatory and respiratory responses to hypoxia are governed by the balance between them.

Parasympathetic impulses affect the stomach and intestines, which in turn, through changes in the blood, affect the heart. After a heavy meal, heart rate and output may increase, but after a light meal the rate may slow; in either situation sleep becomes tempting. During sleep the parasympathetic impulses dominate.

From the higher centers in the brain, nerve impulses indicating excitement, fear, pain, or anger go to the deep brain centers of the sympathetic nervous system control areas in the brain stem and then on to the heart. This activity is part of what we call the "love, fight, or flight" response. Receptors in the skin that are sensitive to temperature also signal the brain to send orders to open skin capillaries and cause sweating or to change the heart rate or output. Other centers in the brain may send instructions to glands of internal secretion like the adrenals to release the powerful stimulant *epinephrine* and its analogs, which control blood pressure, for example. Some of these messengers affect the heart, and may override its basic rhythm.

This scheme also acts as an advance warning system: Veteran racehorses greatly increase both rate and output of the heart in anticipation, many seconds before the start of a race. We humans do the same as we anticipate a difficult or dangerous task, increasing cardiac output (and breathing) before the need actually arises. This epinephrine-effected response is common to many animals.

If these effects on the heart and circulation seem familiar, they are indeed like the increase in respiration in anticipation of upcoming exercise discussed in Chapter 3, "Moving Air: Respiration." There it was described how receptors in the carotid bodies in the neck, reacting to need, stimulate breathing. The carotid bodies can also influence how much blood the heart pumps and thus increase the amount of oxygen-rich blood delivered to the body tissues. On arrival at altitude, in response to hypoxia, the carotid bodies direct the heart to beat faster and more forcefully, putting out more blood per stroke and per minute. This increased cardiac output continues for a week or so before being replaced by the other adjustments. (See Chapter 13, "Acclimatization.")

So essential is a sustained flow of blood that redundant control centers are located in several other places; these can supplement or even take over in case others fail. Some of these small collections of cells are able to sense and can affect blood pressure, heart rate, depth and rate of respiration, and even oxygen transport. They too may be disturbed by hypoxia, but discussion of their functions is beyond the scope of this book.

Starling's Law of the Heart

The heart must pump out what it receives: If blood volume is decreased by hemorrhage or dehydration, and the amount of blood flowing into the heart falls, cardiac output decreases as well. If an increased amount of blood enters the heart, cardiac output initially increases. However, if the amount of blood entering the heart rises too high, cardiac output increases only so far before

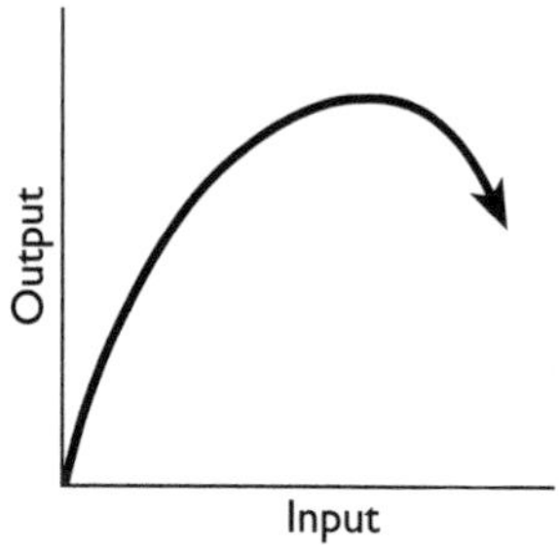

Figure 12. *Starling's law of the heart*

Starling's Law of the Heart

Many brilliant people have studied the heart and circulation since William Harvey's day, and new findings are still frequently described. Wonderful techniques and instruments have been developed since Harvey's simple mathematics and Stephen Hales's measurements of blood pressure. One fundamental "law" was defined in 1918 by Ernest Starling, a brilliant physiologist with wide interests. He and his colleagues showed that the heart could expel more and more blood as it received more and more. But at a certain level (depending in part on the health of the heart), output would falter, and the heart would fail if the inflow continued to increase. Today this corollary seems obvious. Known as the "law of diminishing returns," it applies to many situations in physiology, politics, and economics.

---

it begins to fall, as shown in Figure 12. This "law of the heart," developed by British physiologist Ernest Starling around 1918, is an example of the general law of diminishing returns that also applies to many other processes.

The Effect of Altitude

In addition to stimulating respiration in response to hypoxia, the carotid bodies stimulate the heart to beat faster and a bit harder above 5,000 feet. The work of climbing increases the rate and strength of the heartbeat still more, and at higher elevations may push the heart close to its capacity to respond. This might limit work by older people, whose *maximum achievable heart rate* (MAHR) can be crudely defined as 200 minus half one's age. However, studies at extreme altitude show that in healthy adults it is the lungs rather than the heart that limit work capacity. Maximal breathing capacity also decreases with age, though not predictably. But even at extreme altitude, in most people, other systems falter and fail before the heart.

Cardiac output, both at rest and during exertion, increases as we ascend, but then, after a short stay at moderate altitude, the output decreases to sea level values or even lower. At extreme altitude, toward the summit of Everest for example, cardiac output falls sharply as altitude increases. These decreases in output do not signal congestive heart failure, but more likely are due to a smaller circulating plasma volume. Although the *right ventricle* works harder at altitude due to increased pulmonary artery pressure, the *left ventricle* actually works less.

Coronary Arteries

Heart muscle receives its nourishment and oxygen through the *coronary arteries*, and blood flow through these arteries increases when the heart is called on for more work. Once cardiac rate and output return to or fall below sea level values, coronary blood flow also falls. Does this mean that people with some coronary artery obstruction will tolerate altitude well—or poorly? What it does suggest is that such individuals may tolerate altitude better than one might expect, although they may still be placed at risk by extreme exertion.

Because coronary artery disease tends to be more common in older people, we should ask if the heart affects the tolerance for altitude of the elderly. First, anyone with coronary artery disease should talk seriously with a knowledgeable doctor before planning a climb or any strenuous activity, even at moderate altitude. Going to stay in a mountain resort may be safe and even beneficial for some, but going much higher might cause problems.

Of a group of ninety-seven elderly men and women sojourning to 8,250 feet, 20 percent had pre-existing coronary artery disease but all tolerated the altitude well for at least the five days we followed them. Their blood pressure rose during the first day, but then returned to their sea level values for the next four days. Those with pre-existing hypertension responded similarly but at a higher level. Those with angina at home were no worse at altitude. Several played tennis every day.

This was a small and perhaps biased sample at modest altitude, but another, larger study of people climbing and walking in the Alps showed that fewer men and women had heart attacks at altitude during their walk or climb than would have been expected in a similar group at sea level.

Until the twentieth century, measurements on arterial blood were limited to animals, or obtained by slashing an artery; neither method was satisfactory for studies of the dynamics of respiration and circulation. During an epidemic of pneumonia in 1916, William Stadie wished to see whether the amount of oxygen in blood might predict the outcome in serious cases. Through a small cut in the skin, he inserted a needle a little smaller than a thin pencil into an artery, drew blood, and measured the oxygen content. Ten years later, Joseph Barcroft used this same type of needle to draw arterial blood while at the same time collecting alveolar air to demonstrate that the lungs did not secrete oxygen as some claimed. Arterial punctures are commonplace today, but modern-day needles are much smaller and do less damage to the artery.

In 1940 I had a brief encounter, which did me no credit, with another advance. I was finishing my residency training when two doctors senior to me asked if they might do an experiment on one of my patients. Appalled by what they told me, I refused indignantly, saying I couldn't see any use whatever for what they wanted to do, and they went elsewhere. What they proposed was cardiac catheterization. (See Figure 13.) Both of them, Andre Cournand and Dick Richards, later became my good friends. Their pioneering work has enabled others to watch the working of the heart as it had never been seen before.

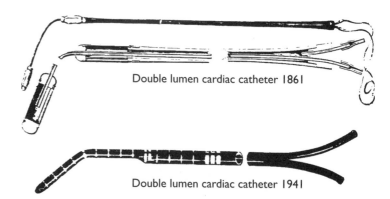

Double lumen cardiac catheter 1861

Figure 13. *Cardiac catheters*

Double lumen cardiac catheter 1941

Cardiac Catheters

In the mid-nineteenth century, two French physiologists, Auguste Chauveau and Jules Marey, devised a double-chambered tube (*catheter*) that they passed through a vein into the right side of the heart to measure the cardiac output of horses (Figure 13, top). Another giant step was taken in 1929 when a young German surgeon, Werner Forssmann, pushed a thin flexible catheter (much like the one Stephen Hales had used on a horse 200 years before) through his veins into his own heart, monitoring the process on a fluoroscope. For this work Forssmann shared the Nobel prize with Andre Cournand and Dickinson Richards, who later perfected the instrument (Figure 13, bottom) and technique and were able to measure not only the dynamics within the heart, but the flow and pressure within the pulmonary artery and the small vessels of the lung. This permitted an intimate understanding of how the heart functions normally or when damaged in some way. And of course it clarified the effects of hypoxia on the circulation of the lung, so immensely important in altitude sickness, and equally so in many illnesses that cause lack of oxygen.

BLOOD

Blood is a vital, complex living tissue. As discussed earlier, its most obvious functions include carrying oxygen from the lungs to the body cells and carbon dioxide from the body cells back to the lungs. Blood is made up of living cells and a liquid component known as *blood plasma*. Plamsa, which normally makes up 60 to 65 percent of blood volume, also contains a range of dissolved substances including *albumin, clotting factors, hormones,* and *electrolytes* (or salts, predominantly sodium and chloride ions). Blood cells include the *red cells* that carry oxygen, the *white cells* that fight infection, and cell fragments known as *platelets* that are vital to blood clotting.

Red Blood Cells and Hemoglobin

Oxygen is carried in blood, not in solution but loosely attached to a protein, *hemoglobin*, which gives blood its reddish color and is the key player in oxygen transport. Throughout recorded history, blood has been associated with life, even more so than has air, perhaps because it is so highly visible and so easily spilled. As noted in Daniel Gilbert's *Oxygen and Living Processes*, in the fifth century B.C. Empedocles wrote that "the blood is the life," and Aristotle believed that the soul depended on the composition of the blood. Their contemporary, Anaxagoras, was more specific: "The blood is formed by a multitude of droplets, united among them," a remarkable statement that seems to anticipate observations made by a Dutch lens-maker 2,000 years later.

In 1674 Anthony Van Leeuwenhoek read his landmark paper to the Royal Society in London, and delighted the members who looked through his little microscopes:

I have divers times endeavored to see and to know what parts the blood consists of and at length I have observed, taking some blood out of my hand, that it consists of small round globules driven through a cristalline humidity of water; yet whether all bloods be such I doubte.

Leeuwenhoek was not the first to use a magnifying glass; single lenses had been known for centuries. But he was the first to combine lenses to make what we know as the compound microscope, which could magnify up to 300 times. He was fascinated by everything small, and estimated the size of the "little animals" he watched (varieties of protozoa), as he did every other object, by comparing it with a grain of sand. His estimation came astonishingly close to 7.5 microns, which we know today is the diameter of the normal, average red blood cell.

The "globules" he saw are not actually round but flattened disks, each shaped like a doughnut whose center has not been completely punched out. These disks are flexible, able to distort into narrower shapes as they pass through tiny vessels. Red blood cells (*erythrocytes*) are packed with a reddish stuff, called *hemoglobin,* that has a very special talent: It can combine easily but loosely with oxygen when the partial pressure of oxygen rises as blood passes through the lungs, and can release oxygen easily to the cells where partial pressure of oxygen is low.

Air and Hemoglobin

Ten years before Leeuwenhoek saw his little cells, Richard Lower, one of the remarkable group of men in the young Royal Society, noticed that blood changed from dark red to a brighter carmine when it was agitated with air. His contemporary Robert Hooke soon showed the Royal Society that an experimental animal could be kept alive when the chest was widely opened, so long as air was rhythmically blown into the lungs with a bellows. Lower, seizing on this, observed that blood also changed from dark to bright red while passing through well-aerated lungs. By this time expansion of the lungs had been explained, but oxygen had not yet been identified, so no closer connection between breathing air and the change in blood was possible.

In 1747 Menghini burned blood and showed that its ash was attracted to a magnet, an observation that a century later led Justus von Liebig to speculate that blood contained some form of iron that carried oxygen, not in simple solution, but bound to a compound within the red cells. Lothar Meyer soon showed this to be true, and in 1865 Felix Hoppe-Seyler crystallized this substance and showed it to his friend Paul Bert.

Bert, considered the father of altitude physiology, also did much of the basic work in the last thirty years of the nineteenth century to establish the relationship between oxygen and hemoglobin. He was remarkably versatile: a lawyer, a plastic surgeon, and a physiologist until, deeply saddened by the death of two young colleagues in a balloon flight, he accepted appointment as governor general of Indochina where he died at age fifty-three.

He had studied under the great Claude Bernard; became interested in blood, oxygen, and high altitude; and in 1878 wrote the seminal book on high-altitude medicine, *Barometric Pressure*. A wealthy patron, Denis Jourdanet, had several decompression chambers built for Bert, in which Bert had himself taken to simulated altitudes much higher than Hooke had gone 150 years earlier. Bert described his symptoms at altitude, showed that they were prevented by breathing oxygen, and advised its use by balloonists for the high flights that had again become popular. Three of these balloonists were part of his laboratory and soon would demonstrate how terribly important this advice was.

The Oxygen–Hemoglobin Dissociation Curve

Paul Bert must also be remembered for his careful studies of how hemoglobin combines with oxygen. Using instruments he designed and ordered to be made for him, Bert exposed measured amounts of blood to different partial pressures of oxygen. He then used a vacuum pump to extract the oxygen that had combined with blood, and was able to plot the relationship between oxygen pressure and the percentage of hemoglobin combined with it. From this he was able to draw the first oxy–hemoglobin dissociation curves (Figure 14).

When Bert drew the rough curves describing this relationship, he was not able to measure some of the other influences (such as temperature, carbon dioxide, and acidity) that affect the shape of the curve. Consequently he could not fully appreciate the beauty of the special S-shape of the normal

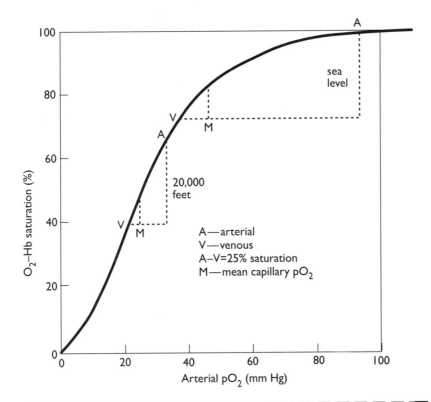

Figure 14. *Oxy–hemoglobin dissociation curve*

Transport of Oxygen by Hemoglobin

In man and most animals, oxygen is carried not in simple solution but in combination with a "respiratory pigment." There are many different kinds of such pigments, but most mammals use one in which molecular iron—hemoglobin (in loose combination with other materials)—grasps oxygen molecules when exposed to a high partial pressure of the gas, and releasing them when the partial pressure falls. The relationship between oxygen pressure and the percentage of hemoglobin combined with it can be plotted in the oxy–hemoglobin dissociation curve. (See Figure 14.)

curve for human hemoglobin. We have made enormous strides since his innovative work and can better realize how admirably adapted to its task is hemoglobin.

When blood is exposed to a high partial pressure of oxygen, it quickly becomes nearly saturated, as its iron-containing hemoglobin molecules pick up molecules of oxygen. This happens in the lungs. When oxygen-rich blood reaches the tissues where oxygen pressure is low, the iron molecules quickly release oxygen, which diffuses into cells. The depleted blood then returns to heart and lungs for another load of oxygen. The S-shape of the dissociation curve shown in Figure 14 illustrates how quickly and completely oxygen is loaded and unloaded, and thus how humans and other animals acquire essential oxygen and tolerate its lack.

Blood's Oxygen Content and Carrying Capacity

Blood carries oxygen almost entirely in loose combination with hemoglobin; very little is in physical solution. Each gram of hemoglobin will bind or carry 1.34 milliliters (ml) of oxygen when fully saturated. Because there are or should be about 15 grams of hemoglobin in each hundred ml of our blood, it follows that each 100 ml can carry fifteen times 1.34, or about 20 ml of oxygen, when hemoglobin is fully saturated. We call this the *oxygen-carrying capacity* of blood, normally described as 20 volumes percent. Changes in blood acidity, temperature, and content of carbon dioxide change the carrying capacity and thus alter its *oxygen content.*

When less oxygen is available, blood is less than fully saturated. Capacity and content are the same only when enough oxygen is available to fully saturate the hemoglobin. Both capacity and content increase when hemoglobin is increased, and if hemoglobin increases in parallel with a decrease in available oxygen, there may be near-normal oxygen content even at altitude. So it is not surprising that an increase in circulating hemoglobin should be one of the ways in which man and some animals accommodate to lower oxygen in the ambient air (discussed in Chapter 13, "Acclimatization").

Blood Acidity

The shape of the oxy–hemoglobin dissociation curve (Figure 14) is affected by carbon dioxide (CO_2) and by the acidity of blood. The former is determined by respiration, the latter by metabolism. The acidity or alkalinity of blood (like any solution) depends on the amount of hydrogen ion (H^+) or hydroxyl ion (OH^-) in solution. The degree of acidity is indicated by the symbol pH, which is the negative logarithm of the concentration of hydrogen ions. A neutral solution (when both H^+ and OH^- ions are exactly balanced) has a pH of 7.0: The lower the pH falls below 7.0, the more acid the solution; alkaline solutions have a pH higher than 7.0.

Our metabolism produces many acidic substances, including lactic acid, fatty acids, nucleic and uric acids, and of course carbon dioxide. These acidic compounds can threaten the stability of blood and the "internal environment" on which, as Claude Bernard said, our free and active life depends. When one realizes how many acids and how few alkaline substances enter the blood, the small range of pH it maintains is all the more remarkable. This equilibrium depends on the stabilizing effect of several important buffers that can "absorb" H^+ or OH^- ions without much change in pH. There are six major buffers in blood, three involving hemoglobin. But of these, the most immediately effective is the *carbonate–bicarbonate buffer*, which is as important in altitude physiology as it is in normal everyday life because of the speed with which it can be altered by exhaling carbon dioxide or by excreting bicarbonate.

Chapter 3, "Moving Air: Respiration," described how carbon dioxide diffuses through capillary walls much faster than does oxygen. Most of the carbon dioxide is carried in blood in solution or as bicarbonate, a compound produced through the reaction of carbon dioxide with water. This reaction is catalyzed by the enzyme *carbonic anhydrase*. There is a high concentration of this enzyme in red blood cells, lungs, and kidneys—places where a shift in acidity can be speedily accomplished by changing the exhalation of carbon dioxide or loss of bicarbonate in the urine. The fact that the carbonate–bicarbonate buffer is found in so many body tissues makes it an important target for useful medications such as the diuretic Diamox (discussed in Chapter 15, "Prevention and Treatment").

Human Hemoglobin

We humans have three different forms of hemoglobin at different times in our lives. The embryo's blood contains a primitive form (P-hemoglobin) that soon changes to the F, or fetal, form, which has an affinity for oxygen much stronger than does the adult form, A-hemoglobin. The stronger affinity for oxygen enables the fetus's blood to take up oxygen more easily from its mother's blood as it passes through the placenta, and thus helps the fetus survive and grow in an oxygen environment comparable to that on top of Mount Everest. F-hemoglobin changes to the adult form soon after birth. Some experimental procedures have been able to convert abnormal human hemoglobins to the F form, a practice which someday may help individuals who are chronically short of oxygen from illness.

The affinity of hemoglobin for oxygen also changes as the blood circulates. The high temperature, acidity, and elevated carbon dioxide levels found within the tissues decrease the affinity of hemoglobin for oxygen. This change, known as a "right shift" of the oxy–hemoglobin dissociation curve, allows oxygen to leave hemoglobin more easily and enter the cells. In the lungs, the lower temperature, reduced carbon dioxide level, and lower acidity increase the affinity of hemoglobin for oxygen. This is known as a "left shift" of the oxy–hemoglobin dissociation curve and makes hemoglobin take up oxygen from the alveoli more readily.

Hundreds of different or mutant hemoglobins occur in humans. The development of more sophisticated methods for analyzing respiratory pigments has enabled identification of many subgroups of these abnormal hemoglobins, but very few are important in altitude physiology.

Sickle Cells

One important mutation of hemoglobin is S-hemoglobin. People with two copies of the S-hemoglobin gene are said to have the *homozygous* genotype. These people, most of whom have West African, South Asian, or Mediterranean ancestry, have sickle cell anemia. An additional group carries one copy of the S-hemoglobin gene (the *heterozygous* genotype) and possess what is called the "sickle trait." The sickling trait, the most common abnormality of hemoglobin, usually causes no problems under normal conditions, although some forms do cause chronic anemia. But when people with the sickle trait go to altitude or become hypoxic from whatever cause, the cells become distorted and tension within the hemoglobin molecule makes it stiff so that the misshapen red cells may stick like burrs in the narrow capillaries. (See Figure 15.) Consequently, any cause of decreased oxygen such as altitude or lung disease can cause problems through obstruction of small blood vessels, most commonly in the spleen and kidney. The sickle cells

Sickle Red Blood Cells

Approximately 10 percent of the population in the United States has a form of hemoglobin whose configuration is abnormal. The most common abnormality includes a molecular configuration that under certain conditions can exert strong stresses within the red cell that distort some cells into sickle or half-moon shapes instead of the normal flat disk (as shown in Figure 15).

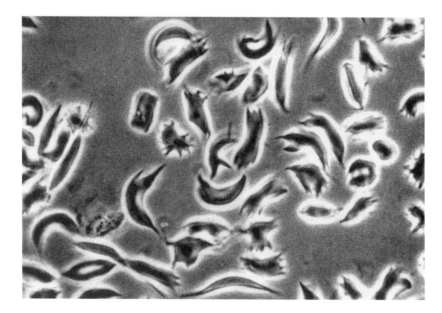

Figure 15. *Sickle red blood cells*

revert to normal with oxygen or descent from high altitude, although damage to the spleen and sometimes other tissues is not reversed immediately, but heals slowly. Interestingly, only alveolar hypoxia causes sickling; carbon monoxide hypoxia apparently does not.

Fortunately sickling is a rare occurrence—but one that can be serious if not recognized. Sometimes the damage caused by the obstructions causes a confusing clinical picture that may lead to mistaken or delayed diagnosis. Simple laboratory tests can solve the puzzle. In the 1950s, when the complications of sickling were not widely recognized, the following case was reported:

A young Caucasian mechanic took a long bus ride from sea level to 7,000 feet and within two hours of arrival developed nausea and severe pain in the upper left quadrant of his abdomen. During the next three days he grew worse, and only after special tests were done was his blood found to contain sickle cells. The cause of his abdominal pain was an abnormally enlarged spleen, which was removed and found to have several infarcts (areas where blood vessels were obstructed, causing death of the affected tissues). The tentative diagnosis of sickle cell disease was proven. He was given supplementary oxygen and slowly improved.

This young man's father, on hearing of his son's illness, drove up from sea level and within three hours of arrival developed somewhat similar symptoms. Tests confirmed the diagnosis of sickle cell disease. He quickly improved with oxygen and descent, and surgery was not done. He stoutly denied mixed ancestry but later acknowledged that "miscegenation in his progenitors was likely."

Another group, perhaps 1 percent of the population, has some mutant form of hemoglobin that combines differently with oxygen. Some forms may pick up oxygen avidly in the lungs and release it in the tissues only when partial pressure is very low. Other forms acquire oxygen slowly but release it more readily. These other mutant hemoglobins are rare medical curiosities with little medical importance; they don't form thrombi or *emboli* (blood clots).

Other Respiratory Pigments

Myoglobin is a special protein closely related to hemoglobin. It has the capability of carrying oxygen and releasing it rapidly when tissue needs are acute. It serves as an emergency supply, capable of releasing a large amount of needed oxygen very rapidly. Myoglobin is found in skeletal and cardiac muscle tissue.

Throughout the animal kingdom, there are many different respiratory pigments, of which hemoglobin is one, with different affinities for oxygen. For example, most invertebrates use a substance that strongly attracts and holds oxygen, while in other species the attraction is rather weak. Tadpole hemoglobin attracts and holds oxygen very tightly, but as tadpoles become adult frogs, this attraction weakens. The blood of animals living at high altitude or in other oxygen-poor environments—such as the marine environment—generally has a stronger affinity for oxygen than does human blood. When the pigment is carried in solution rather than in cells, as is the case with some animals, the "blood" tends to be thick and move more sluggishly than when the pigment is contained in cells. There is persuasive evidence that the choice between solution and cells was dictated evolutionarily long ago by the lifestyle of the animal. Animal variations are of interest to those interested in altitude and hypoxia because they may someday show us other pathways for managing hypoxic illnesses.

Blood Vessels

The essential role of the heart is to move blood throughout the body, and it does so through a network of blood vessels, starting with large-bore (half-inch), thick-walled muscular arteries, which leave the heart to divide and branch into ever smaller arteries and arterioles. These lead into the precapillary vessels, which are especially important because, unlike the capillaries, they have thin muscular walls and are able to contract or relax. From the precapillary vessels, blood flows into the capillaries. As discussed in Chapter 3, "Moving Air: Respiration," it is from these thin-walled vessels that oxygen leaves the blood and enters the body while carbon dioxide leaves the tissues and enters the blood. After leaving the capillaries, the blood flows through veins of larger and larger diameter. Veins are similar to arteries in construction but have much less muscle tissue in their walls. Veins need less muscle than do arteries because they carry blood at a much lower pressure.

Endothelial Cells and Nitric Oxide

The lining (*endothelium*) of the small precapillary vessels can release minute amounts of a powerful agent that was first appreciated only recently (1980) and was labeled *endothelium-derived relaxing factor* (EDRF). It was soon after identified as a simple chemical substance, *nitric oxide* (NO), which is formed in the inner lining of blood vessels. Although the principal action of NO is to relax blood vessels, it has important effects on many other physiological functions. Nitric oxide—not to be confused with nitrous oxide (NO_2), known as laughing gas—may be a simple chemical, but the processes by which it causes its effects are complex.

Minute amounts of NO are produced by the action of a specific enzyme (*nitric oxide synthase,* or NOS) in all endothelial cells in every mammalian organ at a steady basal rate. Various substances *increase* NO release, which relaxes blood vessels, allowing smaller ones to dilate. NO also slows or halts the stickiness and clumping of platelets, thereby helping to decrease the tendency for clot formation in blood vessels.

Endothelial cells also release a family of substances called *endothelins*, one of which constricts blood vessels in direct opposition to NO. The balance between endothelin and NO (and probably other substances as well) governs blood flow and pressure. This balance is particularly important in determining pulmonary artery pressure.

Certain other physiological substances *inhibit* NO synthesis and release, and thus increase vascular tone and blood pressure, increase clot formation, and increase the leakiness of capillary blood vessels. These activities are all important in adjusting to hypoxia through an intricately balanced system.

More recently, NO has been found to play an even more important role—helping hemoglobin to "dictate" how much, and where, oxygen is delivered to tissues. It does so because the binding of oxygen to heme ions also promotes the binding of NO to hemoglobin. When hemoglobin releases oxygen in the capillaries, the shape of the hemoglobin molecule changes and this in turn releases NO in precapillary arterioles and even in capillaries. The released NO relaxes the blood vessels. It is amazing that hemoglobin not only provides oxygen but also "senses" oxygen need and alters capillary flow to provide what is needed where and when.

As for its role in altitude illnesses, NO appears to be a central player in at least one of these—high altitude pulmonary edema, discussed in Chapter 10, "HAPE: High Altitude Pulmonary Edema."

Blood's Multiple Functions

Of course blood has many other functions besides its most important one of transporting oxygen and carbon dioxide. It carries nutrients to feed all living tissues. It can pick up water and carry it where needed, and it can also release water through the skin in sweat. Waste materials (of which carbon dioxide is only one, but a very important one) are carried to kidneys or lungs or even the skin for discharge. Poisonous products are taken to the liver for detoxification. And so on…

The circulatory system is also the highway over which scores of hormones and enzymes are moved. And blood contains many special materials with a host of important tasks, such as those that protect us against infections and that stanch bleeding from wounds without clotting in the blood vessels.

As mentioned earlier, Greco–Roman philosopher–scientists believed that blood "cools the innate heat" of the body—and they were quite right! We might call blood an air conditioner: When we are too hot, the heat-regulating center diverts blood from core to skin, where it may cool by convection, and by increasing water loss in sweat will increase heat loss further by evaporation. Cold diverts blood away from skin to organs that must be kept warm if the body is to survive. The circulating blood is indispensable for keeping the body at an even temperature, which rarely varies by more than a degree; this is more precise than many home furnaces! Even in feverish illness, the flowing blood distributes heat to the skin where it can be carried off.

The brain directs the conservation of water by shutting down urine formation and sweating when too much water has been lost from the blood; conversely, if we try to overload with water, blood facilitates its efficient excretion in urine.

Oxygen transport is such a vital function of blood that it is easy to forget its many other functions. Without white blood cells to fight infection, without platelets to help stop bleeding, and without distribution of hormones and other necessities throughout the body, we would not survive very long.

We now understand how the respiratory and circulatory systems work together to supply oxygen to our body cells—the ultimate users of this vital substance. We have seen how movement of the chest cavity brings oxygen-rich air into the lungs, how that oxygen crosses into the blood, how the blood is pumped by the heart to the body tissues, and how oxygen then leaves the blood and enters the cells. We have also discussed how these processes (in particular ventilation) are controlled to assure a constant level of oxygen (and carbon dioxide) in the blood. We learned how the blood circulates throughout the body, bathes the tissues with oxygen and nutrients, and carries away wastes. We have seen how molecular feedback mechanisms strive to maintain a perfect balance of fluids, salts, gases, and other factors. In subsequent chapters, we will use this understanding to explore how our bodies respond to the challenges of low oxygen levels at high altitude. But first we will examine those ultimate users—cells, the building blocks of life—and how oxygen fuels their every activity.

CHAPTER 5

CELLS: THE ULTIMATE USERS

In my early teenage years a retired doctor friend of my parents, Dr. William Bradshaw, let me borrow his microscope. It was a gorgeous old brass scope with both high and low power lenses, and it fascinated me immediately. I quickly learned to examine paper, cloth, and hair, then moved on to dead insects, feathers, and plants. Once I examined a drop of water collected from a swamp. A whole new world opened up to me! There were all sorts of things in that water, many plants that seemed to move, dots that darted at incredible speed, larger "animals" that moved slowly, and others that swam more rapidly. The more I looked, the more I saw, and the more fascinating the whole enterprise became. My parents gave me a small old book, The Wonder of the Microscope, *which opened up another world in which I saw a whole new range of natural substances to look at, and beyond that horizon a plethora of man-made materials to examine.*

Somewhere in that book or another I saw a picture of the earliest microscope, made by Anton Van Leeuwenhoek in the mid-seventeenth century. This fascinated me, and soon I found a book depicting his microscopes and the "little animals" he described, eventually to the Royal Society of England and the French Academy. He portrayed red blood cells as grains of sand on the beach, and he described the cellular structure of many substances, notably cork.

This was my introduction to the cell, and a rich introduction it was. I was eager to explore anything that would fit on my microscope stage. I was too impatient to see new things to take the time to study any of them in depth, but I certainly covered a wide range. After a glorious summer of exploration and excitement, I returned to school, where the adventure ended for many years. My parents returned the microscope to that dear doctor who had influenced my life so greatly, and I turned to other activities—travel, mountaineering, and studying for my future life.

The movements of air and blood, while vital to survival, are not ends in themselves. Rather, these actions combine to nourish and protect living cells. Our breathing provides oxygen to and removes carbon dioxide from the blood. As it passes through the intestines, the blood also picks up nutrients that we ingest in our food. The blood then carries the nutrients and oxygen to cells, and removes carbon dioxide and other waste products. Blood flow also helps regulate our body temperature. If either respiration or circulation fails to provide oxygen and fuel or to control temperature for more than a short while, cells begin to die. The death of our entire body is not far behind. Of all our physical needs, a steady supply of oxygen is most urgent: Without it, death is minutes away.

Cells are the blocks from which a living organism is built, but unlike bricks they are busily functioning units that live and die and replace themselves. We are made of 75 to 100 trillion cells of many different types and functions. With few exceptions they all have similar components. Only a few of the many elements of the cell are mentioned here, although all are essential and may be affected by oxygen deficit.

A TYPICAL CELL

Although cells with different specialties are somewhat different internally, all consist of a rich soup contained in a thin skin. The soup's "broth" is a watery fluid called the *cytosol*. Dozens of components called *organelles* are suspended in the cytosol; these highly organized compartments each have a specific and essential job. Cytosol and organelles (other than the cell *nucleus*) together make up the *cytoplasm*.

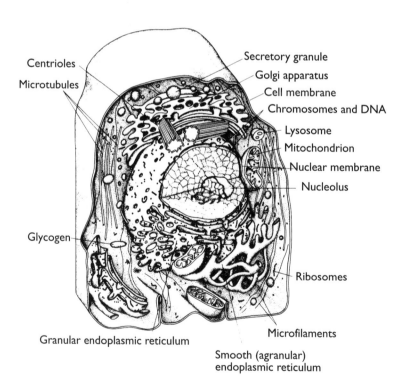

Figure 16A. *A typical cell. (From* Textbook of Human Physiology, *by Arthur C. Guyton. W. B. Saunders Company, 1991. Reproduced with permission.)*

Centrioles
Microtubules
Secretory granule
Golgi apparatus
Cell membrane
Chromosomes and DNA
Lysosome
Mitochondrion
Nuclear membrane
Nucleolus
Glycogen
Ribosomes
Granular endoplasmic reticulum
Microfilaments
Smooth (agranular) endoplasmic reticulum

The protective skin surrounding the cell is called the *cell membrane*. This important barrier separates the fluid inside the cell (the cytosol) from the fluid outside the cell (the *interstitial fluid*). Membrane structure and permeability are crucial to life and powerfully affect how well or poorly we tolerate environmental challenges such as oxygen deficit, heat, cold, or toxic substances. Because it surrounds the cell, the interstitial fluid is the environment in which cells exist, and its composition is important to the proper functioning of the cells. The interstitial fluid is also in contact with blood plasma at the capillaries. Nutrients and oxygen move from blood to interstitial fluid and then on into the cells. Waste products, including carbon dioxide, take the reverse pathway.

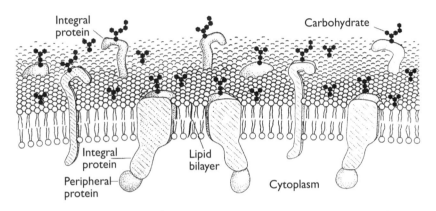

Figure 16B. *Detail of a typical cell. (From* Textbook of Human Physiology. *Reproduced with permission.)*

A Typical Cell

Cells are held together to form the tissues that make up the various structures that define the various organs of the body: spleen, liver, heart, and bone, for example. Each is built of its unique type of cells and supported by fibrous material, all bathed in a common liquid, the extracellular fluid, which maintains a stable environment for the cells. We are made of much more water than solid stuffs, and the constancy of our cells' functions is completely dependent on the extracellular fluid.

The cytoplasm and its contents (organelles, mitochondria, nucleus—see Figure 16A) are contained within a thin, tough *membrane*, a double layer of *lipid* (fat molecules) and scattered protein linked to *carbohydrate* (*glycoside*) molecules. These *glycoproteins* form channels through which water-soluble substances passively diffuse in and out of cells, selectively. (See Figure 16B.)

The cell membrane is as essential to life as are other parts of the cell, because its integrity determines what substances enter or leave the cytoplasm.

When salts dissolve in water, they form charged particles or ions. Many of these ions can cross the cell membrane only through special channels. Some of these channels are open all the time and allow ions to diffuse passively from areas of higher concentration to areas of lower concentration. Other channels open only at specific times. For example, there are calcium channels in the membranes of heart muscle cells that open when the muscle is stimulated electrically. Calcium enters the muscle cells from the interstitial fluid (which has a concentration of calcium much higher than the calcium concentration within the cell), causing the muscle cells to contract. Other molecules, such as oxygen and carbon dioxide, flow freely across the cell membrane from regions of higher to lower concentration. They are said to move by *passive transport*, according to Fick's first law of diffusion. It is worth remembering that Fick's law of diffusion applies to all molecules, be they gas, liquid, or solid.

Some ions constantly need to be moved between the intracellular and extracellular fluid by molecular pumps that can transfer selected ions across the cell membrane from an area of low concentration to one where it is higher. Carrier proteins embedded in the cell membrane pick up a molecule on one side and deposit it on the other. These *active transport* pumps require energy and consume a great deal of oxygen, and therefore are vulnerable to hypoxia. One important example of a carrier protein is the *sodium–potassium pump,* which requires energy to pump sodium ions out of cells and potassium ions into cells. It is responsible for the fact that the interstitial fluid and blood have a high sodium level but a low potassium level while the reverse is true for the cytoplasm. Because water commonly follows salt across cell membranes, the sodium–potassium pump is vital to maintaining both proper salt and water balance within the cell. There will be more later about the reaction of the sodium–potassium pump to hypoxia.

Another important example of a carrier protein is the *glucose transporter*. This membrane protein binds a molecule of the simple sugar *glucose* in the interstitial fluid outside the cell and deposits it into the cytoplasm inside the cell. In some cells, the glucose transporter only works when the hormone *insulin* is present. People whose bodies cannot make insulin develop *diabetes mellitus*. In this disease glucose cannot enter cells. It builds up in the blood and interstitial fluid. Blood sugar levels are high but the cells are starved for nutrients.

HOW CELLS ARE FUELED

The food we eat consists of large, complex molecules including carbohydrates, fats, and proteins. These molecules are digested in the intestinal tract and broken down into simpler compounds: six-carbon sugars, fatty acids, and amino acids. Each type of nutrient contains a large amount of energy originally derived from the sun and waiting to be released. Sugars and amino acids pass through the cells of the intestinal wall directly into the blood. Fatty acids pass first into the *lymph*, and then reach the blood. From the blood, these nutrient molecules pass into the interstitial fluid and on into each cell. Cells use these molecules as structural building blocks. Some cells also store carbohydrates or fats for later energy use.

As a fundamental energy source, glucose is the most important of the six-carbon sugars. Because carbohydrates make up a major portion of our diet, and because the liver can convert fatty acids and amino acids to glucose whenever the need arises, it is important to look in detail at how cells use glucose.

Glucose is taken up by cells through the glucose transporter. Once glucose enters the cell, it can be used in several ways. Some cells, such as those in skeletal muscle and the liver, can store glucose as the complex carbohydrate *glycogen*. (When marathoners "carbo load" the night before a race, they are attempting to top off their glycogen stores. When they "hit the wall" several hours into a race, it may be at least partly because those glycogen stores are exhausted.) Excess glucose in the blood is converted to lipids (fats) by the liver cells and then stored in the *adipose* (fat) tissue.

Much of the glucose that enters cells is used to generate the energy-rich molecule *adenosine triphosphate*, or ATP. The process by which cells extract

Burning Food for Energy

Two centuries ago, the discovery of oxygen was followed by demonstrations that most materials would burn in the presence of oxygen. Burning released heat and light, sometimes a great deal of heat, very rapidly. Over the years, scientists recognized that food was burned by the body much as a candle burns—as long as there is a good supply of oxygen. The nagging question became, how can this happen without torching the body?

Answers were slowly found in the first half of the nineteenth century when Justus Liebig developed equations to support the concept that sugars are "burned" gradually and slowly, step by step, in the tissues (the cells), not in the blood, to produce carbon dioxide, water, and a little heat. Louis Pasteur, studying the fermentation of sugary grape juice into alcohol, suggested that there might be some resemblance between this process and what happens to sugars in the body. At the end of the century, Hans and Edward Buchner isolated the substance in yeast that turns sugar into alcohol; from this phenomenon (fermentation, which has been known since Noah!) came the term enzyme, meaning "in yeast."

Liebig's concept was refined and tested, and finally, in the 1920s, Hans Krebs described an elaborate biochemical process involving citric acid; this process is commonly known as the *Krebs cycle*, in his honor. This chemical pathway burns fuel and thus provides the energy of life.

energy from glucose begins in the cytoplasm. In a series of biochemical steps collectively known as *glycolysis*, glucose is converted to *pyruvic acid*. Only a small amount of ATP is formed in this process, and it is *anaerobic*—no oxygen is required. Glycolysis by itself is an inefficient way to produce energy. We humans can do anaerobic work for only a very short time.

If cellular oxygen levels are low, as they might be in skeletal muscle during peak activity, the pyruvic acid is converted to lactic acid. If lactic acid builds up inside the muscle cell, it can contribute to muscle fatigue. If it leaves the cell, it can increase the acidity of the blood and eventually compromise the function of vital organs including the heart and brain. Assuming that we stop exercising before our vital organs are compromised, muscle cells convert the lactic acid back to pyruvic acid and then use the pyruvic acid in a variety of ways. However, the cells need oxygen to do this. This need for oxygen is one reason we continue to breathe hard after stopping vigorous exercise. The fact that oxygen is in short supply at high altitude is one reason that our ability to exercise is lower there than it is at sea level.

MITOCHONDRIA: CELLULAR POWER PLANTS

Luckily, cells have a much more efficient way to use pyruvic acid than converting it to lactic acid. This process is known as the *tricarboxylic acid* (TCA) *cycle* or *Krebs cycle*, and it takes place in the *mitochondria*. (See Figure 17.)

Mitochondria are organelles within the cytoplasm enclosed by their own membrane. Studded into the membrane of mitochondria are a series of proteins called the *electron transport system* (ETS). When cells have sufficient

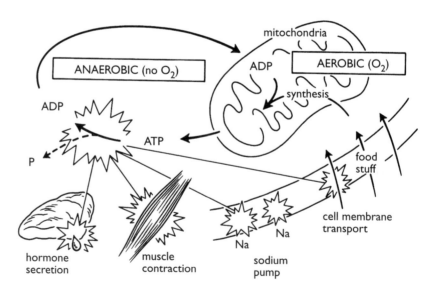

Figure 17. *The Krebs cycle and the phosphagen cycle*

ANAEROBIC (no O₂)

AEROBIC (O₂)

mitochondria

ADP

synthesis

ADP

ATP

P

food stuff

cell membrane transport

Na

Na

hormone secretion

muscle contraction

sodium pump

oxygen, pyruvic acid formed during glycolysis enters the mitochondria, where it undergoes another series of biochemical transformations in the TCA cycle. The products of the TCA cycle are molecules that can donate electrons to the electron transport system, which uses the electrons to capture energy in the form of ATP. The ETS requires oxygen. If sufficient oxygen is present, the mitochondria produce large amounts of ATP from each molecule of pyruvic acid.

Energy released from ATP powers the cells' work; it can be used to power muscle contraction or the energy-requiring membrane pumps. Each molecule of ATP releases energy in a small, uniform quantity so that cells may use the energy effectively and efficiently. Nevertheless, not all the energy released from ATP goes into the work of the cell. Some is released in the form of heat. At first, this might seem wasteful because this heat represents energy lost in the sense that it is not performing work. This heat, however, allows us to maintain the relatively high body temperature that we mammals need for life, and thus performs a vital biological role.

THE NUCLEUS: CELLULAR CONTROL CENTER

The cell nucleus is the organelle that contains the chromosomes. We humans have twenty-three pairs of chromosomes. Chromosomes are made up of *deoxyribonucleic acid*, or DNA. DNA is a two-stranded molecule shaped like a twisted ladder. It carries information in the form of a long array of nitrogen-containing bases, which form the rungs of the ladder. When a cell divides, the DNA copies itself; thus every cell in our body has the same DNA. DNA controls cell function by directing the production of proteins. We call the bit of DNA that carries the information for building a single protein a *gene*.

The first step in building a protein is the stimulation of the DNA of a particular gene to produce a single-stranded molecule known as *ribonucleic acid* (RNA). This process is called *transcription*. The RNA string is made using the DNA string as a template, so it carries the same information as the DNA of the original gene. Once transcription is complete, the RNA leaves the nucleus and enters the cytoplasm.

The Ribosome: Protein Factory

In the cytoplasm, RNA binds to an organelle called the *ribosome*, the site of protein production. Proteins are large, complex molecules made up of small building blocks known as *amino acids*. Humans use about twenty different amino acids to construct proteins. The order in which each of these amino acids appears in the protein chain determines its shape and function. Once the RNA is bound to the ribosome, the ribosome reads the information on the RNA and translates it to create a sequence of amino acids, which are strung together one at a time to build a protein. A change of even a single base in a particular gene could produce a change in the structure and function of the protein produced from that gene—this is what is known as a genetic *mutation*. Genetic mutations can confer advantages or disadvantages to an organism. Chapter 14, "Genetics of High-Altitude Performance," discusses how these mutations might help some human populations adjust more easily to life at high altitude.

Proteins perform a variety of roles within a cell. They may act as structural elements that give a cell its shape. Proteins can also be functional. The cell membrane channels and carriers discussed above are proteins. So are the receptor molecules on the surface of cells that allow cells to respond to hormones and the motors responsible for muscle contraction. Proteins can also function as enzymes and hormones. Enzymes speed chemical reactions and determine which chemical reactions occur in our cells. Hormones are molecules produced by one tissue that reach distant tissues by way of the bloodstream and impact the function of the cells in those tissues.

As our understanding of genes and the control of transcription increases, we are gaining insights into the ways that genetic and environmental influences interact. Scientists interested in how people meet the challenges of high altitude are exploring how genes might impact our response to lack of oxygen, or to cold or heat, as well as to other environmental, physical, or emotional stresses.

HOW HYPOXIA IMPACTS ORGANELLES

We know that mitochondria require oxygen to extract energy from glucose and other nutrient molecules. Without sufficient oxygen, the mitochondria cannot perform this vital function. In the absence of oxygen, cells can still get a small amount of energy from nutrients through glycolysis and the conversion of pyruvic acid to lactic acid, but this anaerobic (literally, without oxygen) pathway supplies very little energy and extracts a high price: Lactic acid builds up, increasing blood acid levels. This process can produce a potentially dangerous condition known as *acidosis*. Many organs are adversely affected by acidosis, but muscle tissue is particularly vulnerable. Both heart and skeletal muscles contract less forcefully when acid levels are high.

Hypoxia impacts other vital cell structures as well. The sodium–potassium pump, the membrane channel responsible for maintaining proper salt and water balance in cells, requires a large amount of energy to do its work. Severe hypoxia can stop the work of the sodium–potassium pump, resulting in damaging swelling of the cells.

Scientists once thought that this phenomenon, brought about by the hypoxia of altitude, might be the cause of the abnormal fluid collection seen in high-altitude illnesses that affect the brain and lungs. This turns out not to be the case. However, hypoxia may impact the sodium–potassium pump in a more subtle way. The epithelial cells that line the air sacs (alveoli) of the lung have their sodium–potassium pumps situated in a way that allows them to move salt and water from the alveoli to the interstitial space and ultimately to the blood. This keeps fluid from accumulating in the alveoli. Hypoxia slows transcription of the gene for the pump, decreasing the number of pumps that the alveolar epithelial cells produce. This loss of pumps diminishes the body's ability to remove water from the lungs. This hypoxia-induced "down-regulation" of pumps may contribute to the accumulation of water in the alveoli seen in high altitude pulmonary edema. (See Chapter 10, "HAPE: High Altitude Pulmonary Edema.")

Other cellular pumps and channels also might be impacted by hypoxia. Normal brain activity and consciousness require that nerve cells pass signals from one to another in an orderly and efficient manner. This process depends on pumps and channels embedded in the cell membranes of brain cells. When a person loses consciousness as a result of severe hypoxia, it is caused at least in part by a loss of function of these membrane pumps and channels.

From Cells to Tissues

So, if all our cells have the same genes, and if genes direct protein production, and if proteins determine cell structure and function, how can we have different types of cells? The most direct answer to this question is that different genes are turned on (*induced*) in different cell types. Liver cells make liver proteins, and heart cells make heart proteins. There are many different cell types in the human body. Scientists classify them into four categories, or "tissue types": epithelial tissue, connective tissue, muscle tissue, and nerve tissue. All four play a role in high-altitude climbing.

Epithelial tissue covers the exposed surfaces of the body. The upper layer of skin (called the *epidermis*) is epithelial tissue, and so are the lining of the blood vessels and the alveoli of the lung. Epithelial tissue lining the blood vessels is known as the *endothelium*. Because of its position in blood vessels and lung, epithelial tissue plays a critical role in the diseases of altitude. Epithelial tissue has no blood vessels, and thus must receive its oxygen from the blood vessels in nearby connective tissue. For this reason, epithelial tissue is particularly susceptible to damage from reduced oxygenation. One example of this is the eruption of bed sores, which form on the skin of a person who lies for too long in one position, cutting off blood supply to tissues near the epidermis.

Connective tissue provides structure, stores energy, and has transport functions. Bone, fat, and blood are all connective tissues that play a role in our ability to climb high. Nerve tissue carries electrical signals from one area of the body to another. Because it has a high metabolic rate and thus needs large amounts of oxygen to function well, the nerve tissue of the brain is particularly vulnerable to the effects of high altitude.

Muscle tissue is capable of contraction and force production. Skeletal muscle allows conscious motion; smooth muscle lines the walls of hollow organs, including blood vessels; cardiac muscle is found exclusively in the heart. All three muscle types are impacted by the hypoxia of altitude. Because they need large amounts of oxygen to do work, skeletal and cardiac muscle may be particularly vulnerable.

We know there are some rare and unusual species of bacteria able to exist in extreme environments that are completely devoid of oxygen. Nevertheless, for virtually every creature on earth, any function performed by the elements within their cells depends on oxygen and, therefore, is at least somewhat affected by hypoxia, whatever its cause. High altitude strikes at the most fundamental processes of life.

There are a good many bacteria for which oxygen is toxic. These anaerobic organisms can cause serious illness. Furthermore, far beneath the earth's surface, a few organisms live entirely without oxygen and multiply extremely slowly. Two miles deep in the ocean dwell other living organisms that depend on sulfur rather than oxygen. These and many other variants are fascinating, but beyond the reach of this book.

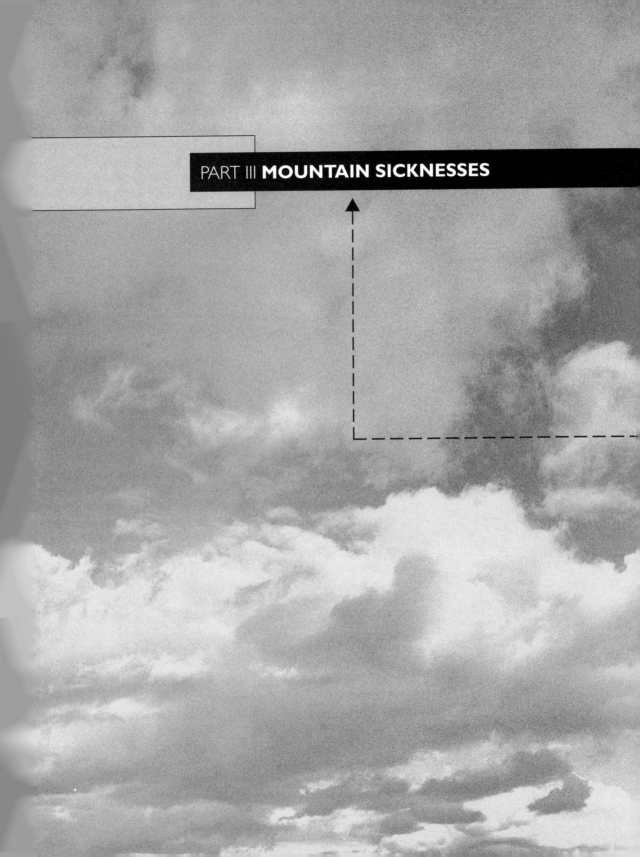

PART III **MOUNTAIN SICKNESSES**

CHAPTER

MOUNTAIN ILLNESS: THE AIR UP HIGH

In 1925 I embarked on my first trip to the Alps, terribly excited at my first climb on a small, rocky spire. We left in darkness. Soon I was tied to a guide and sick to my stomach—not from altitude illness (we were only at about 8,000 feet) but from sheer excitement. During my first experience on the high Himalayas, in 1936, one member of the party became ill at 22,000 feet with a strange combination of symptoms that only many years later did I realize had been high altitude cerebral edema, one of the less common and more serious symptoms of altitude illness. Not until World War II, as a certified flight surgeon in the U.S. Navy, did I begin to learn about high altitude and its dangerous effects on the body.

Back in World War I, pilots managed to fly airplanes higher than they were meant to go, and they were taught to suck oxygen through a pipe stem from a small bottle in the cockpit. Many pilots scorned this precaution as "sissified," and perhaps some died as a result. By the start of World War II, aircraft could routinely go much higher than humans could safely go, and oxygen equipment became mandatory. Training pilots and aircrew in the use of this equipment was a lot easier than training them to recognize when they didn't have enough oxygen, because lack of oxygen is so very insidious, creeping up on one without warning. My major task as a World War II flight surgeon was to teach aircrew how to recognize the subtle signs of lack of oxygen.

After World War II I retired to medical practice and only reentered the mountaineering field in 1950 and 1953, when once again I went very high and once again recognized what was happening at high altitude. Then, in 1960, by a curious set of circumstances, I rescued a man with a bizarre pneumonia-like illness from a high mountain in Colorado; it soon became clear that this was high altitude pulmonary edema and the first case described in English medical literature. (It had been described earlier in South America.) Largely through this experience I was given leadership in a ten-year project studying the effects of altitude at 17,500 feet in the Yukon with a dedicated group of several hundred volunteers and several distinguished scientists.

Over the last thirty years, research into altitude hypoxia—and, belatedly, hypoxia from other causes at sea level—has become chic, and a vast amount of data has been collected. But almost a century ago, Thomas Ravenhill, a physician for a mining company in northern Chile, described patients he saw who developed several kinds of illness, which he blamed on the altitude. He classified them as neurological, cardiac, and "normal" because of the signs and symptoms he saw. He recognized that sending patients to a lower altitude would cure them almost immediately, even enabling a few to return to altitude after a stay near sea level. His work was lost for fifty years; since it resurfaced the classifications that Ravenhill adopted have become the basis of our current definitions. Today we understand more and more of how the human body reacts to the lack of oxygen and how this response is modified genetically and biochemically as well as by various other influences such as dehydration, illness, and fatigue. All of this is outlined in the following chapters, which describe mountain illnesses, chronic and acute, as well as the ordinary causes and effects of hypoxia.

Our forebears wove many myths and legends about the four "elements"—air, earth, fire, and water. Of these, they knew that only invisible, impalpable air was essential to life, but why this was so remained a mystery for many centuries.

What we know today about the air in which we live has been learned slowly and gradually, and recognition of how this relates to experiences on mountains is much more recent. Mountains have been worshipped as the home of gods, feared for the havoc they might inflict, and for many years the highest ones were seldom visited. Two thousand years ago, Chinese General Du Quin advised his emperor not to send envoys to Kashmir because "travelers have to climb over Mount Greater Headache, Mount Lesser Headache, and the Fever hills.... " This warning may have discouraged travelers, but 1,500 years later another traveler (as noted by Fa-Hsien) described a more daunting obstacle:

The lakes in the Snow Mountains are inhabited by poisonous dragons that breathe out poisonous clouds when enraged....

Travelers are often attacked by fierce dragons so that they should neither wear red garments, nor carry gourds with them, nor shout loudly....

We haven't heard much about mountain dragons recently, but such beliefs persisted for a long time. Dragons may have been one reason only a few people ventured into the mountains as hunters, gold miners, or missionaries. In olden days a few intrepid explorers and some invaders crossed high mountains, and they suffered great hardship from cold and altitude. Today dragons are relegated to the deep waters of Loch Ness and Lake Champlain.

In the fourteenth and fifteenth centuries, Mongol tribesmen rampaged across Central Asia and high Tibet, and into Europe, crossing deserts and high mountain passes. Mirza Muhammad Haider, a Mongol chieftain,

described in perceptive detail the hazards of altitude on the high Central
Asian plateau:

> Another peculiarity of Tibet is the *dam-giri* which the Moghuls call
> *yas* and which is common to the whole country, though less preva-
> lent in the region of forts and villages. The symptoms are a feeling of
> severe sickness (*nakhushi*) and in every case one's breath so seizes him
> that he becomes exhausted, just as if he had run up a steep hill with
> a heavy burden on his back. On account of the oppression it causes it
> is difficult to sleep. Should, however, sleep overtake one, the eyes are
> hardly closed before one is awake with a start caused by the oppres-
> sion of the lungs and chest....
>
> When overcome by this malady the patient becomes senseless,
> begins to talk nonsense, and sometimes the power of speech is lost,
> while the palms of the hands and the soles of the feet become swollen.
> Often, when this last symptom occurs, the patient dies between dawn
> and breakfast time; at other times he lingers on for several days....
>
> This malady only attacks strangers; the people of Tibet know
> nothing of it, nor do their doctors know why it attacks strangers. No-
> body has ever been able to cure it. The colder the air, the more severe
> is the form of the malady.

Haider's account is notable in several respects: He gave us an early description
of several important signs and symptoms of mountain sickness, he noted
that it also affects horses, and he clearly recognized that something protected
lifelong altitude residents—which may have been the first unequivocal mention of acclimatization.

Jesuit Missionary Father Alonzo Ovalde, traveling in the Andes near the
end of the sixteenth century, described what others might expect to experience (as recounted in Pinkerton's 1813 *A General Collection of the Best and
Most Interesting Voyages and Discoveries in all Parts of the World*):

> When we come to ascend the highest point of the mountain, we feel
> an aire so piercing and subtile that it is with much difficulty we can
> breathe, which obliges us to fetch our breath quick and strong and
> to open our mouths wider than ordinary, applying to them likewise
> our handkerchiefs to protect our mouth and break the extreme cold-
> ness of the air and to make it more proportionable to the temperature
> which the heart requires, not to be suffocated; this I have experienced
> every time I have passed this mighty mountain.

Father Ovalde's more frequently quoted colleague, Father Jose Acosta, was
more dramatic:

> ...I felt such a deadly pain I was ready to hurl myself from the horse
> onto the ground...and almost immediately there followed so much
> retching and vomiting that I thought I would lose my soul, because
> after what I ate and the phlegm, there followed bile and more bile

both yellow and green so that I brought up blood from the violence I felt in my stomach.... I therefore persuade myselfe that the element of the aire there is so subtile and delicate as it is not proportionable with the breathing of man.

Horace-Benedict de Saussure, a broadly educated philosopher–scientist, experienced great weakness during the second ascent of Mont Blanc (15,771 feet) in 1787. Later, impressed by his sensations on the summit, he recorded his pulse, respirations, temperature, and symptoms on that and other mountains, and wrote:

...the sort of weariness which proceeds from the rarity of the air is absolutely insurmountable; when it is at its height, the most imminent peril will not make you move a step faster.... Since the air [on the summit of Mont Blanc] had hardly more than half of its usual density, compensation had to be made for the lack of density by the frequency of inspirations. That is the cause of the fatigue that one experiences at great heights. For while the respiration is accelerating, so also is the circulation.

De Saussure may or may not have related his fatigue to the discovery of oxygen ten years earlier, but he clearly recognized that decreased air density was a factor, as did Friedrich von Tschudi, who wrote a dramatic account of his nasty experience while exploring the high Andes in 1838–1842:

My panting mule slackened his pace, and seemed unwilling to mount a rather steep ascent which we had now arrived at. To relieve him I dismounted, and began walking at a rapid pace. But I soon felt the influence of the rarefied air, and I experienced an oppressive sensation which I had never known before. I stood still for a few moments to recover myself, and then tried to advance. My heart throbbed audibly; my breathing was short and interrupted. A world's weight seemed to lie upon my chest; my lips swelled and burst; the capillaries of my eyes gave way, and blood flowed from them. In a few moments my senses began to leave me. I could neither see, hear, nor feel distinctly. A gray mist floated before my eyes, and I felt myself involved in that struggle between life and death which, a short time before, I fancied I could discern on the face of nature. Had all the riches of earth, or the glories of heaven, awaited me a few hundred feet higher, I could not have stretched out my hand toward them. In that half senseless state I lay stretched on the ground until I felt sufficiently recovered to remount my mule.

A century later, more and more adventurous men and women were climbing high mountains and, not surprisingly, describing their different sensations. Once the nature of the atmosphere had been described, the causes of mountain sickness could be more closely examined. By the end of the nineteenth century it was generally agreed that lack of oxygen due to decreased atmospheric pressure caused most illness experienced on mountains.

EARLY RESEARCH INTO THE CAUSES OF MOUNTAIN SICKNESS

Two hundred years after Acosta and Ovalde, after the necessity of oxygen for life had been recognized, some discerning individuals put these mountain experiences together with Perier's demonstration that air weighed less at altitude (see "The Barometer" in Chapter 1, "The Air About Us") and agreed that the thinner air on mountains might cause mountain sickness. Thomas Beddoes recognized this in 1818 when he wrote:

> Now in ascending these rugged heights the muscular exertion must expend a great deal of oxygene which the rarefied atmosphere will supply but scantily.... The experiments of Mr. Saussure, Pini, and Reboul, concur in shewing that, independent of its rarefaction, the atmosphere of very elevated mountains contains a far smaller proportion of oxygene than that of lower regions, especially than that of the high vallies of the Alps.

Twenty years later a famous traveler, Alexander von Humboldt (whose account is described in Pinkerton's *General Collection*), after comparing his symptoms on the high Andes to seasickness, expressed the idea as we might today:

> ...the air seems as rich in oxygen in these high regions as in the inferior regions; but [since] in this rarefied air the barometric pressure was less than half the level to which we are normally exposed in the plains, a lower quantity of oxygen was taken up by the blood at each breath.

He was exactly right! However, in the first half of the nineteenth century only a few people thought that lack of oxygen was the major cause of mountain sickness. Distinguished doctors offered a variety of explanations, many of them fanciful, and some worth quoting. In 1853 Stanhope Speer, an English physician, after climbing Mont Blanc, wrote a book listing a score of symptoms and summarized his thoughts about the causes, although he avoided direct mention of the role of oxygen:

> These symptoms [of mountain sickness] may be referred to a three-fold source, viz, a gradually increasing congestion of the deeper portions of the circulatory apparatus, increased venosity of the blood, and loss of equilibrium between the pressure of the external air and that of the gases existing within the intestines.... the causes of mountain sickness are themselves the result of a change from a given atmospheric pressure and temperature, to one in which both are greatly and suddenly diminished.

His contemporary, Conrad Meyer-Ahrens, listed even more symptoms and more explanations in 1898:

> Others [symptoms] are observed, although less frequently, such as vomiting of blood; oozing of blood from the mucous membrane of the lips and skin (due merely to the desiccation of these membranes); blunting of sensory perceptions and the intelligence, impatience, irritability....
>
> When one sees the appearance of mountain sickness correspond to varying altitudes, he asks himself what [causes them]. In my opinion the principal role belongs to the decrease of the absolute quantity of oxygen in the rarefied air, the rapidity of evaporation and the intense action of light, direct or reflected from the snow; the direct action of the decrease of pressure should be placed in the second rank...to which are added others due to the action of light on the cerebral functions, an action which affects the preparation of the blood liquid.

In view of what we know today, it is especially interesting to note that Meyer-Ahrens, a distinguished medical practitioner, included, as an effect of altitude, the blunting of intelligence and sensation.

Early mountaineers described a variety of effects suffered and ascribed diverse causes. For example, 150 years ago quite a few doctors considered the

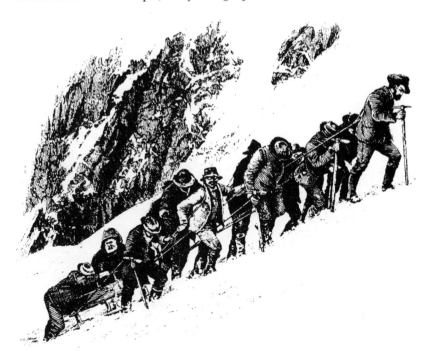

Figure 18. *Dr. Janssen ascending Mont Blanc*

source of the excessive weakness experienced at altitude to be "dislocation of the coxo-femoral articulation (hip joint) from the decreased atmospheric pressure." There is an abundance of tales from the "Golden Age" of alpine climbing (1854–1885), when failure to describe one's symptoms might cast doubt on whether one had reached a summit. Some effects, like bleeding from the eyes or nose that so many experienced in those days, simply don't happen or are rare today.

Studying How Exertion Affects Mountain Sickness

In 1891 a Swiss railway company planned to build a railway to the summit of the Jungfrau (13,600 feet), which affords a spectacular view of the Matterhorn. Dr. H. Kronecker, an experienced physician–mountaineer, was hired to determine whether tourists might suffer from altitude sickness during the ascent. He first made a series of studies in a decompression chamber, taking two people at a time to a pressure equivalent to 13,000 feet in fifteen to twenty-five minutes and then "descending" in twenty minutes, which was the time estimated for the round-trip railroad journey. He examined pulse and blood pressure and ability to exercise, finding that this simulated altitude and rate of ascent caused symptoms in some of the thirty persons studied, and that the effects would be aggravated by exertion. He studied reports from many of the mountain railroads in North and South America, and examined accounts by many mountaineers who had—or had not—suffered from mountain sickness. Kronecker began his work doubting that mountain sickness would be a problem, but his travels and his research studies convinced him that the altitude of 13,600 feet might indeed cause problems for passengers on the proposed railway.

So he recruited seven people (ages ten to seventy) and persuaded them to be carried up the mountain, as they would be in a train. He thought this little experiment would suggest what effect the absence of strenuous exertion would have on passengers. Sixty men took turns hauling the sled and passengers from 5,500 feet to 12,000 feet. The porters worked in shifts but were exhausted by the effort, and several were too sick to continue. The "passengers" felt no discomfort, though most noted increased pulse rates and respiration. Kronecker added, "The most important and striking symptom was the disastrous result of even the least muscular exertion." (The illustration in Figure 18 shows a similar experiment made by astronomer Janssen on Mont Blanc, as he was preparing to build an observatory near the summit; Janssen had the same experience as Kronecker.)

This satisfied Kronecker and the railroad company that the trip would be safe and feasible, provided passengers did not exert themselves at all. As it turned out, the railroad was built only to the Jungfraujoch (11,300 feet) and has been popular ever since—although many visitors do become ill after walking around at the upper station.

LACK OF OXYGEN DETERMINED TO BE THE CAUSE

Before the nineteenth century ended, serious research into mountain sickness had begun. Paul Bert is rightly regarded as the major historical figure in altitude physiology (see Chapter 4, "Moving Blood: Circulation"). His pioneering studies of how hemoglobin carries oxygen, and his first curves showing the relationship of the partial pressure of oxygen to arterial saturation, were certainly as important as his best-known work in decompression chambers and with gas mixtures. These studies proved that lack of oxygen was the principal if not the only cause of mountain sickness, which

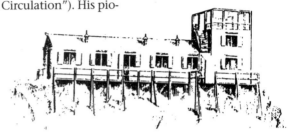

Figure 19A. *Architect's drawing of the Margherita Hut*

The Margherita Hut

Queen Margherita of Italy was an enthusiastic mountain climber, and generously supported Angelo Mosso's research on mountain sickness. On August 18, 1893, the queen and entourage, including her little dog, climbed to the summit of Monte Rosa to dedicate a special altitude research laboratory. (See Figure 19B.) Mosso did most of his studies on the summit of Monte Rosa (15,025 feet) or in the Sella laboratory 4,000 feet lower on the mountain, whereas Paul Bert had done no mountain studies. Mosso exercised soldiers who served as his subjects on the summit and at the base to compare their work capacity as well as to measure respiratory exchanges. Although he had some disagreements with Bert, Mosso's studies of work, the use of carbon dioxide to prevent mountain sickness, and particularly his studies of the brain at altitude in his decompression chamber were complementary to Bert's, and equally important.

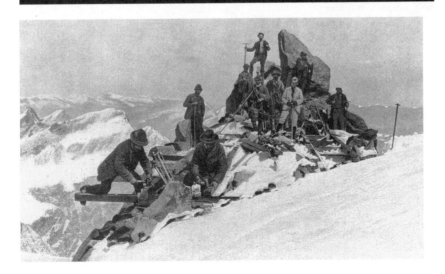

Figure 19B. *Workers starting construction of the Margherita Hut, 15,025 feet*

could be prevented—and remedied—by breathing supplementary oxygen.

Angelo Mosso, a distinguished Italian physiologist and ardent mountaineer, thought otherwise. With the enthusiastic support of Queen Margherita, he established a small laboratory, precariously perched on the summit of Monte Rosa. Near the foot of the mountain he built a larger laboratory, including a small decompression chamber. (See Figure 21.) Mosso studied Bert's book, but cited his own studies to contradict Bert:

> Mountain sickness has been thought a simple asphyxia due to lack of oxygen, whereas in reality, it is a very complex phenomenon, as the arterial blood loses a considerable part of its carbonic acid when the barometric pressure diminishes, and even before the effects due to lack of oxygen appear the phenomena produced by the diminution of carbonic acid in the blood have already manifested themselves.

Two Decompression Chambers

Paul Bert's best-known studies are those done in a decompression chamber built in 1870 to his specifications and funded by his friend, Dr. Denis Jourdanet. (See Figure 20.) After many experiments with animals in a smaller chamber, in 1877 he wrote:

Evidently I could not limit myself to experiments made on animals, however convincing, when I was using practical precepts intended for mountain travelers and aeronauts.

I resolved to begin by experimenting on myself. I had already undergone in my large sheet-iron cylinders, rather considerable decompression to the point of experiencing certain discomforts. I then thought of trying the test again, so as to remove the discomfort by breathing superoxygenated air. I placed beside me a large rubber bag, containing air whose oxygen content was in proportion to the degree of decompression.

Bert made more experiments and effectively proved that breathing his "superoxygenated air" would prevent or relieve the "discomforts" that, as we know, were similar to mountain sickness. Thus he was able to state that lack of oxygen, and not decreased pressure alone, caused mountain sickness. This may have been the first use of a decompression chamber for human studies since Hooke's "barrel" 200 years before!

Angelo Mosso had a similar chamber built around 1890, as shown in Figure 21. This was smaller but had a window and access for instrumentation. He studied soldiers during exercise on Monte Rosa, Italy, and in his chamber.

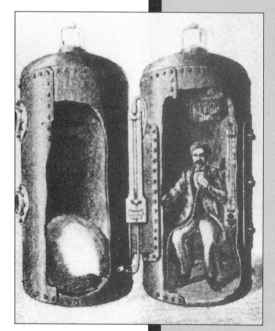

Figure 20. *Paul Bert's decompression chamber*

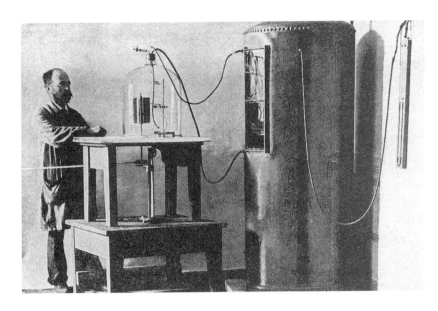

Figure 21. *Angelo Masso's decompression chamber*

He coined the word *acapnia* to describe this condition of "diminution of carbonic acid," which he believed was the major cause of mountain sickness. He buttressed his case by showing that breathing air to which a small percentage of carbon dioxide had been added enabled his subjects to tolerate very high altitude with few symptoms. (This beneficial effect may have been due to the greatly increased breathing caused by the increased carbon dioxide in the chamber air.) Mosso also conducted some daring experiments by taking up in his decompression chamber a man whose brain was partly exposed as the result of an accident, enabling Mosso to observe how the brain became congested at altitude.

Mosso's acapnia theory had few supporters. Paul Bert and Denis Jourdanet, building on the work of others, had conclusively shown that lack of oxygen was the primary cause of mountain sickness. Acapnia, which does occur at high altitude, is not the cause of mountain sickness, but instead a consequence of efforts to adjust to hypoxia.

High-altitude problems are certainly triggered by hypoxia, but what actually happens in the body to cause the signs and symptoms that range from unpleasant to fatal? Other types of exposures, notably to heat, cause symptoms surprisingly similar to mountain sickness, as William Bean described in 1961:

> There is a sense of overwhelming oppression which rapidly takes the spirit out of men.... Trifling work is fatiguing and more burdensome work rapidly leads to exhaustion. A throbbing headache may develop and reach cruel intensity. Dizziness occurs, accentuated in the standing position. Dyspnea may be a problem.... Nausea, vomiting and

loss of appetite are commonplace. Lack of coordination reduces the efficiency.... Apathy may be interrupted by bursts of irritability. Judgment and morale decline.... Unwillingness to continue work or the onset of physical disability may rapidly disorganize a well-disciplined and efficient unit.

These observations suggest that the response to hypoxia is not specific to hypoxia, but in many respects resembles the effects of other stimuli. We know that not everything that causes lack of oxygen (for example, anemia or certain lung disorders) produces all the same symptoms experienced on mountains. One recent study suggests that the combination of a lack of oxygen and lower atmospheric pressure causes more symptoms than either lack of oxygen or decreased pressure alone. The more we learn about human physiology, the more vexing this question becomes.

WHAT IS MOUNTAIN SICKNESS?

As mountain illnesses have been studied more intensively, it has become evident that they fall along a spectrum of altitude-related problems, and they are now less frequently considered as separate, discrete illnesses. Some form of mountain sickness is likely to affect anyone who ascends rapidly above 8,000 feet, but lack of oxygen will affect different individuals differently.

For convenience we describe the signs and symptoms by familiar names and use acronyms as shorthand. The best known and most common has long been *acute mountain sickness* (AMS), or less often *benign acute mountain sickness* (BAMS), or in former times *puna, soroche, damgiri, yas*, and still others. Today we believe that AMS has some neurological elements, and overlaps to a varying degree with the more severe illness known as *high altitude cerebral edema* (HACE). (See Chapter 8, "The Spectrum of High-Altitude Illness: AMS/HACE.") When the thin air of the high mountains afflicts the lungs, the resulting illness is called *high altitude pulmonary edema* (HAPE), which is discussed in Chapter 10. *Chronic mountain sickness* (CMS), discussed in Chapter 11, "Chronic and Subacute Mountain Illness," is an uncommon and a less well understood syndrome affecting longtime high-altitude dwellers.

About ten years ago we began to realize that the convenient scheme for classifying mountain sicknesses built from historic observations and more modern experience was inadequate and not quite accurate. We came to recognize that the three major syndromes of acute high-altitude exposure (AMS, HACE, and HAPE) often occur together, and that the concept of a spectrum—as opposed to a scheme for pigeonholing symptoms—was more appropriate. The more we learned about the signs and symptoms of AMS, the more obvious it became that many of these symptoms were due to changes in the central nervous system, peripheral nerves, arterial constriction, or neurotransmitter levels. So now, rather than distinguishing between AMS and HACE, many of us are instead beginning to use the term AMS/HACE. While HAPE may also occur to some degree in AMS/HACE, it is better to avoid unnecessary confusion and discuss HAPE as a separate entity, as this illness can be the major problem that a sick climber faces at high altitude.

One challenge in the diagnosis of AMS is that people with AMS commonly display nonspecific symptoms including headache, intestinal upset, insomnia, dizziness, and fatigue. Given this list of symptoms, it is easy to see that a sick climber (or even a physician treating a sick climber) could easily mistake AMS for a range of other ailments that might occur at high altitude, such as dehydration, exhaustion, hypoglycemia, or even viral infection. To avoid these mistakes, many physicians who treat people at high altitude employ the definition of AMS as headache plus at least one of the other symptoms listed above in an individual who has newly ascended to an altitude of 8,000 feet or more.

Some of the signs and symptoms of mountain sickness are occasionally seen with hypoxic illness at sea level. We may speculate that some of the hallucinations, delusions, and erratic behavior experienced by individuals with hypoxic illness at sea level may have the same or similar origin as AMS/HACE. Even more intriguing, many manifestations of hypoxia can also be caused by hypothermia, hypoglycemia, some medications, and even alcohol. The similarities between mountain illness and "ordinary" hypoxic illness are discussed in Chapter 12, "Hypoxia in Everyday Life."

CHAPTER

THE BODY UP HIGH: CELLULAR AND VASCULAR RESPONSES TO HYPOXIA

Many years after my teenage studies of microscopic swamp creatures, I visited a research laboratory where a friend showed me a fascinating experiment with the very same tiny animals. He had taken a flock of paramecia and placed them in a long, shallow trough half filled with water. He covered the trough and introduced a slow flow of nitrogen into the water at one end and at the other end a similar slow flow of oxygen. One side of the trough was lacking in oxygen while the other one was rich. It was amazing to see how the paramecia migrated from the low to the high oxygen region of the trough and to notice how sensitive they were to even small differences in levels of oxygen in their environment. This simple experiment provided conclusive evidence that these single-celled animals had an oxygen sensing mechanism.

We now know that many—possibly most—cells of the human body sense oxygen and respond to it in various ways, depending on their structure and function. My colleagues and I saw one example in the mid-1980s, during Operation Everest II. Our studies of single muscle cells showed that at high altitude mitochondria in the cell moved from near the center to near the periphery, presumably induced to move by a microscopic difference in oxygen pressure found within the cell. Given that individual cells respond to variations in oxygen level, it is not surprising that the tissues and organs these cells make up respond as well.

In the *Proceedings of the 1995 Hypoxia Symposium*, neurologist Roger Simon encapsulated the effects of hypoxia on the brain of unacclimatized individuals abruptly exposed to low oxygen: "At sea level when the [inhaled] pO_2 is decreased to 75 percent of normal, complex task performance is altered; at 65 percent, short-term memory is impaired; at 50 percent, judgment is altered; unconsciousness occurs with the pO_2 between 30 percent and 40 percent of normal." These percentages correspond approximately to 8,000, 12,000, 18,000, and 28,000 feet, respectively. The responses of well-acclimatized individuals would, of course, be substantially different.

The mechanics of climbing a mountain—surviving cold and lack of oxygen, overcoming technical difficulties—is a very simple matter compared to the complexities of the mechanisms our bodies enlist to make mountaineering possible. It would be a disservice to the reader to ignore the miraculous and complex currents of activity within the human organism that allow us to go high, but of which we are totally unaware as we climb. Because we, the authors, are so excited by this complex mosaic, we have included a rough approximation of the scientific basis of how the body responds to high-altitude conditions—at least insofar as we understand it today. The reader who becomes befuddled by too much scientific detail can skip much of this without harming his or her comprehension, but we believe the most intriguing nuggets lie herein.

BASIC MECHANISMS OF HYPOXIA AND THE BRAIN

Suppose you put your hand on a hot stove. Instantly a heat-sensitive nerve ending (*receptor*) in your skin initiates an electrical signal that races along a nerve or nerves leading to the spinal cord (this might take a thousandth of a second). In the spinal cord, the nerve ends in a gap (*synapse*) where the signal is converted quickly to a chemical (*neurotransmitter*), which spreads to other, secondary nerve cells. At each of these secondary nerve cells, the chemical neurotransmitter is converted into electrical impulses that flow out along other nerves to other destinations. Some of these messages return directly from your spinal cord to the muscles of your arm, ordering them to immediately withdraw your hand. Other secondary nerve cells carry the pain message to the brain, allowing you to become consciously aware of the stove's heat. All this has taken a tiny fraction of a second.

In the brain, the message of the secondary nerve cells also stimulates additional neurons that stimulate the "fight or flight" mechanism of the sympathetic nervous system. This branch of our unconscious (*autonomic*) nervous system then stimulates an increase in blood pressure and respiration. Some messages also go to the parts of the brain responsible for memory, where the sensation and responses are stored for the future: "Don't touch a hot stove!" Or, like Mark Twain's cat, "don't touch even a cold stove." Every time one nerve cell communicates with another, it does so by means of a chemical messenger or neurotransmitter.

Much of what we know today about the central nervous system involves the manufacture of these chemical messengers and the release of each messenger across the synapse onto its specific site on a nerve ending, much like a key going into a lock. We know that some specific illnesses, for example Parkinson's disease or schizophrenia, are due at least in part to changes in these chemical neurotransmitters. We know too that many medications—and substances that are often abused such as alcohol, heroin, and others—also affect these chemicals.

Chemical and electrical messages are sent throughout our bodies millions of times a day, and we are unaware of the vast majority of them. Those that travel the *autonomic nervous system* control all the essential functions:

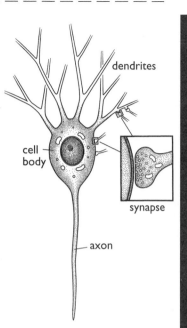

Figure 22. *Nerve cells
and receptors*

Nerve Cells, Axons, and Synapses

The basic nerve cell consists of a large cell body (which includes parts similar to those in other cells), a long tail, or *axon*, and a few or many hairlike branches, or *dendrites*, that extend to other nerve cells. (See Figure 22.) Stimuli generally reach a nerve cell body by way of its dendrites. The cell body then initiates an electrical signal that proceeds down the axon. Axons terminate at a gap, or *synapse*, where they come close to, but do not touch, a second nerve cell. Chemical messengers (neurotransmitters) are released from the axon terminals. They traverse the synapse and bind to and stimulate specific receptors on the second nerve cell. The neurotransmitters are then broken down or are taken up by the nerve cells for reuse.

The second nerve, thus stimulated, may carry its electrical message to another synapse. Here, the second nerve may release yet another neurotransmitter. In this way, information from the most remote parts of our body can reach the brain, and commands from the brain can reach our muscles, glands, blood vessels, and heart. Now and then, by illness, injury, medication, or disuse, a few dendrites from the brain cells are "pruned" and the connected functions inactivated.

One theory of how hypoxia affects the brain is that the chemical messengers in the synapses are altered by lack of oxygen, thus affecting specific responses. There are dozens of messenger chemicals in each synapse. We understand the chemistry of many and are able to change that chemistry by medication or by altering our environment.

breathing, digesting, sweating, shivering, focusing our eyes, balancing when we stand or sit, and many, many others. These functions are automatic and beyond our conscious control.

This rough sketch suggests where the brain and nervous system might be vulnerable to hypoxia, or to other hazards like infection, heat, cold, poisons, or deficiencies of necessary nutrients. Despite many protective loops, such a highly complex bio-electrical system remains vulnerable.

We know that hypoxia affects the nervous system by impacting neurotransmitters long before it damages the nerves themselves. We can hypothesize that distorted messages from the nervous system might cause or aggravate the many signs and symptoms we associate with HACE and HAPE. This does not mean that the other possible causes, such as those operating at the local level in specific tissues or organs (the blood vessels, for instance), are not operative, but it may explain how they are invoked. Given the role that the nervous system may play in high-altitude diseases, it is worth understanding how messages move in the nervous system and how those messages control the activity of other tissues.

VASCULAR RESPONSE TO HYPOXIA

When we first ascend to high altitude, our bodies respond to the drop in oxygen pressure similarly to the way they would respond to any potentially harmful stressor—with stimulation of the sympathetic nervous system and a triggering of the "fight or flight" response. This response, which involves the release of the neurotransmitter *norepinephrine* from nerves directly onto blood vessels, and the release of the hormone *epinephrine* from the adrenal glands into the bloodstream, causes arteries to constrict, increasing the resistance to blood flow and raising the blood pressure. The increased blood pressure may be of particular importance in the pulmonary artery, where it can contribute to HAPE. The heart is also stimulated to beat faster. However, the amount of blood that the heart pumps with each beat (the *stroke volume*) may actually decrease, meaning that the amount of blood that the heart pumps each minute (the *cardiac output*) may be little changed. Exposure to cold, which is certainly not uncommon at high altitude, can further stimulate the sympathetic nervous system and exaggerate arterial constriction. This is probably the mechanism by which cold exposure contributes to HAPE.

Blood Vessel Response to Tissue Hypoxia

In addition to the sympathetic nervous system responses that impact the entire cardiovascular system, hypoxia of any individual tissue has interesting and important effects on the arteries that feed that tissue. To understand these effects, it must be seen how each tissue in the body controls its own blood flow so that each individual tissue receives sufficient oxygen to meet its needs.

Consider the example of skeletal muscle. When a muscle is at rest, its need for oxygen is low, and the smallest arteries that feed it (the *arterioles*) are constricted. The muscle gets the blood flow and oxygen it needs, but no more. When we exercise, the oxygen needs of our muscles increase manyfold. The muscle tissue releases a range of chemicals including lactate, carbon dioxide, and potassium. These chemicals diffuse the short distance to the arterioles that feed the muscle tissue, causing the arterioles to dilate and the blood flow to the muscle to increase. The oxygen needs of the muscle are met. This is a remarkably efficient system for meeting the varying oxygen needs of the many different body tissues. However, this feedback system can cause problems when we climb to high altitude and experience hypoxia. To understand how, we can look at the way two specific arterial beds—those supplying oxygen to the brain and to the lungs—respond to hypoxia.

How Blood Vessels of the Brain Respond to Hypoxia

When the brain is exposed to hypoxia, the arterioles that feed it initially dilate, and blood flow increases. The result, at least for mild to moderate hypoxia, is that oxygen delivery to the brain is maintained at normal levels despite the reduced level of oxygen in a given volume of blood. This response really only represents a matching of blood flow to tissue oxygen needs, and is thus no different from what was described above for skeletal muscle. However, the brain is a very delicate organ and any change in its blood flow can have serious consequences. If brain blood flow is not increased in hypoxic conditions, oxygen delivery to the brain could be compromised. If brain blood flow does increase, it exposes the cerebral capillaries to blood at high pressure. The cerebral capillaries can begin to leak, and this can lead to HACE.

Hypoxia is not the only factor that impacts brain blood flow at altitude. The hypoxia of high altitude stimulates increased ventilation. This reduces the blood carbon dioxide level, causing the blood and cerebrospinal fluid to become more alkaline. (For more on this important response, see Chapter 13, "Acclimatization.") These chemical changes cause the blood vessels feeding the brain to constrict, limiting brain blood flow. However, if the initial hypoxia was not too severe, the increased ventilation will have brought more oxygen into the lungs and raised blood oxygen levels back toward normal, and the brain will no longer need a greatly increased blood flow to meet tissue oxygen needs. This intricate adjustment illustrates the delicate balance that must be maintained between O_2 and CO_2 partial pressures in brain blood vessels.

How Blood Vessels of the Lung Respond to Hypoxia

The blood vessels of the lung respond to hypoxia differently than those of other organs. To understand this response, consider the example of pneumonia. People who have pneumonia may have areas in their lungs where the alveoli get little air during respiration. As a result, these lung areas develop a low oxygen level (that is, regional hypoxia). Physicians have known for years that patients in this situation have a tendency to constrict the branches of their pulmonary arteries that send blood to these diseased lung areas. This response, called *hypoxic pulmonary vasoconstriction* (HPV), results in blood being shunted away from diseased alveoli toward healthy areas of the lung where the alveolar oxygen level is higher and the blood can more readily pick up oxygen. HPV also occurs in response to the hypoxia of high altitude, but with less positive results.

Patients with HAPE have an elevated blood pressure in their pulmonary arteries. Their chest X rays show a patchy pattern, indicating that some areas of the lung have edema fluid while others are spared. (See Chapter 10, "HAPE: High Altitude Pulmonary Edema.") These findings suggest that when people ascend to high altitude and develop hypoxia, some branches of their pulmonary arteries may develop a more robust HPV response and constrict more strongly than others. This regionally high resistance to blood flow increases pressure in the main pulmonary artery, forcing blood through unconstricted pulmonary artery branches and into the capillary beds beyond at higher than normal pressure. The areas that receive this extra blood flow at high pressure are on their way to developing pulmonary edema. When tested in the laboratory, the edema fluid from the lungs of people with HAPE is usually found to have a high protein content. This suggests that people with HAPE have also damaged their pulmonary capillaries in some way, allowing protein that would normally be retained within the capillaries to leak out.

How Edema Develops

Because the two most ominous complications of the hypoxia of altitude are edema of the lungs (HAPE) and edema of the brain (HACE), any discussion of the impact of hypoxia on the vascular system must look in some detail at the process by which edema develops. Edema is the accumulation of fluid in a tissue, generally between the cells, in the interstitial space. Normally, as blood flows through the capillaries of body tissues it gives up oxygen and nutrients to the cells while taking on carbon dioxide and waste products from the cells. In the capillaries of the lung, blood gives up much

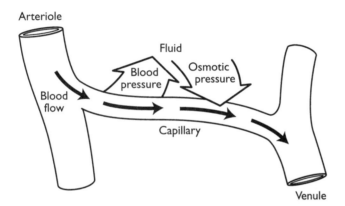

Figure 23. *Fluid movement between tissue and capillary*

Edema: Fluid Accumulation in Tissue

As blood flows through the capillaries, fluid leaves the plasma, enters the interstitial space, and then returns to the plasma, as shown in Figure 23. The major force pushing fluid out of the capillaries is blood pressure. Any change that increases capillary blood pressure (such as *hypoxic pulmonary vasoconstriction*, or HPV) can cause excess fluid to leave the capillaries and produce *edema*—fluid build-up in the tissue. The major force that pulls fluid back into the capillaries is the *osmotic pressure* of protein molecules suspended in the blood plasma. Any change that allows plasma proteins to leak out of the capillaries (such as damage to the capillary wall) can reduce the amount of fluid that reenters the capillaries, causing edema.

of its carbon dioxide to the alveoli and picks up more oxygen from these air spaces. Our bodies facilitate this process by moving large volumes of fluid out of the capillaries and into the interstitial space in the initial segments of the capillary and reabsorbing the fluid back into the capillaries again in the later capillary segments. (See Figure 23.)

The major force responsible for the movement of fluid out of capillaries is blood pressure, and the major force responsible for the reabsorption of fluid back into the capillaries is *osmotic pressure*, produced by the concentration of proteins in the blood plasma. Under normal circumstances, these forces are balanced, so that not much fluid is left in the interstitial space. The spaces between capillary cells are normally small enough so that very little protein can leak out of the capillaries. Any fluid (or protein) that does accumulate in the interstitial space is returned to the circulation by the *lymphatic system*. Any change in the circulatory system that increases the capillary blood pressure or decreases the plasma osmotic pressure can result in the accumulation of fluid around the cells in the interstitial space and cause edema. Consequently, a range of medical problems—including heart failure, liver disease, starvation, and hypertension—can cause edema.

Hypoxia also can cause edema. Within hours of ascent to high altitude, a person experiences a decrease in blood plasma volume, indicating that plasma has escaped the blood vessels and entered the interstitial space surrounding the cells. One relatively benign form of this hypoxia-induced edema is the development of mild swelling, mostly in the face and head in the morning, and the hands and feet during the day. More serious is the excessive accumulation of fluid in the lungs or brain, which causes HAPE and AMS/HACE. A combination of increased capillary blood pressure and excessive protein leakage may contribute to the edema seen at high altitude. However, edema sometimes can occur even when the capillary blood pressure and blood proteins are normal. As discussed below, this results from physical damage to the capillary walls.

CELLULAR RESPONSE TO HYPOXIA

Ultimately, the body's response to high altitude is a result of changes in the function of individual cells. This area of science, known as cell biology, can be both fascinating and frustrating to study. It is fascinating because it involves intricate mechanisms, and understanding these mechanisms may allow us to treat or even prevent HAPE, HACE, and many other diseases. It can be frustrating because these intricate mechanisms often seem to interconnect in unexpected ways, forming a complex, but as yet not fully understood, web of interactions.

It has been shown how the blood vessels of the lung and brain respond to hypoxia. We know that people with HAPE have increased *pulmonary artery pressure* (PAP), which may lead to damage of their pulmonary capillaries, allowing protein and fluids to leak out. Patients with HACE have similar problems in the capillaries that supply the brain (the cerebral capillaries). Unlike the situation in the lung, hypoxia causes *dilation* of the arteries to the brain (the cerebral arteries) and increases blood flow through those arteries. This response brings more blood, and therefore more oxygen, to the brain. But it also exposes the cerebral capillaries to blood at high pressure. As is the case for the pulmonary arteries of patients with HAPE, the cerebral capillaries of patients with HACE begin to leak.

People with HAPE have pulmonary capillaries that are exposed to high blood pressure and are damaged so that they leak protein, while people with HACE have a similar picture in their cerebral capillaries. The forces responsible for fluid movements into and out of the capillaries help explain how pulmonary edema and cerebral edema develop. By delving into the cell biology of artery constriction versus dilation and capillary leakage we can begin to understand the basis for these changes.

Biologically Active Substances

The level of constriction of the pulmonary arteries (and thus the pressure in those arteries) is impacted by both nerve messages from the brain and biologically active substances produced in the lung itself that act locally. Two important examples of these substances are *nitric oxide* and *endothelin*.

First discovered in the mid-1980s and initially named *endothelium derived relaxing factor* (EDRF), nitric oxide (NO) was found to be important in a number of vascular activities. This substance was soon identified as a simple, two-atom molecule, nitric oxide. Scientists then determined that NO is formed in the endothelial cells of blood vessels throughout the body.

NO may be a simple chemical, but its effects are complex. Minute amounts of NO are produced by a specific enzyme, *nitric oxide synthase* (NOS), in all endothelial cells in every mammalian organ at a steady basal rate. Various substances increase NO release, which relaxes vascular tone, allowing small blood vessels to dilate. NO also inhibits the adhesion and clumping of platelets, thereby helping to decrease the tendency for clot formation in blood vessels. Certain physiological substances inhibit NO synthesis and release, and thus (among other things) increase vascular tone and blood pressure, increase clot formation, and increase the leakiness of capillary blood vessels.

Endothelial cells also release a family of substances called *endothelins*, at least one of which has an effect on blood vessels exactly the opposite of nitric oxide: It constricts vessels by increasing their tone and platelet stickiness. The balance between these antagonists (and perhaps others, too) affects blood flow through the smaller vessels.

Nitric oxide has been reported to play yet another role in the precapillaries—essentially "dictating" how much and where oxygen is delivered to tissues. It does so because hemoglobin carries NO and releases it, perhaps by changing red cell shape in precapillary arterioles and in capillaries. The

Viagra: A Nitric Oxide Amplifier

Nitric oxide has come to popular attention because it plays a role in the action of drugs such as *sildenafil citrate*, more commonly known by its brand name Viagra. As anyone who has viewed the TV commercials featuring politicians and sports celebrities knows, Viagra helps some men who have erectile dysfunction achieve erections. While optimum sexual function may not be a high priority for most climbers at high altitude, the way that Viagra works provides important lessons about NO, vasodilation, and high-altitude disease.

How does Viagra work? When NO binds to a receptor on a smooth muscle cell in the wall of an artery, it sets in motion a chain of biochemical reactions that elevates the level of a messenger molecule known as *cyclic guanosine monophosphate*, or cGMP, within the cell. cGMP reduces the calcium level in the arterial smooth muscle cell, causing these cells to relax and the artery to dilate. cGMP is broken down by an enzyme called *phosphodiesterase* (PDE). Viagra blocks the action of the type of PDE that is found in the blood vessels of the penis and lung. It keeps those vessels relaxed, allowing blood to fill a spongy area of the penis called the *corpus cavernosum* and producing an erection. Viagra also blocks PDE in other organs, although to a lesser extent. This is responsible for the side effects that the drug can produce, such as a drop in blood pressure and blue vision.

released NO relaxes the blood vessels, and when molecules of oxygen are released by hemoglobin, NO is scavenged back into the red cell, the vessels constrict, and the blood, moving into the veins and carrying less oxygen, returns to the heart and on to the lungs for another load of oxygen.

As for their role in all altitude illnesses and perhaps in hypoxia from other causes, NO and endothelin appear to be central players. One study of individuals with HAPE shows that inhaling small concentrations of NO (forty parts per million) decreases pulmonary artery pressure dramatically, shifts blood flow away from flooded sections of the lungs to those less perfused, and raises arterial oxygen saturation. Several other studies show that inhaling NO (40 ppm) rapidly decreases PAP and relieves HAPE.

More intriguing are studies showing that individuals who are susceptible to HAPE have less NO in their lungs at high altitude than do non-susceptibles. This has raised a fascinating question: Can HAPE susceptibility be due to a deficiency of NO, or of the NO-synthase that releases NO in the endothelium? Chapter 14, "Genetics of High-Altitude Performance," discusses how our genes might be involved in these differences.

If lack of NO contributes to HAPE and/or HACE, why don't climbers at altitude simply carry a supply of NO? This is impractical because NO is so difficult to administer effectively. Yet there may be another way to take advantage of the link between low NO levels and high-altitude disease. At the time of this writing, Viagra is being tested as a treatment for a serious medical condition called pulmonary hypertension in which patients at sea level (some with hypoxia from lung disease) develop elevated blood pressure in their pulmonary arteries. Clearly, there are parallels between pulmonary hypertension and HAPE. (See Chapter 12, "Hypoxia in Everyday Life.") A very low dose of Viagra, 25 mg every three hours, has proven to be more effective than nifedipine (a drug that dilates arteries) in treating HAPE, and Viagra does not have as strong a tendency to lower blood pressure as nifedipine has. Whether or not the longer-acting analog of Viagra, marketed under the brand name Cialis, will be suitable for HAPE susceptibles to take prior to a high climb remains to be tested.

Reactive Oxygen Species

Another group of biologically active substances that may play a role in the impact of hypoxia on the constriction and dilation of blood vessels are known as *reactive oxygen species*. Reactive oxygen species (ROS)—chemicals such as hydrogen peroxide, free oxygen radicals, and superoxide—are formed in body cells as an unavoidable part of the process by which cells use oxygen to extract energy from nutrients. This process takes place in the mitochondria of the cells and is known as *aerobic metabolism*. (See Chapter 5, "Cells: The Ultimate Users," Figure 17.) However, ROS are highly reactive chemicals that can damage the very cells in which they are formed. Under ordinary circumstances, cells are protected from potential damage by ROS because ROS are quickly broken down in the cells by the enzyme *superoxide dismutase* (SOD) and by small *antioxidant* molecules, including vitamin E.

ROS and High Altitude

Because ROS formation is associated with high levels of oxygen use, it might seem counterintuitive that ROS production would be increased in the thin air of high altitude. However, this may well be the case. As climbers first exert and then rest, their tissues are first deprived of oxygen and then resupplied with it. This pattern is known as *intermittent hypoxia*—reoxygenation—and it may increase ROS production. It is similar to the phenomenon called *ischemia–reperfusion injury* in which the heart muscle of a patient being treated for a heart attack is further damaged by a flood of ROS production when it is resupplied with oxygen after a period of deprivation. ROS also may form at high altitude even without reoxygenation when oxygen-starved mitochondria are called upon to meet the energy needs of intense exercise. Several other elements of high-altitude climbing not directly related to low oxygen—including exposure to ultraviolet light and lack of dietary antioxidants—may also increase ROS levels in the cells of climbers at high altitude.

Elevated ROS levels predispose the climber at high altitude to both HAPE and HACE in several ways. We have seen that levels of the vasodilator nitric oxide are reduced by hypoxia, and ROS can deplete NO even further. Reduction of the vasodilator NO may contribute to the elevated pulmonary artery blood pressure seen in patients with HAPE. NO is also an antiinflammatory. Because the inflammatory response includes an increase in the permeability of blood vessels, reducing NO could also lead to increased protein leakage from blood vessels into the interstitial spaces between cells and contribute to HACE.

If elevated ROS levels lead to HAPE and HACE, should climbers at high altitude simply flood their systems with antioxidants such as vitamin E to reduce these chemicals? There is no clear answer to this question, but caution is probably in order. Low levels of ROS serve several important positive functions in the cells. They are needed for the production of thyroid hormone and for optimal force production by muscle. Perhaps most important, ROS serve as part of the natural cellular defense against infection, and inflammation from lung infections can increase the likelihood of HAPE. In light of this, it is probably not surprising that studies of the use of antioxidants to prevent HACE and HAPE suggest they do not help in staving off mountain sickness.

ROS also may play a role in acclimatization to altitude. We have seen that NO is produced in epithelial cells by nitric oxide synthase (NOS). NOS comes in two forms. One form, known as endothelial NOS or eNOS, functions at low levels at a constant rate to produce the NO that endothelial cells need at all times. The other form is called inducible NOS or iNOS, a much more powerful enzyme that can produce large amounts of NO and which also can be turned on (induced) by specific stimuli. Over time at high altitude, ROS can stimulate or induce iNOS activity, leading to increased NO production. Thus, climbers ascending to altitude may initially experience reduced NO levels but later achieve elevated levels. This NO may block inflammation in the lung and brain and dilate pulmonary blood vessels, contributing to the reduced inflammation and pulmonary artery pressures that occur during the process of acclimatization.

Inflammation and Capillary Leak at High Altitude

Because capillary leak seems to play a role in both HAPE and HACE, and because inflammation can contribute to capillary leak, it is vital to look closely at what inflammation is and how it develops. In general, inflammation occurs in tissues as a local response to injury. The inflammatory response includes a dilation of small blood vessels, which increases blood flow to the injured tissue, and an increase in capillary permeability, which allows white blood cells (leukocytes) to leave the blood vessels and enter the interstitial space to fight infection. While inflammation clearly has a vital role in tissue healing after an injury, it can have a devastating effect when it occurs in the lungs or brain of a climber at high altitude.

ROS, which are increased at high altitude, stimulate leukocytes to release inflammatory chemicals that can damage endothelial cells and increase capillary permeability. Leukocytes and inflammatory chemicals have been found in the lung fluid of some, but not all, people with HAPE. This suggests that inflammation may contribute to HAPE in some situations, such as when the climber has a respiratory infection. Studies on animals also show that exposure to hypoxia can stimulate the production of a protein known as *vascular endothelial growth factor*, or VEGF, by cells in the brain. Because VEGF acts to increase protein leakage from brain capillaries in these animal studies, scientists have proposed that it may play a role in the brain edema of HACE.

Angiogenesis

VEGF may also contribute to HACE in other ways. VEGF is a potent stimulator of blood vessel growth, or *angiogenesis*. Low tissue oxygen levels are known to increase VEGF production, leading to blood vessel growth. This phenomenon is seen in the developing placenta and in the eye of the newborn. The role of angiogenesis induced by VEGF in HACE remains controversial. HACE can develop within hours upon ascent to high attitude, and clearly new blood vessel growth could not occur during this short time. However, the first steps in angiogenesis do involve the weakening of capillaries and capillary leakage. So the initial stages of angiogenesis may play a role in HACE, particularly after several hours of exposure to high altitude. It is also important to note that a range of other chemicals, including *interferon* and *interleukin*, better known for their role in the angiogenesis of cancer, are also released during hypoxia.

Neurotransmitters

So far the discussion has focused on the role of NO as a vasodilator and the possibility that a reduction in NO caused by hypoxia could contribute to the vasoconstriction of HAPE. However, it is important to realize that there are a variety of substances in the human body that act as vasodilators or vasoconstrictors. Many of these substances fall into the general category of *neurotransmitters*—chemicals released by a nerve that stimulate another nerve, a muscle, or a gland.

Some examples of neurotransmitters are *acetylcholine*, which stimulates skeletal muscle; *norepinephrine*, which stimulates smooth and cardiac muscle; and *dopamine*, which acts in the brain and other points in the nervous system. (For an interesting example of how dopamine plays a role in the response to hypoxia, see Chapter 14, "Genetics of High-Altitude Performance.") Because muscle contraction is central to our ability to perform at altitude, it will be used as an example to illustrate how neurotransmitters work.

How Muscle Contracts. Smooth muscle is the tissue that lines the hollow organs of the body, including the digestive tract and blood vessels. The smooth muscle of arteries contracts when the neurotransmitter norepinephrine binds to specialized receptors on the smooth muscle cell surface. Norepinephrine can come either from nerves that are part of the sympathetic nervous system and end at the muscle or from the adrenal gland by way of the blood.

Regardless of its origin, once the norepinephrine has bound to the smooth muscle cell, it sets in motion a chain of events that result in an increase in the calcium level in the cell. Some of this extra calcium is released from storage areas inside the cell, but most enters the cell from the extracellular fluid through specialized channels. Once the calcium level in the smooth muscle cell rises, this sets off another chain of events that culminate in a chemical change to the protein known as *myosin*, the motor within the cell that powers muscle contraction. The chemical change stimulated by calcium, called *phosphorylation*, activates myosin, and the muscle contracts.

Skeletal muscle, as its name implies, is the muscle we use to power the conscious movements of our skeleton. Skeletal, or striated, muscle contraction is initiated somewhat differently than smooth muscle contraction. Skeletal muscle contracts in response to a different neurotransmitter, acetylcholine, which reaches skeletal muscle only from nerves leaving the brain or spinal cord. Like norepinephrine in smooth muscle, acetylcholine binds to specialized receptors on the surface of the skeletal muscle and produces an increase in calcium within the muscle cell. However, in skeletal muscle virtually all of this calcium comes from storage areas within the cell. Calcium causes muscle contraction by binding directly to proteins within the cell that are involved with contraction rather than by causing phosphorylation.

How Hypoxia Influences Smooth Muscle Contraction. Hypoxia is known to cause the release of norepinephrine; other, similar chemicals; and a range of stress hormones into the blood. This could contribute to smooth muscle constriction in the blood vessels of the lungs (as in HPV) and could contribute to HAPE. However, the exact role that norepinephrine plays in the blood vessels of the brain and lung during hypoxia remains unclear. There are a number of other substances, some of which may act both as neurotransmitters and local biologically active substances—endothelin, angiotensin II, neuropetide Y, and substance P—that also may affect the constriction of pulmonary and cerebral arteries. Experiments meant to uncover the role of neurotransmitters in HAPE and HACE are challenging because the response of most animals to hypoxia is somewhat different than that of humans, and as much as climbers wish to understand high-altitude illness, few would be willing to donate a cerebral or pulmonary artery to science! In addition, HAPE and HACE appear in the setting not just of hypoxia but of altitude, cold, and other stimuli as well. Thus, it may be many years before the changes in smooth muscle that occur at altitude are fully understood.

IMPACT OF HYPOXIA ON GENES

To understand how hypoxia influences genes, a few basic definitions are needed. Genes are made up of DNA and found on chromosomes. Very loosely, a gene can be defined as the bit of DNA that carries the code for building a single protein. (See Chapter 5, "Cells: The Ultimate Users.") Humans have about 30,000 genes, but not all of them function all the time or in all cells. (Surprisingly, the Human Genome Project, completed in 2003, found a much lower number of genes than previous estimates of about 100,000 genes.) Indeed, liver cells are different from brain cells because in the two cell types different sets of genes are active. This is why liver and brain cells build different proteins. When a gene is turned on (induced) and makes a protein, we say that the gene is being *expressed*. (See Chapter 14, "Genetics of High-Altitude Performance.")

VEGF and iNOS have already been mentioned as proteins whose production is stimulated by hypoxia. When protein production is increased, it is most likely that the gene that codes for that protein has been stimulated. This is the case for VEGF, but VEGF is not unique in this respect. Hypoxia also impacts the expression of other genes whose protein products may play a role in HAPE and HACE.

The Sodium–Potassium Pump. All body cells have a protein embedded in their cell membranes called the *sodium–potassium pump*. It maintains the proper salt balance inside and outside cells by pumping sodium out of cells and potassium in. Because water generally follows sodium in the body fluids, this also maintains the proper water balance and keeps cells from swelling.

The epithelial cells that line the air sacs (alveoli) of the lung have one side that borders on the alveoli, while the other side borders on the interstitial space and faces toward the lung capillaries, as described in Chapter 5, "Cells: The Ultimate Users." The sodium–potassium pumps work to keep water from accumulating in the alveoli. Hypoxia acts on the gene that codes for the sodium–potassium pump and decreases its activity. This reduces the number of pumps that the alveolar epithelial cells produce, reduces the body's ability to remove water from the alveoli, and may contribute to the accumulation of water in the lung observed in HAPE. (See Chapter 10, "HAPE: High Altitude Pulmonary Edema," Figure 28.)

Other Hormones

Erythropoietin. *Erythropoietin*, or EPO, offers another example in which hypoxia influences gene function. EPO, a hormone produced in specialized kidney cells, stimulates bone marrow to produce red blood cells. Hypoxia, whether produced by ascent to high altitude or by lung disease, activates previously dormant EPO-producing cells. Within these cells, the EPO gene is stimulated so that EPO levels in the blood rise. Increased EPO levels are responsible for the high red blood cell concentration (high *hematocrit*) we see in those who live at high altitude for extended periods and in those with severe lung disease. Interestingly, EPO is produced within minutes of acute exposure to hypoxia, and production is turned off when red blood cells have reached an optimal level.

The effects of EPO can be helpful because a higher number of red blood cells means an increase in the amount of oxygen the blood can carry. However, there are limits to this benefit. An elevated concentration of red blood cells thickens the blood and increases the workload on the heart, which can lead to heart failure for those with severe lung disease. At high altitude, dehydration can reduce the amount of blood plasma, further raising the hematocrit. This blood thickening can predispose the blood to clotting and may contribute to pulmonary emboli (often, blood clots that form in veins, often in the legs, and travel to the lungs) with deadly results. It is also interesting to note that EPO is produced in the brain as well as in the kidney. In the brains of climbers at altitude, EPO may both protect cells from the damage of hypoxia (a potentially helpful effect) and stimulate VEGF production (a potentially harmful effect). (See Chapter 4, "Moving Blood: Circulation.")

Leptin. Over the past decade a number of hormones and neurotransmitters have been discovered that control appetite. *Leptin* is an important hormone that may influence high-altitude performance. Leptin is produced by fat cells throughout the body and is released into the bloodstream when energy stores are high. It travels via the blood and acts at a specific area of the brain called the *hypothalamus* to produce a feeling of satiation and reduce appetite.

Both climbers and the scientists who study them have known for years that those who venture high commonly experience poor appetite and weight loss. Exertion and poor diet play a role. However, recent findings show that people at high altitude have elevated leptin levels, even when they have depleted energy stores. Although the mechanism responsible for this inappropriate production of leptin is not known, it almost certainly involves stimulation of the gene for leptin. What we do know is that high leptin levels could contribute to poor appetite and weight loss at altitude.

Mechanical Stress

The barrier between air in the alveoli and blood in the lung capillaries, known as the respiratory membrane, is very thin. (See Chapter 10, "HAPE: High Altitude Pulmonary Edema," Figure 26.) In fact, it consists of only two layers of cells divided by a basement membrane. From an engineering standpoint, this construction can be viewed as a trade-off. Making the barrier thicker would impede oxygen transfer from alveolar air to the blood. Making it thinner would weaken it to the point where it could fail.

At high altitude, the respiratory membrane is exposed to elevated pressure in the pulmonary blood vessels. Some experts believe that this elevated pressure causes physical damage to the pulmonary capillaries, causing them to leak protein-rich fluid and leading to HAPE.

So, what actually causes HAPE and HACE? There probably is no one answer to this question. Indeed, it is likely that virtually all of the mechanisms discussed here, as well as many still unknown, contribute. To make matters even more complex, any particular mechanism may be more important in some people than in others. For this reason, it is unlikely that science will discover a "magic bullet" to prevent or cure HAPE and HACE in all people any time soon. And so we are left with the time-proven advice: Limit your rate of ascent, descend if you get severe symptoms, and treat severe symptoms with oxygen and general drugs such as *steroids*, which block the inflammatory response, and drugs like nifedipine that reduce pulmonary artery pressure.

THE SPECTRUM OF HIGH-ALTITUDE ILLNESS: AMS/HACE

My first experience with what today I might call cerebral hypoxia was in 1936, many years before various expressions of mountain illnesses had been widely recognized. We had spent several weeks approaching our mountain and relaying camps to within reach of the summit. Most of us were well and strong. The man most experienced in the Alps, but who had never been at high altitude before, was convinced that he was the fittest of the party (even though at fifty-four he was the oldest) and best able to reach the 25,600-foot summit. In fact at 23,000 feet he was severely hypoxic, cyanotic, and quite irrational in his arguments. Several days later when we descended, he still contended that he was the fittest. Not until a few days after we reached low altitude did he resemble his usual self, but he held his conviction for many years. Two years later at the same altitude on a different mountain he experienced a similar episode, and the entire party was endangered while taking him down.

As we were working toward finishing the fifth edition of this book, I had another personal and rather disturbing experience with acute mountain sickness (AMS). I had been invited to Colorado in the fall of 2003 for a fiftieth anniversary remembrance of our 1953 K2 adventure. All the surviving team members were expected, and it promised to be an emotional and probably final reunion. But I was in poor shape. Not only was my vision failing, I had also suffered a severe hemorrhage, lost a lot of blood, and been in and out of the hospital several times. The final blow came when I fell out of bed and landed on my left shoulder and chest, which made it difficult for me to breathe. I'd been getting more short of breath anyway, and the conjunction of these misfortunes made my taking the trip highly questionable. Nevertheless, I was determined to go.

I knew that the altitude—9,400 feet—would be difficult to tolerate, so I arranged for oxygen to be supplied at night. Pete Schoening, the youngest member of our team and the one who saved our lives on K2, was suffering from infiltrates in his lungs, and he, too, would need oxygen at night. (Hypoxic stress is often more severe at night because of body position and because breathing is generally less efficient during sleep, even at sea level.)

We both managed quite well the afternoon of our arrival at the

magnificent house in which we were accommodated. We went to bed hap-
pily, breathing low-flow, supplementary oxygen at a rate of 1.2 liters per
minute. I slept like a stone for two hours, but then woke suddenly, gasping
for air in one of the most alarming episodes of my entire life. I could not
get enough air, my heart was racing at over 200 beats per minute, and my
mind was racing even faster, with no coherent thought—no hallucination,
but no sequence. The oxygen bottle was empty. In the dark of this strange
house I did not know where to turn. For the next few hours I barely sur-
vived, almost wishing for death. I staggered downstairs that morning at
sunrise to find a haggard Pete Schoening, who had suffered an identical
experience. His oxygen had run out and everything happened to him exactly
as it had to me. Neither of us had ever before had problems at altitude, cer-
tainly not at 9,400 feet.

These are only two cases, but they are so startlingly identical that I
can't help but draw a conclusion from the experience. The abrupt loss of
oxygen left us at a high altitude to which we were completely unacclima-
tized, to near-disastrous effect. This experience suggests that if you are go-
ing to a mountain resort at 8,000 or 9,000 or 10,000 feet, and choose to
rely on oxygen at night, make sure you have enough. Alternatively, don't
use oxygen at all, and rely only on acclimatization.

The previous chapters examined the involvement of the central nervous system and tissue edema in mountain illness. When individuals go too high too fast, as it is so easy to do nowadays with the ready availability of means to travel rapidly to high altitudes, they run the risk of falling victim to *acute mountain sickness* (AMS), a syndrome of nonspecific symptoms that can include dizziness, fatigue, insomnia, and headache. The serious and potentially fatal condition *high altitude cerebral edema* (HACE) is a clinical diagnosis based on the presentation of more severe neurological symptoms such as loss of voluntary muscle coordination and hallucination. HACE is considered to be the end-stage of severe AMS. The symptoms of both AMS and HACE are largely neurological, and evidence increasingly supports the idea that cerebral edema plays a role in both conditions. For these reasons AMS and HACE are now viewed as two regions on a continuum of disease severity.

AMS: ACUTE MOUNTAIN SICKNESS

At one end of the AMS/HACE continuum is AMS. AMS is usually mild and lasts only a day or two, but it can be very unpleasant. A patient related this typical story several years ago:

My husband and I have gone skiing in Colorado for many years. We
usually fly from the East Coast to Denver and drive up to the resort at
9,000 feet. By dinnertime I have a splitting headache and feel slightly
nauseated; I can't eat and go off to bed, knowing that I'll toss and turn
most of the night, unable to sleep. Usually the headache is a little better

next morning, and by the second or third day I'm able to ski with pleasure for the next week.

Each time she goes to altitude she is miserable for a day or two, but her symptoms never progress or become complicated by the more serious problems in the spectrum. Over the years she has worked out a strategy that almost eliminates her symptoms.

Symptoms and Signs of AMS

We speak of symptoms to describe what a person experiences or feels, as compared to signs, which can be observed by others. Some people who go to the mountains complain only of headache, while insomnia plagues others. Nausea and vomiting are particularly unpleasant. Shortness of breath is not very bothersome unless AMS is complicated by HAPE. For many people, fatigue and weakness is the worst problem.

Some individuals suffer a whole catastrophe of symptoms. Table 1 shows the frequency of each of the common symptoms experienced by those who had AMS among the 3,158 visitors Honigman surveyed in 1993 at several resorts in the Colorado Rocky Mountains.

TABLE 1	
SYMPTOMS OF ACUTE MOUNTAIN SICKNESS	
Mild headache	54%
Severe headache	8%
Easy fatigue	28%
Shortness of breath	21%
Dizziness	21%
Loss of appetite	11%
Sleep disturbance	10%
Vomiting	3%

Incidence

Not everyone venturing onto the mountains suffers as much as those quoted earlier in this chapter, but roughly one out of every five people going rapidly from low to moderate altitude (8,000 to 9,000 feet) will feel unpleasant effects. Most recover in thirty-six to forty-eight hours.

Speed of ascent and altitude reached usually make the difference between being sick or well, but this is not always true: Some individuals become sick every time they ascend to altitude, while others never experience AMS. Some are sick on one trip, but not on another in similar circumstances. It has been said for years that simple AMS is more common in some regions than in others, and that metallic ores, plants, radiation, or Earth's magnetism play a role. These ideas seem far-fetched, but—who knows?—there are still many things we do not know or understand.

Table 2 shows the percentage of visitors who develop "typical" mild AMS at different elevations as reported by different observers.

TABLE 2
INCIDENCE OF ACUTE MOUNTAIN SICKNESS

Author (Date)	Location	Altitude (in feet)	Percent with AMS
Montgomery (1989)	Colorado	6,765	20
		6,900	25
		8,900	40
Houston (1985)	Colorado	8,500	12
		9,500	17
Dean (1990)	Colorado	9,800	42
Maggiorini (1989)	Alps	6,700	9
		10,000	13
		12,000	34
		15,000	54
Hackett (1976)	Nepal	14,000	42
Honigman (1993)	Colorado	6–7,000	18
		7–9,000	22
		>9,000	27

Most of the authors cited in Table 2 were describing the mild form of AMS, without indicating whether other symptoms were present. Montgomery's subjects were doctors attending medical meetings. Dean's subjects were 100 epidemiologists attending a scientific meeting. Maggiorini collected survey data from many thousands of climbers and walkers. Hackett's subjects were trekkers in Nepal.

Honigman reported data collected with a detailed questionnaire answered by 3,158 people attending a variety of conferences during a two-year period at resorts 6,300 to 9,700 feet high. Some caution is needed in interpreting his numbers because most of those surveyed were males averaging forty-three years of age attending forty-five different conferences, and thus were not typical recreational visitors. The diagnosis of AMS was based on specific criteria agreed to at the Lake Louise Hypoxia Symposium in 1991. (See the sidebar, "Lake Louise Consensus," on page 115). The significant data in Honigman's study are shown in Table 3.

Other data in this survey showed little difference between those who had a few alcoholic drinks after arrival and those who did not, between previous smokers and nonsmokers, or between those who were overweight and those who were not. A small number gave a history of heart or lung

TABLE 3
FURTHER DATA IN HONIGMAN'S STUDY

	Total People	With AMS
Male	68%	24%
Female	32%	28%
Previous AMS	47%	35%
Live near sea level	88%	27%

disease or hypertension, but these conditions made no significant difference in the incidence of AMS. It is interesting that a third of all who said they had previously experienced altitude illness also had AMS on this occasion.

It is somewhat surprising that there is little difference between the sexes in resistance or susceptibility to AMS (although there is a significant gender difference in the incidence of HAPE). It is less surprising to find that incidence decreases with age almost linearly. Gender, age, and physical fitness are discussed in Chapter 17, "Limits to Work at Altitude."

Differences in Studies of AMS

The differences in incidence between different studies are striking and, although no statistical listing of specific symptoms in the Alps has been reported, many observers believe that symptoms are fewer and milder at comparable altitudes there than in the United States. Most Alpine resorts are farther south than most of those in the United States, and therefore slightly lower "physiologically," as explained below.

The most likely explanation for the differences reported in different geographical areas lies in how the data were collected, how mountain sickness was defined, and, more important, the profile of ascent. A half-dozen lists of questions or other criteria for defining AMS and quantifying its severity have been used, with marginal agreement between them. The Lake Louise

Lake Louise Consensus on AMS

In 1991 a group of scientists studying altitude sicknesses proposed a grading system in an attempt to make reporting of altitude-related illness more uniform. According to this consensus, in an individual who has rapidly ascended to an altitude higher than 6,000 feet, the presence and severity of each symptom is scored and the total score gives a grade by which studies by different workers in different places can be compared. It has the advantage of being simpler than several other systems in use, and after a few years has become standard in most altitude research facilities.

Lake Louise Consensus

1. Headache
   - 0 No headache
   - 1 Mild headache
   - 2 Moderate headache
   - 3 Severe headache, incapacitating

2. Gastrointestinal symptoms
   - 0 No gastrointestinal symptoms
   - 1 Poor appetite or nausea
   - 2 Moderate nausea or vomiting
   - 3 Severe nausea and vomiting, incapacitating

3. Fatigue and/or weakness
   - 0 Not tired or weak
   - 1 Mild fatigue/weakness
   - 2 Moderate fatigue/weakness
   - 3 Severe fatigue/weakness, incapacitating

4. Dizziness/ lightheadedness
   - 0 Not dizzy
   - 1 Mild dizziness
   - 2 Moderate dizziness
   - 3 Severe dizziness, incapacitating

5. Difficulty sleeping
   - 0 Slept as well as usual
   - 1 Did not sleep as well as usual
   - 2 Woke many times, poor night's sleep
   - 3 Could not sleep at all

6. Change in mental status
   - 0 Not tired or weak
   - 1 Lethargy/lassitude
   - 2 Disoriented/confused
   - 3 Stupor/semiconsciousness
   - 4 Coma

7. Ataxia
   - 0 No ataxia
   - 1 Maneuvers to maintain balance
   - 2 Steps off line
   - 3 Falls down
   - 4 Cannot stand

8. Peripheral edema
   - 0 No peripheral edema
   - 1 Peripheral edema at one location
   - 2 Peripheral edema at two or more locations

Functional score. The functional consequences of the AMS Self-reported score should be further evaluated by one option question asked after the AMS self-report questionnaire. Alternatively, this question may be asked by the examiner if clinical assessment is performed.

Overall, if you had any symptoms, how did they affect your activity?
   - 0 No reduction in activity
   - 1 Mild reduction in activity
   - 2 Moderate reduction in activity
   - 3 Severe reduction in activity (e.g., bed rest)

Consensus reconciles these differences by defining the criteria for diagnosis, and as more workers apply these, the apparent differences may decrease.

Of course, changes in weather and temperature affect barometric pressure—and thus the oxygen available in the air. The higher the altitude, the greater the effect of even small weather-related changes. In bowl-shaped snow valleys, as are found on many great peaks, the reflected hot sun has a weakening effect, which can be confused with AMS.

In addition, due to the flattening of Earth's atmosphere over the polar regions, the air blanket over Earth exerts less pressure in the high latitudes than nearer the equator: Alaska's Denali (Mount McKinley, 20,300 feet at 64 degrees north latitude) is actually more than 2,000 feet higher *physiologically* than Africa's Mount Kilimanjaro (19,340 feet near the equator).

These and other factors not well recognized may explain the differences found among even well-controlled studies. But individual characteristics are also important. Some people (like the female patient mentioned near the beginning of this chapter) are often sick, while others are rarely or never affected. Recent studies suggest that genetic factors may affect how the body processes oxygen; perhaps someday we may be able to identify a specific gene responsible for mountain sicknesses or resistance to it. Perhaps this factor will prove to be important not only for mountain lovers but for many more who develop illnesses that interfere with oxygen delivery. (See Chapter 14, "Genetics of High-Altitude Performance.")

HACE: HIGH ALTITUDE CEREBRAL EDEMA

Acute mountain sickness usually improves in a few days, but when the symptoms worsen and show indications that the brain is affected, we consider that the condition has shifted along the mountain sickness spectrum to high altitude cerebral edema (HACE). In simpler terms, HACE means swelling of the brain. This condition is quite serious and potentially fatal unless quickly and adequately treated.

Either mathematician René Descartes or philosopher Francis Bacon said, 300 years ago: "The only thing that man cannot completely understand is the very thing man uses to understand the world around him—the mind." We have come a long way since then, but the complexities of understanding the human brain loom even larger as we approach them more closely. The beginning of Chapter 7, "The Body Up High: Cellular and Vascular Responses to Hypoxia," outlines how the brain might be vulnerable to hypoxia.

We are confident that mountain illness is caused to some degree by a disruption of function of the brain or nerves, which is why it is helpful to think of AMS and HACE as a continuum. However, we need to distinguish between the unpleasant but minor discomfort of AMS and what happens when the brain becomes more deeply involved. Someday we may change terminology and speak of the early stage as "cerebral hypoxia," reserving the name HACE for cases where the brain effects are more prominent. It might even be more accurate to call the more severe brain component of mountain sickness "high altitude encephalopathy" (literally illness of the brain), or HAE, because although the brain does swell with edema in serious cases, we cannot yet show that it is edema that causes milder and early evidence of brain hypoxia.

It is also important to remember that *acute* hypoxia, which happens when the inhaled oxygen is rapidly and severely reduced or cut off completely (*asphyxia*) for one reason or another, causes events very different from those resulting from the less severe drop-off at altitude or from most hypoxic illnesses.

Symptoms and Signs

One of the early signs of HACE is *ataxia*, manifested by difficulty with walking, inability to do a simple heel-to-toe test or to put one's finger to the nose, and sometimes inability to control arm or hand motions. This lack of coordination is probably due to malfunction of an area of the brain called the *cerebellum* that is responsible for balance and coordination.

People with HACE do complain of headache but sometimes this is no worse than the headache experienced with AMS. Other problems common in AMS may occur in HACE as well, but neurological problems dominate, and it is these that threaten life.

Often those with HACE experience retinal hemorrhages (see Chapter 9, "Vision and the Eye at Altitude"), but these also occur in people with AMS and in healthy people with no symptoms at altitude, so this condition is not helpful in diagnosing HACE. Vision may be affected by HACE, and examination of the eyes sometimes shows that the optic disc, or nerve head, is swollen and even bulges into the back of the eye. Called *papilledema*, this rare condition provides ominous evidence that the pressure within the rigid skull is considerably increased, quite likely due to edema. Identifying papilledema requires an experienced observer.

People with HACE also have an elevated blood pressure and an increased pulse rate. A very high blood pressure is an ominous sign for the following reason. Cerebral edema raises the pressure within the skull, and this high pressure limits brain blood flow. The body reacts to an inadequate brain blood flow by increasing blood pressure and pushing more blood to the brain. Thus, a very high blood pressure may indicate high pressure within the skull and advanced cerebral edema.

In the high mountains, ataxia—stumbling while walking or having trouble balancing with the eyes closed—is an obvious early indicator of HACE. Mental confusion, vague fears, or delusions may also be present, but these are not always apparent because the patient may deny or conceal them quite artfully, so it takes some time and sensitivity to pick up all the cues. But once HACE is suspected, it is time to act decisively. Descent is the best and most helpful treatment, but often impractical (and sometimes impossible) immediately. (Other treatments are described in Chapter 15, "Prevention and Treatment.")

An interesting example of what lack of oxygen can do to humans was described in 1920. It is particularly fascinating because it happened to two distinguished scientists with special knowledge of hypoxia, physiologist J. S. Haldane and mountaineer–chemist Alexander Kellas. And it took place in a decompression chamber where outside observers at sea level could see and record everything that happened.

> ...it was our intention to remain for an hour at about the lowest pressure possible without impairment of our powers of observation.... AMK and JSH went first into the chamber and the pressure was rapidly reduced to 445 mm (about 14,000 feet) and kept there for a short time for observation.... The pressure was then reduced to 320 mm (22,000 feet).... JSH had great difficulty in making observations or even counting the pulse, and especially calculating the pulse from a twenty-seconds observation, or remembering at what point on the second hand the observation had begun. Writing was also very shaky.... He then handed the note-book to AMK who was extremely blue but felt all right and could still write quite normally.... [The pressure was lowered to 300 mm (about 23,500 feet).]
>
> To all his questions about changing the pressure, JSH replied with apparent deliberation "keep it at 320." Persons outside the window were somewhat impatient and anxious and put up messages on the window, but AMK only smiled and referred to JSH, who invariably gave the same answer.... After one and a half hours JSH consented to an increase of pressure to 340 mm. He then began to regain his faculties and took up a mirror to look at his lips, though some little time elapsed before he realized he was looking at the back and not at the front of the mirror, and consented to coming down. [Later] he had no recollection of the long stay at 320 mm nor of anything else after he handed the note-book to AMK.... AMK was much less affected. He could remember everything, and his handwriting had remained quite steady although his face was extremely blue and presented an alarming appearance to persons who saw him through the window.

This account was written by someone who from sea level watched the whole experiment through a porthole. It is an extraordinary record of serious effects of hypoxia on the brain. Fortunately for the subjects, and for science, both subjects recovered completely. Others have not fared so well.

Acute and Subacute Hypoxia

When hypoxia occurs abruptly, in contrast to gradually, as on a climb, the response is much more dramatic. If cabin pressurization should be lost in an aircraft flying above 30,000 feet, many people would fall unconscious quite rapidly unless they were able to put on their oxygen masks immediately. Similar events occurred during World War II when aircraft were flying very high, and oxygen equipment failed. A pilot taking off from sea level in an unpressurized aircraft and flying directly to 12,000 or 14,000 feet is likely to become confused and to behave erratically, especially at night.

More gradual hypoxia occurs, for example, in carbon monoxide poisoning. Several mountaineers have been found dead or unconscious in their tents after leaving their cookstoves going too long in a tightly sealed tent at altitude.

If the exposure is still more gradual, such as when flying slowly to high altitude or being taken up in a decompression chamber without oxygen, the events are quite different. This is best illustrated in a classic report showing what happened to two veteran scientists, Haldane and Kellas, when they were taken on an experimental low-pressure chamber run.

Some climbers have pleasant hallucinations. Often the victim believes he has a companion walking or talking with him, as several climbers high on Everest have described. Although this kind of confusion has long been blamed on altitude, it took some time to develop the concept that it is caused by physiological changes due to hypoxia of the brain. Here are other examples:

A strong young climber was soloing an easy route at 12,500 feet when he felt, as he put it, "disembodied," as if he were watching himself from a distance. He said aloud, "I hope that fellow is being very careful." He was able to put aside this hallucination by concentrating on it, but when he turned his mind back to climbing, the delusion again seemed real.

Those who survived a particularly tragic climb of over 23,000 feet said they had seen bulldozers and palm trees on the snowcapped summit and that strangers had tried to steal their flashlights. These hallucinations remained very vivid and real for days even after they had reached base camp.

A physician who was an experienced climber wrote me a long letter describing his experience at 14,000 feet. He heard voices talking to him and saw people walking nearby. He recognized these as hallucinations and had sense enough to turn back. Several years later on a different, slightly higher peak he began having more severe hallucinations, which he either denied or did not recognize. He became violent and had to be restrained in order to be evacuated. A tape recording made during the episode shows how deranged he was, but even after hearing this, when recovered, he denied the episode.

These experiences were serious and others have ended badly, but we have little data to show exactly what brain changes are responsible for the effects of cerebral hypoxia and the symptoms of HACE. In people hospitalized with HACE, doctors have been able to image the brain with X rays, *computerized tomography* (CT) scans, *magnetic resonance imaging* (MRI), or, for the last twenty years, *transcranial Doppler ultrasound* measurements. More recently, spinal fluid pressure has been measured and CT scans have been taken in patients with cerebral edema, confirming that the brain is actually swollen in HACE. Some of these patients have clear abnormalities such as fluid in certain pockets of the brain, while others show generalized edema. Fatal cases that have been autopsied show edema and old and new hemorrhages, some of which are very small and others large. But milder cases leave no identifying footprints, at least none that we can see with the tools we use today.

Although the effects of altitude on the brain may be subtle at first, the impact of full-blown HACE can be devastating. One need not go very high to get into bad trouble, often aggravated by failure to appreciate just what is happening.

> *I described the following case in 1978 in* Backpacker *magazine, when the concept of HACE was just evolving: Bill drove from New York to 8,400 feet in Wyoming and a day later set off on a cross-country ski trip that he had done before. Each day the party struggled through deep snow, climbing only a few hundred feet; each day Bill's headache grew worse and he had more difficulty keeping up and fell a lot. On the fifth day (at 10,500 feet) he was near collapse, and next morning when rescue arrived he was deeply unconscious and rigid. In hospital an X ray showed pulmonary edema and a neurological examination was abnormal. He improved slowly, regaining consciousness in forty-eight hours, though still mumbling and irrational; after four days he was almost well. He told me that he recalls "seeing Marilyn Monroe, live and in color, on the hospital walls" until the day he left the hospital.*

That party did not go to very high altitude, but they had to work quite hard. Bill almost died because he and his companions simply did not realize how seriously one can be affected even at relatively low altitude and a slow rate of climb. We know today that strenuous exertion aggravates problems like Bill's, but HACE was not well known then. If the party had turned back a few days earlier, he would have recovered quickly, but had they waited a day longer he probably would have died.

Occasionally HACE can come on rather swiftly. In the following case, described in a local newspaper, the victim may have had some warning, but if so he did not seek help:

> *A thirty-eight-year-old man went to bed asking not to be disturbed, soon after driving to 12,000 feet from sea level. Twenty-four hours later when he did not appear for meals, his room was entered and he was found in a deep*

coma, with rigid arms and legs, weak pulse, dilated pupils, and evidence of pulmonary edema as well. Though hospitalized and intensively treated, he died; autopsy showed cerebral and pulmonary edema that were attributed to high altitude.

Such serious loss of judgment or perception is believed to result from failure in the *frontal lobes*, the part of the brain responsible for higher thinking. At first the effect is mild confusion or uncertainty, which may not be easily recognized, and in fact is often denied.

A little confusion, muttered words, and clumsy finger actions may worsen to real hallucinations and ataxia. Denial, plus ignorance, have almost killed other individuals. More seriously affected victims sink into coma and, if not immediately treated, will die.

Pathophysiology of HACE

What is happening in the body to cause a disagreeable but self-limited case of AMS to progress, sometimes rapidly, to a serious case of HACE? Current thinking suggests that, as its name implies, HACE's symptoms are caused by swelling of the brain. However, the exact cause of this swelling is far from clear. Brain tissue swelling (either swelling of the entire brain or swelling of certain vulnerable areas) could cause pressure to build up within the rigid skull, perhaps compressing some areas more than others, or squeezing capillaries in especially sensitive areas. This would reduce the flow of food and oxygen to those cells. The swelling might be due to changes in the permeability of cell membranes, causing individual cells to swell.

The brain capillaries may leak plasma here and there into the loose supportive tissue between the nerve cells. Because brain capillaries are different from those elsewhere in the body, there is considerable debate over this, and the jury is still out. Focal edema in the cerebellum might cause ataxia or (in the limbic areas) hallucinations. Fluid accumulating in the frontal lobe would affect the higher mental processes of thought.

While the ultimate cause of HACE remains in doubt, there are at least three theoretical explanations for how brain swelling develops at altitude.

The *vasogenic theory* attributes overall swelling of the brain to fluid leakage through the thin membranes that constitute the blood–brain barrier between blood and brain tissue. This could be caused by the opening of the tight junctions between the cells lining the capillary blood vessels, or it could be due to the dilation of the small arterioles leading to the brain capillaries. This would increase blood pressure and flow in the brain capillaries.

The *cytotoxic theory* blames HACE on swelling of the individual cells in response to various insults, among them lack of oxygen or nutrients, or to toxins. For instance, a failure of the sodium–potassium pump in nerve cell membranes could cause salt and water to build up within nerve cells.

The *angiogenesis theory* rests on the fact that any tissue made severely

> ### Endothelial Cells
>
> The endothelial cells lining tissue capillaries (shown in Figure 24A) do not have tight junctions between them and may separate when pressure and/or flow in the vessels is increased, leaving a minute gap (exaggerated here as a cleft). This can allow fluid to leak into the tissues as edema, notably in the legs, hands, and face, that is characteristic of mountain sickness, and also of exercise and other unaccustomed situations. Endothelial cells in some locations also have a potential "vesicular channel" that allows passage of certain molecules, selectively.
>
> In contrast to those lining capillaries in the tissues, endothelial cells in the lung and brain capillaries (shown in Figure 24B) have tight junctions, and do not separate easily. Gas molecules pass through them by diffusion, and do not require "vesicular channels."

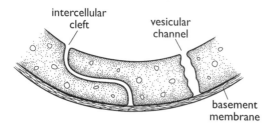
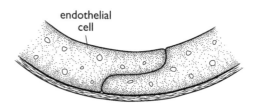

Figure 24A (left). *Endothelial cell of tissue and capillaries*

Figure 24B (right). *Endothelial cell of lung and brain capillaries*

hypoxic releases a protein that sharply increases capillary leakage, destroys some capillaries, and causes local edema. Following this, vascular endothelial growth factor (VEGF) stimulates the formation of new capillaries in the hypoxic tissue. While HACE develops far too rapidly to be caused solely by the rebuilding of new capillaries in the brain, it is certainly possible that the initial stages of this process do contribute to HACE. For more information on the possible roles of angiogenesis and capillary leaks in the development of HACE, see Chapter 7, "The Body Up High: Cellular and Vascular Responses to Hypoxia."

By measuring the pressure of the *cerebrospinal fluid* (the fluid that surrounds the brain and spinal cord), we find that pressure within the skull increases during severe mountain sickness, as shown in Figure 25. This increase can be caused by swelling of brain tissue or by hemorrhage from blood vessels, or even by dilation and leakiness of blood vessels. One hypothesis suggests that parts of the brain may swell more than others, or that localized hemorrhage may occur in especially sensitive areas.

Blood Clots, Cerebral Hemorrhage, and Brain Damage

Stroke, or *cerebrovascular accident* (CVA), is caused either by a blood clot (*thrombus*) in a crucial vessel or a hemorrhage in one or perhaps several areas.

The Brain in Its Hard Case—The Skull

Measuring the pressure of the cerebrospinal fluid (CSF) in patients with HACE has shown that the worse the symptoms, the higher the CSF pressure is likely to be. Furthermore, computerized tomography (CT) and magnetic resonance imaging (MRI) studies of patients with HACE have shown generalized swelling of the brain. In the 1980s, Peter Hackett's team on Denali airlifted a few climbers with HACE to the hospital, where they took CT scans of their brains. These showed more swelling in the white than in the gray matter (which is the largest portion of the brain, and where the higher mental functions originate) as well as in a deeper layer of basal ganglia that takes care of housekeeping functions (respiration, digestion, etc.). The white matter lies beneath the gray matter and contains over 10 billion nerve connections that service every part and every function of the body. It is especially these nerve connections (synapses) that may be affected by swelling.

If the brain accumulates only a little excess water and in only a few places like the white matter (especially the *corpus callosum*—the band of white matter that connects the two brain hemispheres), it might unevenly compress the ventricles, or the midbrain. These are the areas where many of the nervous stimuli originate that trigger symptoms like nausea, vomiting, hyperventilation, rapid heart rate, elevated blood pressure, weakness, insomnia, and other manifestations.

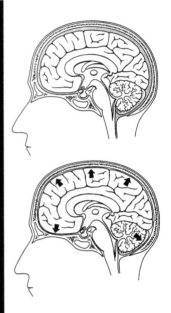

Figure 25. *The brain in its hard case—the skull*

A thrombus may form when the blood, already thickened by an increased number of red blood cells, becomes even thicker from dehydration. In the brain, very small hemorrhages or clots are occasionally silent and their effects are not obvious.

Symptoms of severe HACE have been confused with or complicated by one of several kinds of damage to the blood vessels. Because it is difficult to tell, except with special tests, whether such an event is due to hemorrhage or blood clot, and because both can produce similar signs and symptoms, both are popularly called "stroke."

Minor, brief, and transient neurological signs are called *transient ischemic attacks* (TIA) and may happen at any time anywhere; they may be advance warning of a larger stroke. They may cause brief symptoms on a mountain. Some of these might be considered part of the HACE complex, while those more lasting may be due to hemorrhage or clot formation that can occur at any altitude at any time.

Interesting possibilities are suggested by records for two patients whose "strokes" were probably due to altitude:

A healthy sixty-year-old businessman went on a tour that flew to La Paz, a thirty-minute flight from sea level to 14,000 feet. On leaving the plane he behaved and talked erratically but made no complaints. His uncharacteristic behavior persisted during the next day, but he denied any symptoms.

He was drowsy, slept a lot, and seemed to have trouble with memory. After forty-eight hours the tour leader looked at him and called a local doctor, who gave him some medicine for AMS. He did not improve and his wife took him back to the United States, where he was hospitalized eight days after he had become ill. A complete examination showed small symmetrical hemorrhages in the globus pallidus, small areas on each side of the brain. He did not improve and was unable to run his business, and after some months was forced to retire. He sued the tour company for failure to warn of the risks of that altitude, and won the case, but the verdict was reversed on appeal.

A fifty-six-year-old woman was driven in eight days from near sea level to 14,000 feet. There she slept deeply and next day was ataxic and soon slipped into coma. Though she had no headache, nausea, or vomiting, her companions thought she had AMS. She was still ataxic and confused when she awoke. When she became much worse, they took her down to low altitude. She seemed to recover after descent, flew home to Japan, and returned to work. She appeared apathetic and dull, however, and twenty-six days after onset, a complete workup showed small bilateral and symmetrical hemorrhages in the globus pallidus, almost identical to those in the preceding case. Her affect remained flat and after a year she stopped work when an MRI study showed no change in the lesions.

These two cases are especially interesting because damage in a small brain area called the *globus pallidus* can affect the higher centers, much as does damage to the larger frontal lobes themselves, causing what is called a *frontal lobe syndrome.* This syndrome includes impaired judgment and understanding, apathy or loss of interest in everyday things, and general slowing down of thought. Perhaps transient effects of hypoxia on the globus pallidus might explain some of the cognitive changes that can occur at high altitude.

A twenty-nine-year-old man flew to 9,000 feet and during the next week climbed to 14,000 feet, where he felt nauseated and lethargic but insisted on continuing. At 16,000 feet, nine days after starting his trip, he became unconscious and was evacuated with evidence of pulmonary edema and severe neurological damage. In the hospital he remained unconscious for ten days and still had evidence of brain damage six weeks later.

This man's judgment and realization of danger must have been seriously impaired when he persisted in going higher even as he grew sicker. These cases illustrate how difficult it is to differentiate what we mean by diffuse brain swelling due to hypoxia and "typical HACE" from damage due to a stroke that may be unrelated to altitude.

It is important to remember that other causes of unconsciousness and convulsions can and do occur on mountains; just because a patient is at altitude does not automatically mean the diagnosis is HACE.

A healthy twenty-five-year-old man took thirteen days to reach 16,000 feet on a South American peak. During the next four days, on the way to 17,500 feet, he developed abdominal pain, fatigue, vomiting, fever, and diarrhea. However, he said later that at 18,500 feet "he was still the strongest member of our group.... There was no warning.... When I woke up, nothing worked for me too well, I couldn't think well, and I couldn't talk too well...." During the next two days he was helped down to 13,800 feet, where he waited for helicopter evacuation for a few days, and his temperature went very high. He lost consciousness during the flight and remained in the hospital for several months.

Two years later this patient still had difficulty walking and using his hands. Although his mental functions are otherwise normal, he also has problems with speech. These neurological ailments are unlikely to improve much and it is probable that they were due to a combination of infection and stroke.

Blood Clots in Limbs

Bleeding and clotting are affected by hypoxia, but to a lesser degree than by dehydration. We do not see or hear of the frequent nosebleeds, "bleeding from the eyes," and bleeding gums that were described in climbing accounts in the last century, but why this is so is not clear. Blood clots are frequent at high altitude due to hemoconcentration and the proliferation of red blood cells. However, several studies of fibrinolysis and the clotting mechanism at altitude have not yet clarified our understanding of the situation. They occur most often in the arms and legs, especially in people who have been lying in a tent for days while waiting out a storm high on a mountain.

The year was 1953; the mountain, K2. We had been climbing for many weeks and were well acclimatized and fit. Our red blood cell counts probably had increased a great deal, making our blood thicker and somewhat more prone to clot. At 25,000 feet we were pinned in our tents for ten days by a severe storm. Our stoves did not work well, so we had difficulty melting water to drink, and we became very dehydrated and weak. One of the stronger climbers developed pain and swelling in one leg, which I recognized as thrombophlebitis; the second leg became involved and soon small bits of clot broke off and were carried to the lungs. He was critically ill and his only hope lay in getting down to lower altitude. During a desperate effort to carry him down, all of us fell and he was carried away by an avalanche.

Lasting Brain Damage

The increasing number of people going to high mountains prompts many to ask whether some will have long-lasting or even permanent brain damage. It is an important question with implications for those who remain at sea level. It is also hotly debated! Many who go to the highest mountains without bottled oxygen are reluctant to believe they may become or already have been permanently damaged. Others might blame their business or personal failures on altitude hypoxia. Depressions, broken relationships, even athletic defeats, aging, writers' cramp, and so on could be attributed to their time at altitude.

There is not a lot of hard data on the prevalence or severity of permanent neurological changes in those who go to altitude. We do know that neurological changes are often seen in aging, and that these may be attributable to decreased blood flow and oxygenation to the brain. There are also, unfortunately, many individuals who remain brain damaged after asphyxia, cardiac arrest, or any accident or illness that shuts off oxygen or blood to the brain for more than four or five minutes. These are extreme examples of how hypoxia can have a lasting impact on the brain. There are also cases of a few individuals who show lasting neurological signs after severe sickness on a very high mountain. Others may have had small strokes and show residual changes, like the two individuals with globus pallidus damage described above. A few climbers who returned from Everest without mishap have shown small lasting effects manifested by slowed finger tapping (a test of reaction speed). Recent CT scans done on two veterans of many Himalayan climbs suggest that their brains may have shrunk very slightly, although no changes in performance remain.

For me, the question of permanent neurological damage remains unanswered. My bottom line? I suspect that there may be some lasting damage for a few mountaineers who go repeatedly to great altitude without supplementary oxygen. Is this likely enough to make one hesitate? Considering the many other risks in everyday life, and remembering the great rewards of mountaineering, I would accept this risk.

Because the brain uses 15 percent of the oxygen consumed by the body, but makes up (in an average adult) only 2 percent of the body's total weight, it is not surprising that the brain is so very vulnerable to hypoxia, despite a redundancy of protective mechanisms. Like other living tissues, the brain can swell with edema; its vessels may bleed or leak plasma from capillaries. Perhaps even more common and equally harmful, the electrical networks and the biochemical neurotransmitters, unique to the nervous system, can be affected in numerous places, with ripple effects throughout the body. Joseph Barcroft, who described his work in elegantly simple words, said: "Hypoxia halts the works and wrecks the machinery." The wonder is that we can survive serious hypoxia unscathed—if indeed we do!

VISION AND THE EYE AT ALTITUDE

In 1968, during the Mount Logan High Altitude Physiology Study, a young climber became unconscious soon after being flown to the 17,500-foot laboratory. He was airlifted to a hospital, where he recovered rapidly from what was considered to be a severe form of altitude sickness. The internist noticed a number of hemorrhages in the retina of each eye, and tests for diabetes, kidney disease, leukemia, or other possible causes did not explain them. I was unsure of what this meant, but a few weeks later one of the scientists, also flown to the high laboratory, was also found to have a few scattered retinal hemorrhages. This seemed more than coincidence, so I added retinal studies to the Logan protocols, and over the next few years found that many of the mountaineers had similar hemorrhages.

We published several reports about these high altitude retinal hemorrhages, calling them HARH. In 1969 General Inder Singh of the Indian Army Medical Corps wrote two articles about altitude sickness among Indian troops flown or driven rapidly from low to high altitude during the Sino-Indian border conflict of 1962. Among other things, he noted engorgement of the retinal veins, swelling of the optic nerve head (papilledema), and "vitreous hemorrhages" in several of the sickest soldiers, but he may have confused "vitreous" with "retinal." Singh's men were very sick and the eye pathology was attributed to edema of the brain (which he found in two brain biopsies).

By contrast, many of the individuals we saw on Mount Logan with HARH were not very sick and would not have been aware of the retinal hemorrhages had we not examined their eyes. We did not see hemorrhages in the vitreous, but only in the retina—behind the retinal limiting membrane, to be exact.

During the next few years on Mount Logan we took hundreds of photographs, examined retinal capillary leakage by fluorescein injection with strobe photography, and tried to correlate these hemorrhages with other symptoms, time at altitude, exertion, and other influences.

We found that half of the thirty-nine subjects most completely studied at 17,500 feet showed HARH. Our data showed that strenuous exertion did increase the likelihood of retinal hemorrhages but probably was not itself the cause. We did not find any relationship between number of hemorrhages and symptoms of AMS.

Some subjects had only a few small hemorrhages while others had large and frightening pools of blood. Papilledema was rare, although the optic disc was engorged in several persons. Both retinal veins and arteries were distended and tortuous, and blood flow was significantly greater and faster than at sea level.

The leakage occurred from the smaller vessels but we could not be sure whether from the arterial or venous end of the capillaries. We saw "cotton wool spots," which indicate lack of blood flow (retinal ischemia) in a small area, in one of the thirty-nine persons. Fluorescein injection showed leakage in 40 percent of the individuals we studied, strongly suggesting that the capillaries were more permeable or more subject to tearing than normal. In our series only one or two people noticed any effect on vision, but one individual with a hemorrhage in the area of central vision (the macula) did describe a small blind spot. Many hemorrhages disappeared during the weeks at altitude, and others were gone at the end of the altitude stay. As has been true with other cases I have seen since then, the central blind spot in the individual with a macular hemorrhage took several years to clear.

The eye is often called a window to the brain because its nerves and blood vessels are so intimately connected to those in the brain. The eye is also the lens through which pass images of the world around us. Both "window" and "lens" may be disturbed or disrupted at high altitude or by hypoxia at any altitude. As it turns out, retinal hemorrhages do appear to be commonplace at altitudes above 12,000 to 14,000 feet, and may or may not reflect similar hemorrhages in the brain.

Because they are increasingly examining the eyes of climbers on expedition, doctors have come across an increasing number of reports of visual events attributed to altitude. These are largely anecdotal, but occur with sufficient frequency to deserve a closer look. Many of the visual changes are difficult to explain, and in almost every case are based on what the individual describes, and without objective corroboration.

This chapter looks at several of the effects that hypoxia (and perhaps hypobaria) have on vision. They prove difficult to evaluate, but are very important if they do in fact represent changes within the brain.

Not surprisingly, this comparatively new field has spawned a number of research ventures, many by veterans, but even more by eager youngsters who want the opportunity of going to a high mountain and producing a research report.

HARH: HIGH ALTITUDE RETINAL HEMORRHAGES

From 1967 to 1979, the Arctic Institute of North America sponsored an altitude research laboratory at 17,500 feet on Mount Logan, Canada's highest peak. It was there, in 1968, that retinal hemorrhages due to high altitude were first noted. They were then studied and described over the next few years. Supplementing inspection of the retina through an ophthal-moscope with retinal photographs revealed hemorrhages of many different sizes—from single, small, flame-shaped hemorrhages to many or large blobs of blood. In addition, the veins and arteries, and occasionally the optic nerve itself, were dilated or swollen. These *high altitude retinal hemorrhages* (HARH) were described in a number of papers, which led to many further studies.

Since then many doctors have looked for HARH on mountain expeditions and a few times in decompression chamber work. The reported incidence has ranged from 15 percent to 90 percent, and HARH have been observed at as low as 11,000 feet and as high as 25,000 feet. Many confounding circumstances such as exertion, speed of ascent, hydration, or experience of the observer make it difficult to determine incidence more precisely.

Most would agree that HARH do not permanently affect vision, with the exception of those that occur in or near the macula. These need special mention. In some personal correspondence, ophthalmologist–mountaineer Mike Wiedman wrote:

> Peripheral HARH and retinal hypoxia do not permanently affect visual function. But macular hemorrhage threatens permanent partial visual loss. By the very nature of its random occurrence, macular hemorrhage can recur with repeated hypoxic exposure.

Wiedman suggests that simply by chance alone, a macular bleed could occur again and add to the damage. He has seen many victims of macular hemorrhages, few of whom recovered full vision. Wiedman feels that those who have had macular hemorrhages should be wary of going to altitude again, although this decision depends somewhat on the completeness with which macular vision recovers. He also believes that all HARH are accompanied by small hemorrhages in the brain. A few conservative doctors agree and advise that if someone has had HARH, he or she would be unwise to go very high again—advice that few mountaineers are likely to accept or heed. But if a macular hemorrhage appears, descent would be prudent—just to prevent further damage.

Capillary Leakage

The question of capillary permeability changes at altitude has been debated, not only in relationship to HARH but within the whole spectrum of acute mountain sickness/high altitude cerebral edema (AMS/HACE) and high altitude pulmonary edema (HAPE). Leakage from the small vessels throughout most of the body can occur through gaps in the lining of the blood vessels. The endothelial cells lining the retinal capillaries resemble those in the brain and lungs, having tight junctions between them. It is possible that increased capillary blood flow and pressure (caused by dilation of the smallest arteries that feed the capillaries) may open these tight junctions in a few places and allow leakage. It is probable that nitric oxide

(NO) (discussed in Chapter 4, "Moving Blood: Circulation") is involved in retinal circulation.

In contrast to the capillaries in the brain, those in the retina are not supported by *glia*, supportive cells that surround and protect brain capillaries from overdistention. For this reason, retinal capillaries may be more susceptible to leakage due to increased blood flow. There is a report of an examination of the eye of a doctor who died of HACE that shows that the retinal hemorrhages came from small veins.

Do Hemorrhages Occur Elsewhere in the Body?

Leaks in retinal blood vessels raise some intriguing questions. First and foremost is whether minor bleeding occurs elsewhere in the body at altitude. Because the eye is seen as the window of the brain, we must wonder, as Wiedman does, "If small vessel hemorrhages occur in the retina, can the brain be far behind?" It is a distressing thought, but we cannot answer with any assurance. Patients who die of altitude illness often show hemorrhages in the brain, but these are extreme cases.

Splinter hemorrhages beneath the fingernails at high altitude have been described, but these might well have been caused by the trauma of climbing or cold. Traces of blood have been found in urine of people after ascent to moderate elevations, but this is not common, or at least has not often been mentioned along with other occasional changes observed in kidney function. One wonders whether the many reports of bleeding from the eyes, gums, and nose often mentioned by Victorian-age mountaineers could be somehow related to increased capillary fragility.

Clinical Importance

It is worth repeating that most HARH are not important clinically, that they cause little change in vision at the time of onset or later, except for those in the macula, and that they disappear without treatment. Accounts of blindness or blurred and double vision at high altitude are almost surely due to other causes. The importance of HARH is what they might be telling us about what happens elsewhere in the body. Although other ophthalmologists and climbers disagree, Mike Wiedman says:

> I've been sermonizing for twenty years and on five Everest expeditions about HARH being a prognosticator of cerebral hemorrhages....
> I would advise climbers that there is a probability of concurrent brain damage when HARH are seen. The brain hemorrhage may be of uncertain extent but easy odds are that it is there.... If mountaineers wish to go on with such full disclosure, that's their prerogative.

That might be one way to reduce congestion on the world's highest mountains, and it might also dampen enthusiasm for going anywhere above

15,000 feet! Right now it is appropriate to warn climbers about the lasting effects of macular hemorrhage, but we do not yet know enough to connect HARH firmly with brain hemorrhage or damage.

Other Causes of Retinal Hemorrhages

It is important to remember that retinal hemorrhages (RH) do occur in many other conditions besides hypoxia of high altitude, and this should be kept in mind even when altitude seems the obvious cause.

Severe carbon monoxide poisoning can cause RH, perhaps because it causes tissue hypoxia rather than through a direct impact on the small blood vessels. But RH are seldom present in chronic obstructive pulmonary disease (COPD), even though hypoxia often causes other signs and symptoms. RH aren't seen in cyanotic congenital heart disease, or even in congestive heart failure, despite hypoxia, unless caused by a complicating illness like hypertension or diabetes.

Many illnesses of blood vessels or of the blood itself result in RH, and in fact RH are sometimes the first evidence of a condition like leukemia, severe anemia, high blood pressure, or even diabetes. Hypertension can also damage vision through RH, but seldom as extensively as does diabetes. Adult respiratory distress syndrome (ARDS) or severe infection or toxic shock can also cause RH, perhaps through hypoxia or changes in the mechanism of blood clotting or vascular permeability.

OTHER EYE PROBLEMS

In 1939, as World War II was beginning, Ross McFarland, a pioneer in aviation medicine, published several important articles showing that visual acuity in dim light (night vision) decreases rather markedly above 5,000 feet, and is reduced by more than half a few thousand feet higher. This decline results from changes in visual purple (the retinal pigment in rods), which needs a good supply of oxygen.

A forty-five-year-old engineer and active climber (who did his doctoral research in arterial blood flow) began to have episodes of flickering and often dimmed vision during strenuous exertion, most often on a mountain. He had no headache and, for a time, no other symptoms. The episodes became more frequent and more serious, at times making him almost completely blind and slurring his speech. On one climb he became partially paralyzed. Since these alarming symptoms invariably disappeared when he went down, he did not seek advice until the episode of paralysis scared him! A complete workup showed nothing whatever to explain the episodes, and he had no neurological signs. He recalled that as a youth he had had occasional episodes of flickering vision (scintillating scotomata, in 'medispeak') and had been told he had a form of migraine. These brief episodes ended and he had none for twenty years. After his neurological workup revealed nothing abnormal, and considering the old diagnosis of migraine without headache, he was told to take one aspirin a day; he resumed climbing and had no further episodes. After several years he stopped the daily aspirin and almost at once the vision problems recurred whenever he exerted strenuously as in climbing.

It is likely that this patient has what is called *acephalgic migraine* (migraine without headache, commonly vision related), as Dr. Walter Alvarez has described in several hundred cases. Dozens of climbers have reported symptoms similar enough to suggest the same diagnosis; some have taken and benefited from preventive aspirin.

Does migraine affect or predispose a person to altitude illness? The answer is not known, but migraine is thought to be due in part to excessive constriction or dilation of the smaller arteries in the brain and by changes in oxygen or carbon dioxide in the blood. Perhaps more significant, people with a migraine tendency who go to altitude may not be able to distinguish migraine from severe AMS. One colleague known to us suffers badly from both but cannot tell which is which!

This case is probably different from another episode of sudden complete or almost complete blindness on a high mountain. This occurs at sea level too and is named *amaurosis fugax,* attributed to a brief (ten-minute) reduction in blood flow to the retina, or perhaps to the *occipital* (visual) part of the brain. It probably is not accurately blamed on altitude but might be called *altitude amaurosis* because it disappears with descent. Ten years ago an ophthalmologist related an unusual case:

A woman developed transient blurred vision in one eye only at 20,000 feet in the Himalayas. She stopped climbing for an hour or so and everything returned to normal. She began climbing again and within a half hour or so, the blurring in the same eye returned, and disappeared when she halted. She repeated this a third time, and then decided to go down. There were no aftereffects; she's a very perceptive observer and her story is fully credible. But what was it?

Dimming vision is an early warning sign of hypoxia, at any altitude. Often it is the only warning that the individual may recognize, because the other effects are so subtle. Occasionally climbers at high altitude notice double vision—which can be rather disconcerting while making difficult moves. This is most likely due to fatigue plus hypoxia, bringing out a slight imbalance of the small muscles that move the eyes. Most of us have some imbalance anyway, but this normally does not affect vision because the brain is easily able to fuse the two images. But stress, like fatigue and hypoxia, weakens this central fusing ability, much as alcohol does, causing one to see double.

The popularity of *radial keratotomy,* surgery done to improve nearsightedness, has led to reports of blurred vision at altitude that have been blamed on the operation. During the tragedy on Mount Everest in 1996, one of those who nearly died was a pathologist who had become "almost completely blind" as he descended, after a harrowing night of exposure. This was attributed to his radial keratotomy. However, Geoff Tabin, a distinguished mountaineering ophthalmologist, writing for the *American Alpine Journal,* explains:

> The tiny cuts made like spokes radiating from the center of the cornea weaken the cornea, and altitude hypoxia causes slight swelling around the edges of the cuts, further flattening the cornea.... This in turn causes a slight refractive error...which in an older climber, (together with) the change toward farsightedness, causes blurry vision.

Other climbers have had no difficulty at altitude after radial keratotomy, and the newer techniques eliminate this problem because the cuts are made quite differently.

Is glaucoma affected by altitude? There is not enough evidence to make a confident statement. The few studies that have been done show little or no change in the intraocular pressure in the normal eye. However, the optic nerve is very sensitive to changes in its oxygen supply, and if glaucoma has already affected the nerve, this damage may be aggravated by increased pressure in the eye at high altitude. This suggests that individuals with glaucoma should be carefully monitored before and after a climb, and perhaps consider enjoying lower mountains.

The good news is that the diuretic Diamox, a medication used to prevent and treat high-altitude disease, is a useful agent for decreasing intraocular pressure. Indeed, it may be used for glaucoma. It is just as effective at altitude, and decreases symptoms of AMS as an added benefit. The bottom line? High altitude will not cause glaucoma but may increase slightly any preexisting damage due to glaucoma. Diamox protects against this small risk and may be helpful. There is also the possibility that extensive retinal hemorrhage in the glaucomatous eye could cause a retinal detachment; perhaps this is some cause for concern, but no such occurrence has yet been reported.

Cataracts are very common among high-altitude residents—partly due to the strong ultraviolet light and partly due to poor nutrition, particularly lack of vitamin A.

Some experts also fear that there could be damage to the cornea if contact lenses are worn for a long period at very high altitude. The cornea receives its only oxygen supply from outside air, which would be excluded by most contact lenses except the gas-permeable soft lenses. One problem with contact lenses (worn by many climbers) is dehydration, which inhibits tear production so that the cornea under the lens dries and may be damaged. The other problem is the difficulty of cleaning contacts in very cold weather, increasing the risk of corneal infection and even ulcer.

Snow blindness is more frequent the higher you go, but it is not so much an altitude problem as one related to any snow-covered landscape. It is a painful form of conjunctivitis (inflammation of the outer "skinlike" covering of the eyeball) caused by too much ultraviolet light. Most often, it happens when a person does not wear appropriate protective glasses on a bright sunny day while on snow, but it is a real risk in fog or under thin clouds, which allow UV light to be reflected off the snow. And UV light is more intense the higher you go. We cannot stress too strongly the importance of good sunglasses, with side shields, on a high snowy mountain or, indeed, on any snow-covered landscape. Snow blindness is not limited to altitude.

Viagra has some unexpected effects on vision, and because small doses of that drug are being used more often to treat HAPE, we can expect more reports on the visual effects of Viagra. It is well documented that Viagra, taken at sea level, causes difficulty in discriminating blue–green differences, along with other effects. There is some evidence that repeated use of Viagra may cause small, lasting, harmful changes in vision.

CHAPTER

HAPE: HIGH ALTITUDE
PULMONARY EDEMA

It was New Year's Eve 1960 in Aspen, Colorado. I was closing my office about 6 P.M. when the telephone rang. A young voice asked, "Are you the doctor?" He told me that his friend was stranded in the backcountry, quite ill, and asked if I would rescue him.

Having hitched a ride, the young man arrived at my home an hour later to describe the situation in more detail. He and his friend had climbed from Aspen (8,400 feet) up and over the 12,000-foot Buckskin Pass. The friend became very short of breath and could not go on, and somehow the two managed to descend 1,000 feet, where they spent the night. The next morning the companion was worse and the young man skied twenty miles down to the road, where he telephoned me.

It sounded to me like a case of pneumonia, but clearly the victim had to be rescued because a storm was predicted. I tried to gather a rescue party. It was New Year's Eve. After some difficulty, I tracked down a few friends and a snowmobile, and we agreed to meet at the road head at dawn. The operator of the snowmobile, who was late (and understandably angry at being found in bed with a woman who was not his wife!), towed us as far as he could. We skied the rest of the way and three hours later reached the patient.

He was very weak, coughing, and short of breath. We loaded him on my children's toboggan and got him to the hospital late that evening. There I started him on oxygen and antibiotics. Next morning he was surprisingly well. Evidence of fluid in his right lung could still be heard and seen by X-ray, although the film was not at all typical of pneumonia or heart failure. I asked the opinions of several other doctors, but no one could be sure of a diagnosis. I sent the patient home with a tentative diagnosis of heart failure. Several cardiologists agreed, but were uncertain.

Soon after, Dr. Paul Dudley White, probably the leading cardiologist of the day, visited me. After hearing the story, he said, "I don't see any evidence of heart disease in your workup. I think it has something to do with altitude. You should publish this."

I wrote up a short note in which I included several anecdotes about mountaineers who had died of a similar condition high on a mountain and had been diagnosed with pneumonia. The paper was published by the prestigious New England Journal of Medicine. *Almost immediately I received a flood of letters from around the world describing similar cases among mountaineers. This was apparently the first description of such a case published in a widely known journal. Similar cases occurring in South America had been described in the Spanish literature, and Dr. Herbert Hultgren had published a comparable case history in the* Stanford Medical Bulletin, *but without follow-up.*

I presented this case at a few medical meetings, and a consensus developed that this illness was pulmonary edema caused by altitude. In the fall of 1962, while I was Peace Corps director in India, I heard that Indian troops were experiencing severe altitude illness after being flown from near sea level to around 18,000 feet to meet the Chinese invasion. I visited the All India Medical Center and spoke to the chief of medicine. He either could not or would not tell me much, but as I was leaving he asked if I was related to Dr. Charles Houston. When I admitted that indeed I was he, the chief brightened and said, "Over here we call this Houston's disease." After the war, Indian physicians published several important articles describing altitude illness and continue their research today.

In 1991 I went to the Himalayas and walked from 7,000 to 14,000 feet in a few days. It was a hard trip, and when we arrived I was quite tired and abnormally short of breath. That night I slept poorly and coughed a lot. By morning I suspected HAPE, but I had come a long way to do an interview for the BBC, and I told myself I would tough it out! We did the interview. The second night I was worse, but next morning managed to go down and began to improve after descending several thousand feet. I was fortunate. My advice to anyone is to go down as soon as a diagnosis of HAPE is evident, but in this case I disregarded my own counsel. So here is a clear example of "do as I say, not as I do"!

Looking to the past, we find that high altitude pulmonary edema (HAPE), like other mountain sicknesses, has been around for a long time. One of the earliest descriptions was written by the Buddhist missionary Fa-Hsien (A.D. 334–420) while crossing a pass some 12,000 to 14,000 feet high:

> Fa-Hsien and the two others proceeding southwards, crossed the Little Snowy Mountains. On them the snow lies accumulated both winter and summer. On the north side of the mountains, in the shade, they suddenly encountered a cold wind which made them shiver and unable to speak. Hwuy-Ring could not go any farther. A white froth came from his mouth and he said to Fa-Hsien, "I cannot live any longer. Do you immediately go away, that we do not all die here"; and with these words he died.

The party had been traveling for many months, and one would expect them to be well adjusted to altitude. The emphasis on cold suggests that Hwuy-

Ring probably died from a combination of hypothermia and what we now recognize as HAPE, as discussed in Chapter 18, "The Mountain Way." The combination of cold and altitude has a double impact on the mountaineer; this is particularly important on Denali (Mount McKinley) in Alaska, one of the coldest mountains, where HAPE is quite common. Even on the Alps, the unacclimatized who hurry may pay with their lives, as Angelo Mosso described in his book *Life of Man on the High Alps*:

> In 1891 a member of a scientific party on Mont Blanc had to leave unexpectedly and a young physician rushed up from the valley to take his place. He continued to the summit and returned to the shelter a few hundred feet lower. A few hours later he developed a severe headache and nausea. He tossed all that night, unable to sleep, and next day began to cough profusely. His condition deteriorated, his mind wandered, and after writing a farewell letter to his brother, he sank into coma and died less than three days after arrival.

Autopsy showed what we now recognize as pulmonary edema. This appears to be the first well-documented case of HAPE. One of the cases Thomas Ravenhill described in 1913 was typical of HAPE, which he considered cardiac in origin:

> An Englishman...arrived by train—a fifty-two-hour journey from sea level.... He seemed in good health on arrival, and said he felt quite well.... He woke next morning feeling quite well with symptoms of normal puna. As the day drew on he began to feel very ill indeed.... He became very cyanosed, had evident air hunger.... He seemed to present the typical picture of a failing heart.... He coughed with difficulty. He vomited at intervals.... Towards morning he recovered slightly and as there was luckily a train he went straight down.... I heard later that when he got to 12,000 feet he was considerably better and at 7,000 feet he was nearly well. It seemed to me that he would have died had he stayed at altitude another day.

Ravenhill was mistaken in calling this heart failure; if the patient had a true heart problem he would not have recovered so quickly. The description is characteristic of fluid accumulation in the lungs, the condition we call HAPE, which is less common but more serious than AMS.

Although it has some of the features of fluid disturbance that contribute to acute mountain sickness/high altitude cerebral edema (AMS/HACE), HAPE is different enough to place it slightly apart. And because the lung is more easily examined and probed than the brain, we know quite a lot more about how HAPE develops and why, even though some of the pathology still eludes us.

HAPE is the most common of the serious altitude illnesses. Travel has become so fast and easy that millions can go—and do go—much too rapidly from low to dangerous altitudes, making HAPE, because it can develop so quickly, an even greater risk. It is true that mountain illnesses have stricken travelers for centuries. But in times past, when it took weeks or months to get to high mountains, or, in the more recent past, when it took several days to get to a resort in the Rockies and weeks to the high Himalayas, these problems did not happen to more than a few.

BASIC MECHANISMS OF HAPE

The function of the lung is to supply oxygen to the blood, which delivers it to all the cells of the body. What follows is a short technical summary of what we know or think we know about the physiology of HAPE. The non-scientific reader will find explanations for the unavoidable medical terms in the glossary at the back of this book. Chapter 3, "Moving Air: Respiration," describes the process of breathing, and this section reviews a few salient features of the passage of oxygen from lungs to blood.

The 300 million tiny air sacs (alveoli) at the ends of the branching airways of the lung have a total surface area roughly equivalent to that of a tennis court. So many capillaries surround them that it is as if the alveoli are exposed to a sheet of flowing blood. Here oxygen moves from the alveoli to the blood, while carbon dioxide moves from the blood to the alveoli.

Blood enters the pulmonary artery (which carries low-oxygen blood) from the right ventricle of the heart at a pressure of about 25 torr. As the blood flows into the many branching pulmonary arterioles, this pressure falls sharply. Consequently, as blood enters the capillaries of the lung, its pressure is about 7 torr and normally remains at this level in the pulmonary veins carrying oxygenated blood back to the left ventricle of the heart.

When we are at rest, some of our pulmonary capillaries are collapsed and carry little or no blood. When the amount of blood pumped by the heart rises, the thin-walled capillaries in the lung are protected from excessive flow and pressure by a feedback mechanism that opens up unused capillaries. This mechanism, called *recruitment*, allows the lungs to accommodate the large increases in blood flow that occur during exercise without elevating pulmonary capillary pressure. Blood flow through the pulmonary vessels also is impacted by the oxygen level in the alveoli. When the partial pressure of oxygen in the alveoli is low, the muscular pulmonary arterioles and precapillary vessels constrict, increasing *pulmonary artery pressure* (PAP). This is just the opposite of what happens to arteries in much of the body, which dilate when blood oxygen is low. Thus, at altitude, or whenever oxygen pressure in the alveoli decreases, PAP rises.

Brownie Schoene and Peter Hackett, studying altitude sickness on Denali in the 1980s, collected fluid by bronchoscopy from deep in the lungs of climbers with HAPE, as well as from healthy climbers. They found that fluid from HAPE victims was high in protein and white blood cells, suggesting that HAPE might be due to capillary inflammation and leakage. However,

Passage of Gases—Lungs to Blood

Each alveolus is surrounded by capillaries that bring low-oxygen blood close to the alveolar air, which is higher in oxygen and lower in carbon dioxide. As capillary blood rushes past the alveolar wall, oxygen diffuses in and carbon dioxide out, so that arterial blood returning from the lung to the heart is in equilibrium with alveolar air, whatever it may contain. Diffusion of oxygen takes place across the alveolar wall, which consists of a single layer of *epithelial* cells and their basement membrane. It then moves through a loose interstitial space that is collapsed or nearly so under normal circumstances. The oxygen then crosses the basement membrane and the single endothelial cell layer lining the capillary before it enters the capillaries and binds to hemoglobin in the red blood cells. The alveolar epithelial cells are tightly joined to one another, as are the capillary endothelial cells, and each is bonded to its basement membrane. (See Figure 26.) Despite these layers, the pulmonary membrane is very thin and imposes little resistance to gas diffusion, while tightly containing air on one side and blood on the other.

After rapid ascent to altitude, the capillary endothelium leaks fluid from the blood into the interstitial space. Under normal circumstances, the small amount of fluid that leaks from the capillaries into the interstitial space is returned to the blood by the lymph vessels. But if the leak is excessive, as it might be at high altitude, plasma and some red blood cells accumulate first in the interstitial space and eventually in the alveoli themselves.

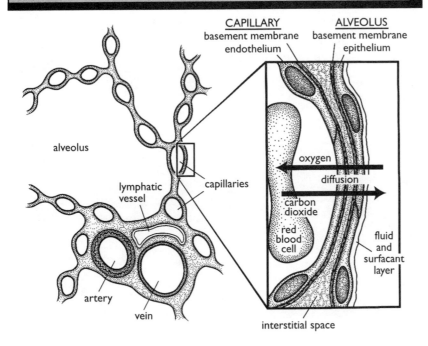

Figure 26. *Passage of gases—lungs to blood*

more recent evidence shows that HAPE can occur with no measurable in-flammation. John West, a leader in high-altitude physiology, believes that increased pressure actually tears the walls of the pulmonary capillaries, allow-ing plasma and red blood cells to leak through. (For more on the response

X rays of Lungs with HAPE

The stethoscope can tell us when even a little moisture is present in the air passages of the lungs. If fluid does accumulate, as the X ray in Figure 27A shows, most of the fluid will be scattered in several places, usually more in the middle area of the lung (the right lung in Figure 27A) rather than near the *hilar* area (root of the lung). Figure 27B shows a computer-enhanced X ray of another case, showing the accumulation of fluid more clearly. The X ray is usually so characteristic that it should not be mistaken.

For those not familiar with conventional chest X rays, the well-aerated lung shows as dark gray or black, while moisture shows as white. The heart shadow and vessels leading from it, as well as the ribs, the diaphragm, and the liver, are also white.

In the patient whose computer-enhanced X ray is shown in Figure 27B, the patches of edema are more clearly defined. This patient's heart is somewhat enlarged, and the pulmonary artery (upper right of the heart) is more prominent than normal.

These two X rays are typical of moderately severe HAPE at 9,000 feet, which cleared very rapidly after descent, oxygen treatment, and rest.

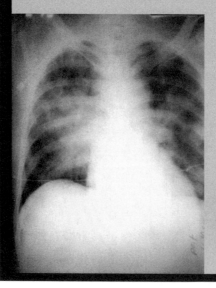
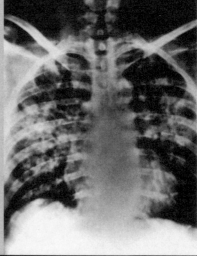

Figure 27A (left). *X ray of characteristic HAPE*

Figure 27B (right). *Computer-enhanced X ray*

of pulmonary blood vessels to high altitude and the controversy around the role of inflammation in HAPE, see Chapter 7, "The Body Up High: Cellular and Vascular Responses to Hypoxia").

Normally the alveoli are kept dry by a mechanism called *standing gradient osmosis*. Sodium pumps on the side of the alveolar cells facing the interstitial space pump sodium from the cells into that space. Water follows the sodium from the cells into the interstitial space. On the other side of the alveolar cells, the side next to the alveolar space, any water that is present in the alveoli moves from the alveolar space into the cells to compensate. The net effect is that any water that leaks into the alveoli gets moved from the alveolar space to the interstitial space. This fluid is quickly drained away from the interstitial space back into the blood vessels by the lymphatic vessels. However, if too much fluid floods the interstitial space, lymphatic drainage cannot keep up and fluid accumulates there, slowing the passage of gases. If this process proceeds too far, fluid begins leaking into the alveoli. This is what happens when an abnormally high pressure in the terminal arterioles (the tiny arteries leading to the capillaries) is transmitted to the capillaries.

Both alveolar and capillary walls are thin and thus can be torn or ruptured by high pressure. At high altitude, when an increase in capillary pressure causes an increase in the permeability, or perhaps even the tearing, of the alveolar wall, the result is HAPE. Lung capillaries also can leak when subjected to certain biologically active substances.

SYMPTOMS AND SIGNS

A person with HAPE presents a more serious picture than the individual who suffers from AMS. He or she looks miserably sick, not merely uncomfortable.

Increasing weakness and shortness of breath are out of proportion to effort, and *cyanosis* (bluish nails and lips) is deeper than expected at that altitude. (Remember that bluish nails, lips, and ears are common even in healthy people at altitude, and cold can cause the skin to look blue.) At altitude, cyanosis is due to generalized deficit of oxygen in the arterial blood, as compared to an oxygen deficit only in the skin in cold weather at lower altitudes.

A slight cough grows worse, and if the sputum is frothy or pink, or sometimes bloody, the case is more serious. Pulse rate is rapid and blood pressure may be a little high. Slight fever and a small increase in the infection-fighting white blood cells are common. More important: The patient looks quite ill. Audible crackles (rales), gurgling, and wheezes can be heard in the lungs, often without a stethoscope and even across the room.

Sometimes people with HAPE also exhibit ominous signs of the HACE portion of the spectrum: headache, confusion, and ataxia—the staggering walk of HACE. In a person who has come up too rapidly to altitude, this combination of symptoms should be considered dangerous and treated urgently because rapid deterioration is not uncommon. Until the late 1960s, people presenting these symptoms were diagnosed as having flu or bronchopneumonia, were inadequately treated, and often the correct diagnosis came too late.

Be alert, though. All the above signs can arise from several other causes, including infection, any of which may be as serious as HAPE and should always be considered in the differential diagnosis.

Remember too that by far the most frequent cause of lung edema at any altitude is increased venous pressure due to a failing heart that is unable to handle blood arriving from the lungs. Backed-up blood begins to flood the lungs, leaking into the alveoli, and flagrant pulmonary edema follows. These events are caused by weakness of the heart muscle, specifically of the left ventricle, or to a badly leaking heart valve, and they are more likely to occur after years of high blood pressure (systemic hypertension). In HAPE, however, the heart functions normally, except in the uncommon subacute or chronic mountain sicknesses described in Chapter 11, "Chronic and Subacute Mountain Illness."

It may be helpful to look at a representative case. One early report has often been cited because it was so typical and so graphically described by the victim's companion:

Over a five-day period, W. B. climbed to 16,000 feet carrying a heavy pack. He was far more short of breath than others in the party, did not eat, and began to cough. His companion later said, "He obviously had fluid in his lungs." Despite penicillin it was harder and harder for him to breathe, his cough got more severe and frequent, and as his companion wrote in his diary, "Over the next hours his breathing became progressively more congested and labored. He sounded as though he were literally drowning in his own fluid, with an almost continuous loud bubbling sound as though he were breathing through liquid." His breathing grew much worse during the night, he became limp, and he died on the second day of illness.

This sad episode, so characteristic of HAPE, happened two years before HAPE became well known; the autopsy was reported as showing "fulminant bilateral pneumonia." Such cases continue to occur; some people still die, but many more know what to do when they are affected:

A fifty-two-year-old man flew from Pittsburgh to Denver and at once drove to 9,000 feet. Next day he consulted a doctor because of severe headache, inability to sleep, lethargy, and increasing shortness of breath. On examination he looked poorly and had scattered moisture (rales) in both lungs, but no other abnormal findings. His chest X ray was typical of HAPE; he was given oxygen for a short time with benefit, and then drove back to Denver (5,000 feet); he had recovered by the time he arrived.

This man was lucky or wise, or both, and today his is a more common scenario, like others that end more happily now that the risks of mountain sickness are better known. Even so, HAPE is still a danger, on low as well as very high mountains, and it still kills the heedless and uninformed, like this man:

> A commercial pilot and his wife flew from his home near sea level to Colorado and drove to a ski area at 9,500 feet. He skied hard the next day but tired easily, and on the third day fell a lot and went home early. During the night his breathing became increasingly labored, and early in the morning his wife managed to take him to the medical clinic. In the car he stopped breathing. Though resuscitated and flown to intensive care, he died eleven days later with pulmonary and cerebral edema and subsequent pneumonia.

This death would never have happened if the victim or his companion had paid attention to his condition—and to what his flight training should have taught him about altitude. In this particular instance, the victim also showed signs of HACE in the ataxia that made him fall so often and in the poor judgment that blinded him to how bad his condition had become. We frequently see evidence of brain hypoxia in patients with severe HAPE. Sometimes the diagnosis is more difficult:

> A healthy, though inactive, 39-year-old man flew from Miami to Mexico City (7,500 feet) where he spent three nights before flying to Bogota (8,400 feet). He taught a class the day after arrival and telephoned his wife that evening, saying he felt fine except for a little shortness of breath. Next morning he was found dead, lying on top of his bed with his glasses on and a newspaper on the floor. He seemed relaxed and there was no evidence of a struggle. Autopsy showed pulmonary edema, and slight arteriosclerosis of a coronary artery. At issue was whether this was due to altitude or to cardiac arrest. Such a sudden death from HAPE is rare, and very uncommon as low as 8,400 feet. In addition, because he had been above 5,000 to 7,000 feet for seven days (including flight times), I considered HAPE slightly less likely to have caused his death than a sudden cardiac episode. Peter Hackett thought HAPE somewhat more probable.

Characteristics

Herb Hultgren reviewed medical records at a clinic in a mountain resort, and described the characteristics of 150 individuals proven to have had HAPE at the 9,000-foot-high area during a three-year period. This is probably the best available picture of HAPE at moderate altitude, so it is summarized here in Table 4.

A diagnosis of HAPE was made based on the clinical picture plus rales (the sound of fluid in the lung heard with a stethoscope) and/or X ray. Listening carefully to the lungs was at least as accurate for diagnosis as was X ray, but because rales often persist for days after full recovery, the X ray

TABLE 4
CHARACTERISTICS OF 150 INDIVIDUALS WITH HAPE

Mean age	34.3 years
Gender	84% males
Onset	3–4 days after arrival
HACE	14%
Temperature	99°
Fever	20% over 100°
Rales	85%
X ray positive	88%
Bilateral	52%
Right only	34%
Blood pressure >150	17%

is helpful in demonstrating progress—not to mention differentiating HAPE from another problem like pneumonia.

HAPE is a dangerous illness, and it is not rare. Fortunately, it is easily cured when treated early, and, above all, preventable. The more people know about its cause (in this case, altitude) and the more attention they pay to prevention, the lower will be the number of HAPE cases. Prevention of all forms of altitude illness is so important that it is described separately in Chapter 15.

Incidence

Because it is difficult to determine the number of people at risk, we can only approximate the percentage of visitors to mountain areas who develop HAPE. In addition to altitude, there are many other contributing factors, such as speed and method of ascent, level of exercise, and individual susceptibility. Extensive data collected from Mount Kenya, the Mount Everest region, the Indian Himalayas, Peru, Colorado, and the European Alps suggest that anywhere from 0.01 percent to 4.5 percent of the people who go to high altitude develop HAPE. One report from the Sino–Indian war in 1962 gave an incidence of 15 percent. Most cases occur after twenty-four to forty-eight hours at altitude, mainly above 10,000 feet. These disparate findings illustrate the difficulty in interpreting information collected in different ways by different individuals in different situations.

At a resort in Colorado at 9,000 feet, Jack Reeves made a careful study of the frequency of HAPE during winter and summer months, matching this to barometric pressure and temperature. He found a small but statistically significant difference: Of all the patients who saw a doctor for any reason in one resort area, the percentage who had HAPE was a little higher in winter

HAPE in Alveoli

The alveolar space normally contains gas made up of oxygen (O_2), carbon dioxide (CO_2), nitrogen, and water vapor—but no liquid. When alveolar oxygen partial pressure falls, blood pressure in the pulmonary artery rises, and this pressure is transmitted to the precapillaries, causing dilation of the capillaries themselves. This causes serum to leak into the interstitial space, and when this cannot be drained rapidly by the lymphatics, it leaks further into the alveoli. If excessive fluid accumulates in the interstitial space (shown in Figure 28), diffusion of oxygen into the capillary is impeded, further increasing pulmonary artery pressure, and worsening oxygenation of blood and tissues.

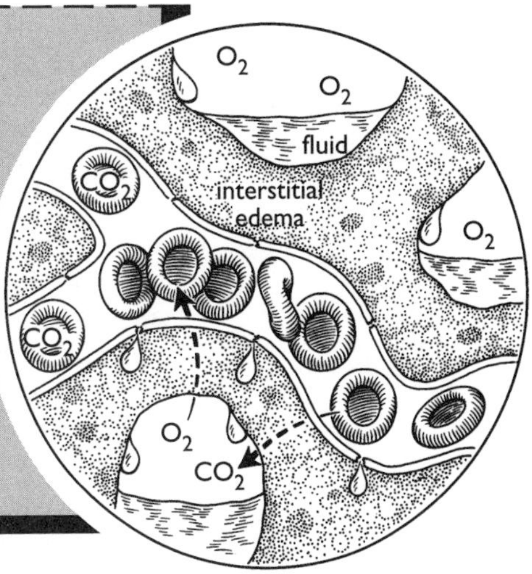

Figure 28. *HAPE in alveoli*

than in summer, and on colder than on warmer days. This was not true of AMS: Weather made no difference. This apparent effect of cold is not entirely surprising because animal and some human studies have shown that pulmonary artery pressure increases slightly (even at sea level) while breathing cold air, or even when the face is exposed to severe cold. The increase is small but might make a difference in the cold, windy air on a very high mountain, especially to an individual whose pulmonary circulation is more vulnerable than normal.

As a very rough estimate, based on the unfiltered information collected from many areas, one might estimate that about 2 percent of all those who go to moderate elevation (above 8,500 feet) will develop clinical HAPE. Most are treated and recover, some descend and recover quickly, but, as many of the reports collected at Colorado resorts show, a few unacclimatized visitors die from HAPE each year. Many are hospitalized at least briefly. Deaths due to HAPE occur on every mountain range, and at altitudes from 8,500 feet and higher.

Unlike AMS and HACE, there is a distinct gender difference in the incidence of HAPE: Several studies show that five or six times as many men as women develop HAPE under comparable conditions. Without much more information about attendant circumstances and the numbers of each gender at risk, it is anyone's guess why this should be true. Data defining influences like activity level, speed of ascent, and others simply are not available much of the time. The menstrual cycle appears to have no influence on HAPE, but the data are inadequate.

There also is an age gradient: Children are more vulnerable than adults, especially children resident at altitude returning after a brief stay nearer sea level. Strenuous exertion soon after arrival increases the risk. Even a mild respiratory infection like a cold or flu seems to increase the likelihood of HAPE.

Most people, even the unwary who take risks by climbing too fast, never experience HAPE. On the other hand, some individuals are hit often. Several studies in the Alps, for example on Monte Rosa (15,200 feet), have shown convincingly that certain people are "HAPE-susceptible," while others are not. We call them HAPE-S, and they are at risk whenever they go to moderate altitude. Of many possibilities, no explanation has been proven.

Twenty years ago a young doctor–mountaineer developed HAPE at a modest altitude, recovered immediately on descent, but over the next few years had several more episodes during similar climbs. A complete and thorough study provided no explanation. Since then he has frequently noticed the warning indications of impending HAPE when he goes above 11,000 to 12,000 feet. He always recovers promptly after descending to lower altitude. With adequate time for acclimatization he has climbed above 20,000 feet without any evidence of HAPE. There is still no explanation for his susceptibility, and he has not routinely taken the HAPE preventive nifedipine.

This well-informed and intelligent physician, active in altitude research, has learned to handle his problem and could probably take appropriate measures if, for some reason of weather or injury, he were unable to get down before his HAPE became severe. Others may not be so fortunate and should carry appropriate medication.

A few HAPE-susceptibles may have an old lung infection or injury or multiple small emboli to the lungs, either of which might predispose them to this disorder. A score of individuals have developed HAPE due to congenital absence of one pulmonary artery, and several have died before the diagnosis was made. Perhaps others with minor congenital or other abnormalities in their lungs retreat to lower altitudes when they begin to have symptoms, and remain undiagnosed.

Recent work suggests that nitric oxide deficiency may predispose an individual; this is discussed in Chapter 4, "Moving Blood: Circulation." Whatever the reason, we now recognize that there is a cohort of individuals highly susceptible to HAPE, for whatever reason. By lowering the pulmonary blood pressure, Viagra, administered in small doses, has proven to be more beneficial than nifedipine in treating HAPE. It may also be that a long-acting form of Viagra, now on the market under the brand name Cialis, may be advisable for HAPE-susceptibles to take before going to an altitude where HAPE is a possibility.

Precipitating Factors

Many anecdotes and case reports suggest that even a mild respiratory infection like a cold or flu increases the chance of HAPE, but there is no firm evidence one way or another. As for exertion, there is no doubt: Strenuous effort or prolonged hard work greatly increases the possibility—and the severity—of HAPE. This is almost certainly because exertion increases pulmonary artery pressure, even at sea level, and the added pressure at altitude may tip the scales.

Cyclists in a long and difficult race at 8,000 to 9,000 feet showed evidence of interstitial or even early alveolar pulmonary edema by X ray, but so too did a comparable group of ten cyclists racing at sea level. Several cases of pulmonary edema occur each year among thousands of runners in the grueling 97-kilometer Comrades' Marathon in South Africa, run at low altitude. Is "exertional pulmonary edema" a manifestation of excessive blood flow in portions of the lung, and unrelated to hypoxia? Although there are no perfect animal models of HAPE, it is interesting and perhaps significant that racehorses, pushed to the limit, cough bloody sputum and develop lung edema that can—and sometimes does—kill them.

Acclimatization does protect against HAPE, but not completely: Even after weeks at moderate altitude, veteran mountaineers, working too hard high on the mountain, have succumbed. A few climbers have died of HAPE on Everest at an altitude higher than 20,000 feet, despite having taken weeks to get there. Very strenuous exertion in extreme conditions almost certainly can precipitate such fatalities, as it does at much lower elevations.

Reentry HAPE

So-called re-entry HAPE is a curious twist on the more general condition that affects some acclimatized individuals who have lived at altitude for many months or even years. A small percentage of them occasionally develop serious HAPE when they return to that altitude after a week or two near sea level. Cases have occurred after only one or two days at lower altitude. As is the case with HAPE, children are more likely than adults to develop reentry HAPE, a phenomenon for which no explanation has been found. As with ordinary HAPE, those who have had this problem once are more likely to have it again and should take extra precautions. Although the percentage of residents so affected is small, it is real, and there may be an important clue here that we are overlooking.

Some expeditions attempting high mountains use a strategy that calls for climbing high on the mountain slowly enough to acclimatize, and then returning to base camp for a period of rest before rushing back to summit. You might think this procedure would predispose climbers to reentry HAPE upon return to high camp, but it does not seem to. Perhaps months rather than weeks of residence at high altitude are needed to set the stage for reentry HAPE.

But this does not tell the whole story: There are no reports of re-entry HAPE among Tibetan natives, whereas there are cases among high-altitude Andean natives.

Other Types of Pulmonary Edema

Another type of pulmonary edema, Adult Respiratory Distress Syndrome (ARDS), results from severe trauma or toxic shock. ARDS is not like HAPE, either clinically or as seen by X ray, and the attendant circumstances should preclude its being confused with HAPE. The prognosis is much worse. Nitric oxide and its antagonist endothelin-L are deeply involved in ARDS.

Many toxic substances cause lung edema, as for example in the 1984 pesticide factory explosion in Bhopal, India, or chlorine gas attacks in World War I. Indeed, pulmonary edema often is a terminal event in many deaths caused by diseases of the cardiovascular or respiratory systems. These situations are very different from HAPE. Any kind of lung edema causes hypoxia; in HAPE it is the hypoxia, but only alveolar hypoxia, that provokes the edema.

The various causes of pulmonary edema produce characteristic X-ray or CT scan images. Any radiologist should be able to diagnose HAPE by X ray alone, and in most instances can differentiate it from pneumonia. However, some atypical pneumonias caused by unusual organisms may look something like HAPE. Just remember that HAPE strikes healthy individuals who have rapidly arrived at altitude.

PATHOPHYSIOLOGY

The basic cause of HAPE is pulmonary hypertension and the chain of events initiated when pulmonary artery pressure (PAP) increases above tolerable limits. Oxygen lack, specifically in alveolar air, increases PAP; exertion and cold magnify the increase; HAPE does not occur unless PAP is high. In many circumstances PAP can rise very high without causing pulmonary edema.

How is HAPE different from brisket disease (the accumulation of fluid in the neck tissues of cattle at altitude), and from other forms of mountain sickness in humans such as chronic, subacute infantile, and adult mountain sicknesses? (See Chapter 11, "Chronic and Subacute Mountain Illness.") In all of these, pulmonary artery pressure is high, but in the ailments other than HAPE heart failure rather than lung edema results. Although we cannot fully explain why this is so, the differences may depend on how quickly and how high the pulmonary artery pressure increases. In HAPE some lung areas receive too much blood and others too little. This nonuniformity is normal under everyday conditions, but when excessive (as at altitude), oversupplied areas flood and fluid accumulates. Blood leaving lung areas that are flooded with fluid carries oxygen at less than full capacity because the fluid acts as a barrier to diffusion of oxygen from the alveoli to the blood. This has been demonstrated by lung perfusion studies of patients with HAPE.

The uneven distribution of blood flow results in areas of the lung that are overperfused and in effect underventilated, while other areas are underperfused but normally ventilated. The imbalance between ventilation, V, and blood flow or perfusion, Q, is described as V/Q mismatch or V/Q

inequity. When there are areas in the lung where ventilation is excessive relative to perfusion (elevated V/Q), some of the ventilation is wasted and the work of breathing is unnecessarily increased. When there are areas in the lung where the perfusion is excessive relative to the ventilation (reduced V/Q), blood does not become fully oxygenated as it passes through the alveoli, and the arterial blood oxygen level suffers. In some medical conditions V/Q inequity results from scattered obstructions due to blood clots (*thrombi*) or smaller particles (*emboli*) lodging in smaller vessels.

In the mid-1970s Dr. Herbert Hultgren suggested that overperfusion of certain areas of the lung could cause flooding, and that these areas might flood the alveoli as well. These scattered areas are fairly characteristic of the shadows seen on X rays.

Evidence supporting the patchy overperfusion theory advanced by Hultgren in 1966 can be summarized today as follows:

1. Although PAP at altitude is high, in HAPE neither the left nor right ventricle is found to be dilated or failing.
2. X rays show only patches of increased density, indicating localized edema; this is very different from the X ray of congestive heart failure. Swelling of the liver, fluid in the abdominal or chest cavity, elevated venous pressure—all signs of a failing heart in brisket disease and chronic or subacute forms of mountain sickness—are not present in HAPE.
3. Recovery from HAPE—when treated early by descent or oxygen—is complete and usually rapid.
4. Congenital absence of one pulmonary artery causes overperfusion of the normal lung at even moderate altitude (6,000 to 8,000 feet) and precipitates HAPE. Similarly, a large, unilateral pulmonary embolus causes pulmonary edema at any altitude.
5. Patchy edema similar to HAPE can be produced in animals by injecting into their lungs tiny glass spheres to simulate emboli.

The magnitude of pulmonary artery pressure increase is not predictive of the likelihood or severity of pulmonary edema. For example, residents of Leadville, Colorado (10,000 to 11,000 feet), have a slightly higher PAP than a comparable population at sea level, and some of the school athletes there actually increase their PAP during strenuous exercise to a level higher than the systemic blood pressure without showing edema. A high PAP is found among natives living in many mountainous areas—but data from different studies are somewhat conflicting. High-altitude Tibetan natives do not have a PAP as high as the Aymara at comparable elevations in the high Andes.

When fatal cases of HAPE are autopsied, micro-thrombi as well as larger clots are found scattered throughout the lungs. Although it is likely that many of the clots occurred after death, some may have contributed to elevated PAP and worsened HAPE.

SUMMARIZING HAPE

Over many years of painstaking research, scientists have put together many parts of this puzzle. Today this much is known about HAPE with a high degree of certainty:

1. HAPE occurs only when PAP is elevated and when the capillaries leak. However, PAP may be high without causing HAPE.
2. Hypoxia increases PAP by causing some of the smaller precapillaries (which have muscular coats) to constrict, thereby changing the distribution of blood in parts of the lungs. But only lack of oxygen in the alveoli increases PAP; other types of hypoxia do not.
3. HAPE is the result, not the cause, of constricted blood vessels in the lung, which increases PAP.
4. Vasoconstriction and vasodilation are caused by substances, among them nitric oxide and endothelins, released from the cells lining blood vessels. Other direct stimuli also alter PAP.
5. Some high-altitude natives (Aymara) have elevated PAP; other ethnic groups (Tibetans) do not. PAP increases with exertion in both groups. HAPE does occur, but only rarely, in high-altitude natives going to even higher elevations.
6. Some residents at high altitude who descend to low altitude for a short time (one to ten days) are subject to HAPE when they return to altitude.
7. Some individuals are more susceptible to HAPE. These HAPE-S individuals may have a genetic defect contributing to this susceptibility.
8. In some individuals HAPE can be caused by a congenital absence of a pulmonary artery and possibly by multiple small pulmonary emboli. These people may get HAPE at altitudes as low as 5,000 feet.

Obviously there is still a great deal to discover about HAPE, as there is about all altitude illnesses. What makes the quest to understand altitude hypoxia so fascinating is that it provides flashes of insight into the many causes of oxygen lack at sea level. These benefits, almost more than those related to mountaineering, were what led to the writing of this book.

CHAPTER 11

CHRONIC AND SUBACUTE
MOUNTAIN ILLNESS

We scientists like to catalog things, and once this is done, to subdivide the classifications. Sometimes this is helpful, sometimes not. The way we classify mountain illnesses has changed little since Ravenhill named the four types of mountain sickness in 1913. Some decades later Carlos Monge, Sr., described a variant of altitude illness that he called chronic mountain sickness, *or CMS, and which today bears his name. Monge and Barcroft had a historic disagreement over whether European visitors or Andean natives were better able to adapt to high altitude. From this collegial but intense debate—which both sides won—emerged our understanding of CMS, an over-exuberant response of the red-blood-cell-forming mechanism that causes the blood to become sluggish, straining the heart.*

I have not seen an unambiguous case of CMS, or Monge's disease. To me, CMS seems to be what Lewis Carroll called a portmanteau term in that it can mean whatever you want it to mean. In actuality, the diagnosis is clear cut, as we shall see, but there has been a tendency among medical professionals to add subcategorizations to the diagnosis.

Changing world demographics and territorial infighting have brought significant population shifts to the high mountains of South Asia. Since China annexed Tibet in 1951, there has been an influx of several hundred thousand low-altitude Han Chinese into High Tibet, an influx that has increased rapidly since 2001. A number of infants, either born at altitude or taken to altitude before the age of one, have developed a condition similar to Monge's disease, which has been called subacute infantile mountain sickness (SIMS). *Like CMS, the disease is progressive and fatal unless the child is taken to sea level.*

The Pakistani and Indian governments have been fighting since the mid-twentieth century to control Kashmir, a high-altitude region in the Eastern Himalayas. Troops are stationed on each side of the twenty-mile gap, at altitudes of 18,000 to 22,000 feet, where they exchange desultory artillery fire and accumulate mountains of waste material that will be there forever. It is a senseless demonstration of man's stupidity! And it has brought to light a new disease called subacute adult mountain sickness. *This affliction is similar to CMS, but occurs after only a few months at altitude, even*

though acclimatization may seem to be complete. As in the case of subacute infantile mountain sickness, the disease is fatal unless the soldier is taken to lower altitude, where recovery takes a few weeks or months.

Lowland dwellers who travel to the mountains commonly find themselves outperformed athletically by high-altitude natives, at least initially. Over time, the lowlanders acclimatize and improve their performance. But high-altitude natives, especially those whose ancestors have dwelt in the mountains for many generations, still seem to have an adaptive edge over most lowlanders. When it comes to acclimatization and adaptation (discussed at length in Chapters 13 and 14, respectively), a climber who lives at low altitude may draw the conclusion that more time at altitude is always better. However, this is not necessarily true. Chronic and subacute mountain sickness, serious illnesses that can cause heart failure, can strike people, both natives and long-term visitors, who have been at high altitude for many years. As is the case for HAPE, subacute mountain illness is characterized by high pressure in the arteries of the lung, which leads to swelling and gradual failure of the heart. CMS is a potentially deadly complication of mountain living that shares many elements with subacute mountain illness. It can begin after years or even decades at high altitude. It can strike the most acclimatized individual, and is even a threat to those whose ancestors have been mountain dwellers for scores of generations.

CMS: CHRONIC MOUNTAIN SICKNESS

In 1927 Carlos Monge, Sr., described a new illness that he called "erythremia syndrome of high altitude," which is now known as chronic mountain sickness (CMS), or Monge's disease, in his honor. His patient was a 38-year-old man who had come up from sea level and had worked at 14,200 feet for one year. He complained of multiple aches and pains, easy fatigue, insomnia, and mental confusion; his blood showed half again the normal red cell and hemoglobin content. All his symptoms disappeared after a time at sea level, but returned when he went back to altitude.

Symptoms and Signs of CMS

Over the next seventy years, many similar cases were described, and CMS is now a well-recognized though uncommon disease. Experts do not agree completely on the diagnostic criteria for CMS. Nevertheless, there is consensus that CMS is a disease that occurs in people who have lived at high altitude for an extended period, that it is characterized by an abnormally high level of red blood cells (*polycythemia*) and an abnormally low blood oxygen level (*hypoxemia*), and that it improves or vanishes with descent.

People with CMS complain of headache, dizziness, breathlessness, fatigue, memory loss, and sleep difficulty. These are the direct or indirect consequences of hypoxemia. Typically the victim is so cyanotic that his skin looks purple, with flushed cheeks and often curved, blue nails. He also experiences muscle and joint pains and sometimes pain in the chest. When examined by a physician, a patient suffering from CMS is generally found to have polycythemia and, often, signs of pulmonary hypertension and heart enlargement on his or her chest X ray and ECG. The patient's hemoglobin (normally 14 grams) may be as high as 22 grams, with a hematocrit (normally 50 percent) between 60 and 80 percent. The hypoxic ventilatory response (HVR) is blunted, as it is in most long-term altitude residents, which is not unusual. Death from right heart failure is likely unless the patient goes to sea level, where he or she recovers slowly. Unfortunately, the problem recurs on return to altitude.

Monge's initial work on CMS was focused on showing that the disease could develop even in people free of other respiratory disease. However, because preexisting chronic respiratory illness can predispose a person to CMS, some experts now distinguish primary CMS (which occurs in people free of other respiratory disease) from secondary CMS (which develops in those who already have a chronic respiratory illness). As discussed below, constriction of the pulmonary arteries in response to hypoxia (hypoxic pulmonary vasoconstriction, or HPV) and the increased pulmonary artery pressure (pulmonary hypertension) that it produces are commonly part of CMS. Because pulmonary hypertension can strain the right ventricle of the heart and lead to right heart failure, physicians in China often distinguish three types of CMS: polycythemia without right heart failure; right heart failure without polycythemia (also called high altitude heart disease, or HAHD); and mixed CMS, which includes both polycythemia and heart disease.

Risk Factors for CMS

CMS occurs wherever people live at high altitude, but some people are more likely to develop this disease than are others. Males who were born or have lived continuously above 12,000 feet for many months or years are affected four times as often as females. A few typical cases have been described at 10,000 feet, as have a few at 7,500 and 6,500 feet, although these are questionable. Without the four diagnostic criteria—cyanosis, arterial desaturation, pulmonary hypertension, and blunted ventilatory response—excessive red cell production may be only an overexuberant response to altitude, or the result of an undiagnosed lung or other disease.

Children have as much as twice the risk of adults, and premenopausal women are protected somewhat compared to men and postmenopausal women. Sea-level dwellers who move to high altitude are generally at greater risk than are high-altitude natives. In the Himalayas, CMS is less common among Tibetans (whose ancestors have presumably lived at high altitude for several thousand years) than it is among members of the Han Chinese ethnic group (whose ancestors moved to high altitude much more recently).

At elevations above 13,000 feet, less than 0.5 percent of ethnic Tibetans but more than 1.5 percent of ethnic Han Chinese develop CMS. Once CMS develops, it is likely to be progressive. Thus, in any given population, adults with severe CMS are likely to be older than those with mild disease.

CMS also seems to be somewhat more common in the Andes than in the Himalayas. This is taken as evidence that Himalayan dwellers (particularly Tibetan natives) may be better adapted genetically to life at high altitude than are Andean natives. But as discussed in Chapter 14, "Genetics of High-Altitude Performance," these sorts of "between group" comparisons are tricky. The environment in the Andes differs from that in the Himalayas in several ways, and a simple comparison of Andean versus Himalayan natives could fail to distinguish environmental from genetic causes for differences in disease rates in these two locations. For instance, one of the reasons that people live at high altitude in the Andes is to work as miners. The sort of mining done in the Andes can expose workers to high levels of cobalt, a toxin known to stimulate erythropoietin (EPO) production and polycythemia. In fact, some Andean dwellers with CMS are known to have elevated blood cobalt levels compared to control subjects who were free of CMS. So it is not unreasonable to propose that cobalt may contribute to CMS development for some Andean natives, although genetic adaptive differences between Andean and Himalayan natives could exist as well. It is also interesting to note that CMS rates are high in Colorado, another location where high-altitude life and mining have been historically linked.

Pathophysiology

CMS can be viewed as a disease of maladaptation to the hypoxia of high-altitude life. As discussed in Chapter 7, "The Body Up High: Cellular and Vascular Responses to Hypoxia," and as will be examined more closely in Chapter 13, "Acclimatization," the kidney responds to hypoxia by increasing EPO production. EPO stimulates the bone marrow to increase red blood cell production. The resulting elevated red blood cell count partially compensates for hypoxia by increasing the oxygen-carrying capacity of the blood. However, an excessively high red blood cell count can increase blood viscosity. This increases the resistance to blood flow, raises the blood pressure, and puts added strain on the heart. People with CMS develop greatly elevated red blood cell levels. These contribute to the pulmonary hypertension and heart failure of CMS.

Chapter 10 discussed how the blood vessels of the lung respond to hypoxia by constricting (hypoxic pulmonary vasoconstriction, or HPV). HPV is highly adaptive to regional hypoxia—a condition that develops, for example, when parts of the lung are infected with pneumonia while other areas remain relatively normal—because it shunts blood away from diseased and toward healthy lung areas and optimizes blood oxygenation. However, at high altitude, the entire lung is hypoxic. HPV throughout the lung can contribute to HAPE in the short term. Over many years it can raise pulmonary artery pressure. This strains the right side of the heart, causing it to enlarge and eventually to fail, which is just what happens to individuals who develop CMS. HPV also contributes directly to pulmonary hypertension, causing a thickening of the walls of the pulmonary artery. Changes in the pulmonary artery walls, which can be particularly severe in children with CMS, contribute further to the pulmonary hypertension and heart failure.

Hypoxia may well be the proximate cause of CMS. But while everyone who lives at high altitude is exposed to hypoxia, not everyone develops CMS. There is, as yet, no way to predict with compete confidence who will develop CMS and who will be spared. However, some facts are beginning to emerge. Chapter 13, "Acclimatization," looks at the importance of a brisk increase in ventilation in response to hypoxia (the hypoxic ventilatory response, or HVR) in compensating for and adapting to high altitude. With time at high altitude, the HVR normally does become somewhat blunted. People with CMS, however, seem to have an abnormally low HVR, probably caused by a loss of sensitivity to hypoxia in the carotid body and brain. This low HVR could add to the hypoxia of altitude and contribute to the development of CMS. A low HVR is probably not, by itself, enough to explain the devastating body changes associated with CMS. The finding that people with CMS are more likely to have abnormal breathing during sleep suggests that poor night ventilation may also contribute.

Prevention and Treatment

The most obvious treatment for CMS is descent to the lowlands. Unless the disease is very far advanced, this increases the blood oxygen level and decreases the elevated red blood cell count over the course of several weeks. The heart enlargement and pulmonary hypertension of CMS may reverse to normal as well, but this can take several years. If descent is not possible, bloodletting (*phlebotomy*) can temporarily decrease the red blood cell count and reduce strain on the heart. One reason premenopausal women are protected from CMS may be that the blood loss of menstruation acts as a check on polycythemia. Another reason may revolve around female sex hormones. Female sex hormones are known to stimulate respiration, and a progesterone derivative has been used to increase ventilation and blood oxygen while decreasing polycythemia in postmenopausal women at altitude.

Other than living in the lowlands and avoiding the obvious environmental causes of lung disease (smoking, for instance), there is not much that a person can do to avoid CMS. Women of the Han Chinese ethnic group who dwell at high altitude in the Himalayas often choose to descend to low altitude to give birth. They may then leave their child with relatives at low altitude for one to five years to avoid the high risk of pulmonary hypertension and resultant heart disease that sometimes occurs in very young children brought to high altitude.

SUBACUTE MOUNTAIN SICKNESS

From the above discussion of CMS, it is clear that prolonged exposure to the low oxygen levels of altitude can produce pulmonary hypertension and, if untreated, heart failure. There is enough variability in (and confusion about) the terms used to describe altitude-related cardiac disease that occurs only over time that it might be helpful to discuss some other terms that are used to describe subgroups of high altitude heart disease. Even animals are not immune to chronic cardiac disease. An interesting cardiac problem known as brisket disease affects cattle at high altitude.

SIMS: Subacute Infantile Mountain Sickness

In the late 1980s two types of mountain sickness with associated heart failure were identified as "subacute." The first, described in 1988, was called subacute infantile mountain sickness (SIMS). SIMS is an uncommon but serious condition seen in infants of low-altitude ancestry who are exposed to altitudes over 8,500 feet for longer than a month. It begins with the development of pulmonary hypertension and leads to right ventricular cardiac failure. Early signs are lethargy, poor feeding, and sweating; subsequent symptoms of heart failure include cough, insomnia, difficulty breathing, decreased urination, and edema.

The only victims so far reported have been infants of Chinese parentage taken to Tibet, or born in Tibet at altitude, who developed characteristic right heart failure within a few months after birth. Later, some children aged two or three were found with a similar condition. These infants often died unless taken to sea level, and autopsy showed increased muscularization of pulmonary arterioles, as well as right ventricular dilation and hypertrophy attributed to severe pulmonary hypertension. Kept at altitude, the children were not responsive to heart medication but sometimes recovered—slowly—when taken to sea level.

This childhood heart failure is due to excessive increase in pulmonary artery pressure, causing dilation and failure of the right ventricle. As such, it is similar to the disease that Chinese physicians call high altitude heart disease (HAHD).

Subacute Adult Mountain Sickness

In 1990 reports surfaced of a similar condition that appeared in adult soldiers after months of living in combat zones in the high Himalayas, even though they had ascended slowly enough and apparently had acclimatized well. The patients developed massive edema of the legs, swelling of the liver, fluid in the chest cavity, and dilation of the heart, especially the right ventricle. However, pulmonary resistance was not exaggerated, and resting pulmonary artery pressure was only slightly above normal. Significantly, however, this pressure rose very high during exertion. Because these soldiers had to work hard for many hours in adverse conditions, it is probable that *episodic* pulmonary hypertension led to right heart failure. When taken to low altitude, they lost fluid rapidly, and their hearts returned slowly to normal. Neither they nor infants with subacute mountain sickness showed an increased hematocrit. It seems likely that subacute adult mountain sickness is a variant of the infantile form.

Brisket Disease in Cattle

Although there are no good animal models of acute mountain sickness/high altitude cerebral edema (AMS/HACE) or high altitude pulmonary edema (HAPE), there is much to be learned from the effect of altitude on certain strains of cattle. When particular breeds native to low altitude are taken above 8,000 feet, many develop a form of altitude illness called "brisket" disease, because they accumulate fluid in loose tissues under the neck (the brisket), in the liver, and in the chest cavity. This edema is due to heart failure—the right side of the heart, unable to pump adequate blood to the lungs against the high pulmonary artery pressure, dilates and then fails. Brisket disease is quite a different kind of maladjustment to altitude than is HAPE, and it is fatal unless the animal is taken down to low altitude. Some strains of cattle have a genetic predisposition to brisket disease, which might have some interesting implications for humans.

> When I lived in Colorado a rancher called me about two valuable young bulls he had just brought up to 8,200 feet: Both had developed brisket disease; did I know anything about this? Actually, I had attended a meeting on the subject organized by Hans Hecht, so I said happily that I would cure his bulls. At the ranch his cowhands threw one of the patients; I shaved his legs, but my electrocardiogram was a flat line. A cowhand said wryly, "Doc, I think yo' patient's daid." The struggle had caused cardiac arrest! I decided to treat the other without an EKG and that one recovered! But for a long time afterwards, when I suggested doing an EKG on a patient, the response was: "I don't know, Doc. I heard what happened to Werk Cook's bull."

Chronic exposure to the low oxygen levels found at high altitude can have harmful effects on the cardiovascular system, including elevated pulmonary artery pressure and excessive production of red blood cells. An individual may develop one or both of these problems. He or she may even have a pulmonary artery pressure that is normal or nearly normal during rest, but which increases dangerously during exercise. These individual differences have led to some confusion about the names we should apply to these diseases and their particular diagnostic definitions. However, all can agree that the constellation of symptoms caused by chronic exposure to low oxygen includes either heart failure or a high risk of developing heart failure—in particular, failure of the right ventricle, which pumps blood into the lungs. The greater the number of people living and working at high altitude, the greater the number at risk for these chronic diseases of the mountains.

HYPOXIA IN EVERYDAY LIFE

In 1942, when I first began working in the U.S. Navy's altitude training unit, I was fortunate enough to find a copy of Paul Bert's book Barometric Pressure, *a magnificent encyclopedia of all that was known about oxygen, high altitude, and mountain sickness toward the end of the nineteenth century. It included voluminous data from laboratory and decompression chamber studies, and some of the pioneering work in oxygen transport by hemoglobin. Also in the training unit library were innumerable and even more interesting works written by climbers and explorers over the preceding several hundred years describing their experiences on high mountains. This was a treasure trove; the books I found there were almost the only works on high altitude and altitude illness available in those years. I was also able to find* Respiratory Functions of the Blood, *written by Sir Joseph Barcroft in 1925, a highly readable collection about oxygen transport based largely on his own work in Cerro de Pasco in the Andes and in the laboratory.*

Barcroft posed one question that has stayed with me ever since: "How can the lessons learned at high altitude be applied to the bedside?" It seemed logical then and even more so today that lack of oxygen at sea level might cause problems similar to those encountered under decreased barometric pressure. Although this question has been largely ignored, it is one that has fascinated and influenced me throughout my career as a physician.

Why should altitude sickness concern anyone other than climbers and trekkers and other mountain visitors? Not very many people ever go above 4,000 to 5,000 feet unless they live in the mountains, so who is listening? Well, the fact is that almost all of us experience hypoxia at some time during our daily lives even though we often don't realize it. Many millions cope with serious hypoxia from illness, for months or years. This chapter discusses some of these other causes of oxygen lack and explains why they are in fact so important to many sea-level dwellers.

Fortunately, our oxygen transport and utilization system (see Chapter 3, "Moving Air: Respiration") makes mild hypoxia almost unnoticeable. In fact many people become slightly hypoxic during sleep—even at sea level. There are many environmental, respiratory, circulatory, and tissue conditions

TABLE 5
CAUSES OF HYPOXIA

Environmental	Ventilatory	Circulatory	Histotoxic
High altitude	Airway	Heart failure	Cyanide
Air pollution	obstruction	Anemia	poisoning
	Alveolar defect		Tissue toxins

that cause clinically important signs and symptoms—and even death—from hypoxia. It is convenient to classify these as shown in Table 5.

RESPONSES TO HYPOXIA

We react to hypoxia from any cause in two ways. The first we might call emergency measures, the "struggle responses," which are slight or marked depending on the cause and degree of hypoxia. These are the first efforts our body makes to restore oxygen to normal levels.

If hypoxia persists, these emergency measures evolve into what we call acclimatization, a series of adjustments that enable us to tolerate considerable oxygen lack, and to climb very high. This process of acclimatization is discussed in Chapter 13, "Acclimatization."

TABLE 6
STRUGGLE RESPONSES

- Increased rate and depth of breathing
- Increased heart rate and output
- Increased circulating red blood cells
- Decreased plasma volume
- Decreased blood flow to nonessential tissues
- Enzymatic changes permitting some anaerobic work

ENVIRONMENTAL HYPOXIA

The preceding chapters discuss how decreased atmospheric pressure on mountains, together with individual characteristics, causes various altitude-related sicknesses. This section describes how other environmental changes increase the effects of hypoxia, just as infection, injury, or damage to different organs complicates chronic shortage of oxygen.

Flying

By far the most frequent cause of brief everyday hypoxia is flying. Although they might reach altitudes of 30,000 to 45,000 feet, the cabins of commercial aircraft are kept at a pressure equivalent to an altitude of between

5,000 and 7,500 feet, depending to some degree on the actual altitude above Earth and the duration of the flight. On a long flight you may be at this altitude for twelve hours or more. For the average passenger flying for a few hours at a cabin altitude of 5,000 to 7,500 feet, the effects are rather mild. A sensitive person may notice slight shortness of breath; occasional irregular breathing; "Cheyne–Stokes," or periodic breathing; and some feeling of uneasiness or discomfort. Those who have a tendency to hyperthyroidism and thus use more oxygen, or those with a mild anemia or a pulmonary–cardiac condition that slightly decreases their blood oxygen, may notice the altitude more. It is likely that oxygen lack contributes to what we call "jet lag" after long trips. It is also worth mentioning that alcohol has an effect on the brain similar to lack of oxygen, and consequently, as we say in the mountains, when you are at altitude "one drink does the work of two" because it raises the physiological altitude slightly.

Cabin altitude varies in commercial aircraft. The flight course is influenced by weather, which in turn affects the outside atmospheric pressure. The structure of the aircraft puts a limit on the pressure difference between the cabin and the outside air. If and when supersonic travel becomes common, we will see more problems resulting from the greater altitude at which these aircraft must fly. Very long flights also may fly high and keep cabin altitude higher than usual.

Bill Gram told me of sitting next to a woman with a severe kyphoscoliosis (a spinal deformity) that compressed her chest so badly that she had real difficulty breathing. Not surprisingly, she tolerated the reduced pressure in the aircraft very poorly, and might have had serious difficulty had the flight lasted much longer.

I carry a small altimeter with me on most flights, and this leads to many pleasant and informative discussions with crew and now and then a passenger. I've asked six commercial pilots (four-stripers) about the following story I've heard: If overly boisterous and noisy passengers or incessantly crying babies annoy the other passengers, a pilot may "bump the cabin altitude up" a few thousand feet, putting people to sleep! Two senior pilots said yes, they sometimes do this and it works. Two others had never heard of it. One said cabin pressure was automatically set (which is true) and cannot be changed by the crew (which is not true). The sixth said he too knew it could be and was occasionally done but was not included in any manual!

There are other factors in air travel that are significant to a passenger's health. One is infection, as anyone who, after a long flight, has returned home with an upper respiratory infection is aware. A more serious infection is tuberculosis. There are several documented instances in which a passenger with active tuberculosis has infected several other people traveling on the same airplane. There have only been two cases in which a passenger, traveling from equatorial Africa, infected a fellow passenger with Ebola or Lassa fever.

Much attention has been paid to the possible effects of cosmic radiation, which occurs at higher levels at higher altitudes. Consequently, it seems reasonable to suspect that aircraft flying at 45,000 or 55,000 feet may expose the people on board to higher and perhaps slightly dangerous amounts of cosmic radiation. There are few reliable controlled studies on the long-term effects, but several studies do suggest, for example, that women are more likely to incur an ovarian cancer after working as flight attendants for many years. Decreased sperm counts have been reported in males flying repeatedly for long periods. This type of data needs rigorous control studies before being fully accepted.

Other risks associated with flying are worth mentioning. The obvious one is for individuals with a sickle trait, sickle cell anemia, or one of the blood disorders in which the red blood cells are made more fragile by lack of oxygen. There are a number of well-documented instances in which a person with unsuspected sickle disease or a similar condition has had a major crisis after flying for several hours. Any individual with a personal or family history of one of these blood disorders (see Chapter 4, "Moving Blood: Circulation") should consult a doctor about the possible risk of flying a long distance in a pressurized cabin. Of course, breathing oxygen during the flight would eliminate that risk. There are occasional episodes of heart attacks during air travel, but the incidence during air flight seems to be no greater than at sea level.

Almost everyone who flies is aware of changes when the aircraft is ascending or descending, felt in the ears or the sinuses, sometimes in a sensitive tooth, and often in the amount of gas in the intestinal tract. These symptoms are due to pressure changes rather than lack of oxygen, and few have lasting effects, although fluid accumulation in the inner ear during a rapid descent can cause problems if the ears are not cleared. Because of the pressure changes, patients who have recently undergone abdominal or open chest surgery should probably not fly because pressure changes could have damaging effects.

Space Flight

Humans are now regularly going into space, far above 100,000 feet, where there is zero atmospheric pressure and essentially not a single molecule of gas. Several approaches to preventing hypoxia among astronauts have been tried. One, used on the Apollo 1 mission in 1967, ended in tragedy during a training session when the tiny cabin was flooded with pure oxygen, which permitted a conflagration of combustible materials. After trying several strategies, NASA has decided on the protocol that maintains the atmosphere in the shuttle, and other space flight vehicles, at sea-level pressure, adding oxygen to maintain a concentration of 21 percent, and removing carbon dioxide. It seems likely that this strategy will prevail in most future space travel. In space, of course, a loss of pressure could be—and at least once (during the Apollo 13 mission in 1970) nearly was—catastrophic.

Common Gases

We take 25,000 breaths a day, inhaling and exhaling more than 10,000 liters of air. That air contains oxygen, nitrogen, and other gases. It also may contain bacteria, viruses, pollen or other particles, dust mites, tobacco smoke, auto exhaust, and other pollutants.

Among the many causes of environmental hypoxia are gases that are natural components of or contaminants in the air we breathe. Many gases are toxic, but they can also produce acute hypoxia by displacing oxygen in the volume of inhaled air or at the molecular level in the blood. Contaminants may cause hypoxia secondarily through alveolar damage, producing a type of interstitial or alveolar edema that is different from high altitude pulmonary edema (HAPE).

Each year in the United States some 1,500 people die from *carbon monoxide* (CO) poisoning, and 10,000 more require medical care. Even more are affected in less developed countries where means of heating or cooking are more primitive. Incomplete combustion of any substance like wood or fossil fuel will produce CO. Stoves, automobiles, space heaters, and especially combustion in confined places like shacks, parking garages, fishing shanties, and tightly woven tents cause problems from carbon monoxide hypoxia. It is probable that many people unknowingly are exposed to brief, minor carbon monoxide poisoning, which causes a few symptoms blamed on other things. But others aren't so fortunate:

> *Five members of a family died from carbon monoxide poisoning in their home, apparently after a car engine was left running in the attached garage.... The bodies were found scattered about the house in a Maryland suburb.*

Carbon monoxide can be highly poisonous and kills from hypoxia by displacing oxygen in hemoglobin. Because it reduces the amount of oxygen carried by the blood, CO poisoning shares some common features with hypoxia. CO also interferes with muscular activity, including heart muscle, because it combines with myoglobin as strongly as it does with hemoglobin, thus further compromising heart activity in individuals who have coronary artery disease.

> *Commuters on congested highways like the Los Angeles freeways may spend an hour or more twice a day sitting in slow traffic where exhaust fumes are particularly bad. For some with early or mild coronary artery disease, this exposure is enough to cause angina.*

The effects of CO poisoning, which gradually and furtively overwhelm the victim, are just as subtle as hypoxia itself.

One young man conducting research in the Andes went too rapidly to altitude. Experiencing mild AMS, he decided to go to bed early, but not before lighting his propane stove to warm his small, poorly ventilated room. The next morning he was found dead, and autopsy showed CO poisoning and pulmonary edema.

There have been reports of mountaineers camped at 15,000 feet or higher who made the mistake of keeping their tent doors closed while cooking. If the tent material is not highly breathable, CO can accumulate, and in a few cases climbers have been found dead from the very subtle hypoxia as the stove slowly burned out.

More than half of atmospheric CO is formed from oxidation of *methane,* which is produced in huge volumes in cattle feed lots, rice paddies, termite nests, and rotting biomass such as marshes.

Methane is inert and kills by displacing air in the lungs. Methane itself is a rare cause of hypoxia, but some unwary people have died from methane inhalation after falling into manure pits. Methane in the atmosphere is twenty times as effective as carbon dioxide (CO_2) in trapping infrared light and thus increasing the greenhouse effect, even though there is less than half as much methane as CO_2 in the atmosphere.

Like methane, *carbon dioxide* kills by suffocation, displacing air in the lungs. A sensational disaster occurred in 1987 when a flood of CO2, released suddenly from Lake Nyos in Cameroon, flowed down a valley and instantly suffocated 1,700 people and thousands of cattle. Less dramatic episodes have occurred near other African lakes. Occasional deaths have been caused by pools of CO2 or methane in dug wells or in desert "sinks."

Propane and natural gas cause suffocation (asphyxia), and other commercially available gases also contain carbon monoxide. *Liquid nitrogen,* used for instant freezing of many materials, has had fatal effects when used in inadequately ventilated space. *Gaseous nitrogen,* used commercially in containers where all air must be excluded, has killed careless workers. The evaporation of solid carbon dioxide (dry ice), like nitrogen, can be fatal for workers handling it in a poorly ventilated area.

Inside a refrigerated and closed truck, two men were transferring vials of frozen sperm from one container to another. The containers carried solid carbon dioxide (dry ice), and during the transfer—which took an hour—the dry ice vaporized. The carbon dioxide accumulated, and when the driver opened the door, he found the two men dead.

Air Pollutants

The contaminants in our air that result from industrial and agricultural activities are not usually direct causes of hypoxia, but they can lead to or aggravate existing lung ailments. According to the U.S. Environmental Protection Agency, the most common air pollutants are ozone, nitrogen dioxide, sulfur dioxide, particulate matter, and carbon monoxide.

We have already seen how carbon monoxide, formed by the incomplete combustion of carbon fuels, can kill at high doses. The low-level CO in the air we breathe, produced mostly by automobiles, can aggravate heart ailments and contributes to the formation of smog and ground-level ozone.

In the stratosphere *ozone* is considered beneficial because it protects us from the sun's harmful ultraviolet rays. At ground level ozone is produced by the reaction of automobile and industrial emissions products (nitrogen oxides, CO, and volatile organic compounds) driven by heat and sunlight. Even at low levels, ozone can cause serious problems, including lung inflammation, aggravated asthma, reduced lung capacity, and increased susceptibility to respiratory illnesses like pneumonia and bronchitis. Repeated exposure to ozone can cause permanent lung damage.

In the presence of heat and light, nitrogen dioxide and sulfur dioxide can react with other compounds in the air to form particulate matter, which can damage lung tissue, aggravate asthma, or worsen respiratory illness. *Nitrogen oxides* are also involved in the formation of ozone.

The most effective—and most preventable—way to introduce pollutants into your lungs is by smoking. Cigarettes contain over forty different cancer-causing chemicals (carcinogens), and tobacco use is the leading cause of preventable death in the United States. Smoking causes 87 percent of lung cancers and most cases of emphysema and chronic bronchitis. Cigarette smoking activates *proteases*—enzymes in the lung capable of breaking down the complex proteins that make up lung tissue. As discussed below in more detail, these enzymes are ordinarily kept in check by inhibitors. Some individuals have an abnormally low level of the protease inhibitors. If these individuals smoke, they are at great risk of developing lung damage that will lead to emphysema.

VENTILATORY HYPOXIA

Ventilatory hypoxia can be caused by any illness or damage that interferes with the flow of outside air through the airways into the lungs, or with the diffusion of oxygen from the alveoli into blood. Problems can occur at any point along the respiratory pathway: in the respiratory control center in the medulla, as may follow head trauma; along the nerves activating the chest muscles and diaphragm, as in several kinds of neuromuscular disease; or in the lungs. The chest can be injured and unable to move adequately. The airways can be partially obstructed by spasm or infection.

Lung Damage

Lung tissue itself is very delicate and easily damaged. Chronic bronchitis over time often leads to *emphysema,* in which the alveoli are first dilated, then torn and combined into larger sacs with less surface area for oxygen diffusion. This reduced area for diffusion causes hypoxia. As emphysema

> ### *Normal and Emphysematous Alveoli*
> The most common cause of chronic hypoxia in everyday life is chronic obstructive pulmonary disease (COPD). This condition develops over many months or years, usually initiated by inflammation of the bronchi (airways), which has progressed to chronic bronchitis. Repeated severe cough, increased difficulty exhaling, and perhaps alveolar wall damage lead to stretching of alveolar walls, tearing, and gradual formation of larger cystlike air sacs from several alveoli (shown in Figure 29). Emphysema may also, less often, be congenital, or develop without obstruction. As the number of individual alveoli decreases, the surface area available for gas transfer decreases and hypoxia gradually worsens. Patients respond roughly in two different ways: by increasing ventilation ("pink puffers") or by increasing hemoglobin ("blue bloaters").

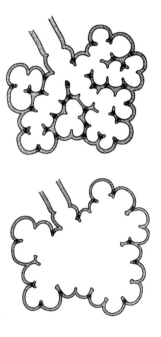

worsens, the resulting hypoxia stimulates greater effort to breathe—and when this is not enough, hypoxia increases still further. Exertion becomes difficult, subtle mental changes gradually appear, and the deterioration all too frequently becomes irreversible. Usually this change happens gradually so that signs and symptoms like those experienced in mountain sickness are not apparent.

Figure 29. *Normal (above) and emphysematous alveoli (below)*

COPD: Chronic Obstructive Pulmonary Disease

The name says it all. Chronic obstructive pulmonary disease (COPD) is something of a catchall phrase describing problems due to obstruction by increased airway resistance; inflammation of the bronchial passages; the spasm and inflammation of airways (asthma); and changes in the size and structure of the alveoli. It is the most common lung disorder, a slowly worsening condition that impedes the flow of oxygen into alveoli and to the blood. Although cystic emphysema occurs, the term COPD usually refers to the common combination of chronic bronchitis and emphysema.

About 16 million people in the United States have COPD, and in 1998 roughly 117,000 died from associated pneumonia, respiratory failure, or other complications such as right heart failure due to pulmonary hypertension. Smoking causes roughly 80 to 90 percent of COPD cases and 5 percent of cases are caused by a hereditary deficiency of the "lung protector" enzyme *alpha-1-protease inhibitor*, known as AAT. Whatever the cause, COPD often becomes a slowly progressing and expensive disability.

COPD is of special interest to us because of the different responses the body makes in its attempt to achieve normal oxygenation. Patients with COPD can be divided roughly but picturesquely into the "pink puffers" and the "blue bloaters," depending on the response. There is some overlap.

"Pink puffers" automatically overventilate all the time, thereby bringing

more oxygen into the alveoli—but losing some carbon dioxide in the process. The resultant *alkalosis* is compensated by the kidney. This is the same way a healthy individual responds when going to moderate altitude. Overventilation allows these individuals to maintain a reasonable blood oxygen level unless some infection intervenes, but they may have difficulty going to the mountains, and sometimes even in commercial air flight.

By contrast, *"blue bloaters"* do not overbreathe; in fact they may actually breathe less than a normal person. Instead they increase the capacity of their blood to carry oxygen by increasing the number of red cells and the amount of hemoglobin. Blood becomes slightly thicker and moves more sluggishly, so there is a tendency to clot formation. Over time the increased load, together with increased pulmonary artery pressure, leads to enlargement of the right ventricle and heart failure. This "blue bloater" adjustment strategy is an exaggeration of how healthy people respond to moderate altitude by making more hemoglobin. Their condition resembles chronic mountain sickness (Monge's disease; see Chapter 11, "Chronic and Subacute Mountain Illness") and follows the same course. Not surprisingly, "blue bloaters" do not tolerate altitude and often cannot fly without supplemental oxygen.

It is interesting to compare a few of these problems with the normal responses of healthy individuals going to altitude, summarized in Table 7.

TABLE 7
ARTERIAL BLOOD OXYGENATION IN CERTAIN CONDITIONS

Cause	Arterial O_2 (in torr)	Arterial CO_2 (in torr)	Hemoglobin (gms/100 ml)
Sea level (normal)	88	42	15
10,000 feet	56	33	16
20,000 feet	41	21	16
25,000 feet	37	13	18
Pink puffer	70	37	15
Blue bloater	50	51	17
CMS	47	34	20

A few patients with certain forms of congenital heart disease combine several responses and, like "pink puffers," are able to engage in near-normal levels of activity. Some aspects of their tolerance resemble the acclimatization developed by healthy high-altitude residents and long-term visitors to high altitude.

This classification of COPD sufferers is obviously oversimplified, but is useful as an introduction to comparing normal and pathological responses to altitude. However, we must be careful not to overemphasize the analogies between normal acclimatization to altitude and accommodation to chronic illness. Natural acclimatization to thin mountain air involves many small balanced changes that are rarely as extreme as the desperate measures needed to cope with COPD.

Damage to Alveolar Walls

Interstitial lung disease (ILD) is a general term covering a number of lung disorders. The walls of the air sacs in the lung become inflamed, and scarring (*fibrosis* or *alveolar proteinosis*) occurs in the tissue between the air sacs (*interstitium*). The lung becomes stiff and breathing becomes difficult. Fibrosis causes a permanent loss in the tissue's ability to transport oxygen by thickening the alveolar membrane. Anything that disrupts diffusion from alveoli to blood may lead to clinically significant hypoxia. The delicate alveolar–capillary membrane is described in Chapter 4, "Moving Blood: Circulation."

Disturbed Breathing During Sleep

Many people tend to breathe unevenly during sleep and notice it little if at all. However, in the extreme case this may become a problem. Misnamed Ondine's Curse and often called Pickwickian syndrome (a literary misnomer), disturbed breathing during sleep can have serious effects. Normally, the breathing is automatically controlled when awake or during sleep, and several fail-safe mechanisms ensure normal ventilatory exchange. But anatomical obstruction due to weakening of the muscles of the soft palate causes *intermittent upper airway obstruction* (IUAO)—a big name for simple snoring. Some patients are partially obstructed enough during the night that arterial oxygen saturation fluctuates markedly. Sleep is disturbed by the struggle to breathe, and the hapless victim is sleepy all day. This sleep disturbance has been blamed for a good many automobile accidents, and in some states legislation requires drivers who have had a few sleep-related accidents to have sleep studies done before regaining their driver's license. It is a real problem that occurs more frequently than we realize.

In severe cases of snoring, preventive measures should be considered, to avoid eventual pulmonary hypertension and failure. Breathing low-flow oxygen may not change breathing patterns, but it prevents a fall in oxygen saturation and minimizes the long-term effects on pulmonary artery pressure.

A device employing a technique called *continuous positive airflow pressure* (CPAP) produces a steady flow of air through a small tube in the nose to provide a slightly higher pressure in the airway; this may be enough to prevent the soft palate from obstructing the airway. A mask can also be used. Surgery to modify the nasopharynx may be helpful if the cause is anatomical. A dental device to prevent the jaw from relaxing and allowing the tongue to block the airway is quite effective.

Sleep Apnea

A less common sleep disturbance stems from some malfunction of respiratory control, which causes irregular breathing with long pauses—similar to the periodic breathing common at high altitude. This condition is *central apnea*. Its cause is not fully known, but it can be brought on by an injury or a disease that affects the brain stem and interferes with brain mechanisms that control breathing. Central apnea is rare and usually diagnosed in patients who are already severely ill.

Whether central or peripheral, sleep apnea causes brief but repeated periods of mild arterial oxygen desaturation, which over time can cause pulmonary hypertension and even right heart failure. Victims of advanced sleep apnea, like "blue bloaters" with COPD, share some features of patients with Monge's disease.

It is interesting that during the periods of sleep apnea, systemic blood pressure increases slightly and falls back to normal on wakening. But over many years the systemic blood pressure during the day gradually increases and stays high, so that years of sleep apnea may be one more, though infrequent, cause of hypertension and its associated problems.

Sleep problems are important at any altitude. Recent studies have shown that when sleep is so frequently interrupted that the individual gets no period longer than a few minutes of unbroken sleep, some of the higher mental functions falter: Judgment, decision making, even reflex actions are impaired the next day. Obviously these skills are especially important high on a mountain, where they are already affected by hypoxia and where survival depends on them. Sleep at the highest camps is seldom sound, often interrupted every few minutes by wind, noise, and discomfort. It seems likely, even probable, that sleep disruption has contributed to some of the dreadful errors made at altitude.

Clearly, disturbed sleep, and specifically sleep apnea, can become a serious medical problem of everyday hypoxia. Unfortunately, the diuretic Diamox, which is so beneficial in treating the periodic breathing of altitude, has little or no effect on either obstructive or central sleep apnea.

SIDS: Sudden Infant Death Syndrome

Sudden Infant Death Syndrome (SIDS), the sudden and unexplained death of an infant under one year of age, is one of the leading causes of death among infants. The exact cause of SIDS is unknown. Until recently it was thought to be due to episodic sleep apnea, causing respiratory arrest, often after several premonitory "near misses."

There is increasing evidence that SIDS is often due to an abnormality in the part of the brain, the *arcuate nucleus*, that senses oxygen and carbon dioxide levels and controls breathing and waking during sleep. Babies with this abnormality are susceptible to sudden death, which could be triggered by an event such as lack of oxygen, excessive carbon dioxide intake, overheating, or infection. Normally, sleeping infants sense inadequate air intake, and the brain triggers waking and crying and a change in heartbeat to compensate. If this protective mechanism is flawed, the baby could succumb to SIDS if it is overheated, is not getting enough fresh air (the head under a blanket or face pressed against soft bedding), or is recovering from a respiratory infection. The risk factors for SIDS include exposure to second-hand cigarette smoke, prematurity at birth, low birth weight, or inadequate prenatal care. An important factor seems to be sleeping position: Infants who sleep on their backs are less susceptible, although this is not the whole answer. As with any cause of severe hypoxia, a baby may survive a "near miss" from SIDS but sustain brain damage. Failure to gain weight and size normally, together with fussiness and daytime somnolence, should at least lead to a suspicion of sleep apnea.

Automatic breathing begins the moment the child is born but is uncertain and erratic at first, sometimes with sighs and even short apneic periods. This unevenness smooths out rapidly. Infants are thought to have a blunted hypoxic ventilatory drive in the first few days or weeks, and thus some may not respond briskly or promptly to brief hypoxia. Whether this is related to SIDS is unknown, though not likely.

Cystic Fibrosis

In *cystic fibrosis* (CF), a recessive genetic defect results in abnormality of the glands that produce sweat or mucus. CF patients form a very thick mucus which accumulates in the intestines and lungs, causing malnutrition, poor growth, susceptibility to respiratory infection, breathing problems, and ultimately permanent lung damage. Repeated accumulation of this viscous material in small airways causes hypoxia and slowly leads to thickening of the alveolar–capillary membrane, pulmonary hypertension, and recurrent infection. With unremitting daily care, some patients may reach adulthood, but infection is a constant risk. Hypoxia can contribute to stunted growth and may have other effects. CF is not a rare cause of hypoxia: One out of every 2,400 Caucasian infants (but one of every 17,000 African-American infants) is born with the defect; many die young from infection and hypoxia.

A few other hereditary enzyme deficiencies have been identified that lead to chronic lung problems. They are uncommon and as yet not curable except by lung transplant.

New research is looking to treat cystic fibrosis with drugs that inhibit the enzyme *elastase*, which breaks down the protein *elastin*. Elastin, a flexible fiber that imparts elasticity, is found in many tissues throughout the body, particularly in tissue of the arteries, lungs, intestine, and skin. In the lung, elastin is vital for allowing the alveoli to stretch and recoil with each breath.

Scientists have known for some time that the specific gene that is abnormal in CF codes for a cell membrane channel through which chloride can pass. People with CF have a nonfunctional form of this protein. This compromises the ability of their cells to handle salt and water, and ultimately leads to the thick lung secretions described above. Because lung cells are accessible via the respiratory system, scientists have tried to treat CF by inserting a normal copy of the chloride channel gene into a non-disease-causing virus and introducing that virus into the lungs by aerosol spray. Unfortunately, they have not yet succeeded in getting the normal gene to enter enough lung cells and produce functional protein. People whose lungs are severely damaged by CF may face lung transplant as a final treatment option.

Asthma

In most cases asthma is an allergic reaction to an inhaled allergen, such as pollen, animal dander, or dust. The immune response is triggered, and airways become inflamed and constricted by bronchial muscle spasms, leading to wheezing and coughing and difficulty breathing. Asthma attacks usually are short-lived, though recurrent, and often part of the combination of problems that lead to COPD. Asthma is a frequent cause of intermittent episodes of hypoxia with many of its symptoms. Treatment usually includes inhaled steroids to reduce inflammation and bronchodilators to relax the muscles lining the airways.

People with asthma have trouble breathing because their constricted airways offer too much resistance to air flow. However, airway diameter is not the only factor that contributes to air-flow resistance. The viscosity of the air plays a role as well. For this reason, some patients with mild asthma do better at moderate altitude because the air is not only cleaner, but also thinner. Thinner air is less viscous, offers less resistance as it moves through the respiratory passages, and requires less exertion to breathe.

Toxic Gases

Silo filler's disease causes hypoxia by the corrosive effect of oxides of nitrogen formed in fermented silage; it is rare thanks to farmer education programs. Many other vapors cause hypoxia by directly affecting the lungs. In World War I, chlorine and mustard gas, a blistering agent that attacks the eyes and lungs, killed or permanently disabled thousands; other toxic gases have occasionally been used against people since then. In 1984 many thousands died, and many more were lastingly injured, when a pesticide factory in Bhopal, India, exploded, releasing methyl cyanate that caused pulmonary edema, killing by respiratory hypoxia. In 1989 the Iraqi military released bombs containing blistering agents on Kurdish villages in northern Iraq, killing thousands.

Submersion

Submersion is a frequent cause of death. The human brain is irreparably damaged after six or at most ten minutes of *anoxia* (complete absence of oxygen). How, then, have a number of children and adults survived, unharmed, after complete submersion for an hour or even longer?

Diving mammals often stay submerged for more than an hour, and can see, think, and swim actively without breathing. This ability is attributed to the dive response, which immediately halts breathing when a dive is started, and soon diverts blood away from nonessential to vital organs. Conflict between the need to conserve oxygen and the demands of swimming muscles is resolved by drawing oxygen from saturated myoglobin (an oxygen-binding protein similar to hemoglobin found in muscle) and from the hemoglobin in the red blood cells. Diving mammals generally have larger supplies of myoglobin and larger blood volumes than do land mammals. Oxygen demand is also met for a short period by changing metabolic fuels and "going anaerobic." This strategy is used by some animals that stay submerged for long months in winter. The anaerobic debt must be quickly repaid when oxygen is again available.

Humans are different. Long submersion is survivable only in water that is near freezing temperature. Central reflexes usually halt breathing at once, or else the victim will inhale water and drown. During the first ten minutes of accidental submersion, the diving response protects the brain by redirecting oxygenated blood to it and to the heart and a few similarly essential sites, and by shutting off blood to skin and extremities and soon to kidneys and liver. If submersion continues, the heart slows markedly (reducing its demand for oxygen), and blood flow to the brain soon decreases.

After several minutes in ice-cold water, hypothermia due to passive heat loss further slows the demand for oxygen and decreases metabolism; the victim becomes unconscious. Children lose heat faster than adults due to their greater ratio of surface area to body mass. Thus the first defense is the dive response, and the second and final is hypothermia. Survival is much more common for children than for adults.

Some studies suggest, however, that passive cooling may not be rapid enough even in children to protect the brain; other currently unknown factors may be operative. Not many such victims are fortunate enough to survive, but if so, most are not brain damaged. If a person is retrieved from cold water submersion with a low body temperature and no heartbeat, emergency medical personnel will probably not be able to restart the heart until they first warm the body to near normal temperature. Thus, the first-aid maxim "not dead until warm and dead" is fitting in the case of cold water submersion anoxia.

Hyperventilation

Under normal circumstances, our urge to breathe is caused more by small increases in blood carbon dioxide level (the hypercapnic response) than by decreases in blood oxygen. A swimmer may hyperventilate to increase the period of time over which she can hold her breath for a sprint or long underwater swim. This advantage is derived more from reducing blood carbon dioxide than from loading a small amount of extra oxygen into the blood. However, hyperventilation poses a potential danger. Subsequent breath-holding will cause the carbon dioxide level to rise as the blood oxygen level falls. But, because hyperventilation has significantly reduced blood carbon dioxide, blood oxygen can fall to a dangerously low level before the hypercapnic response is activated. The diver does not receive the signal that he or she needs to breathe and, because of hypoxia, loses consciousness and drowns.

CIRCULATORY HYPOXIA

Any interference with the carriage or delivery of oxygen can be described as circulatory hypoxia. The two types of circulatory hypoxia are anemic and stagnant hypoxia. In anemic hypoxia, either the hemoglobin concentration is low or the heme group has been rendered ineffective in binding oxygen (CO poisoning). Conditions that can produce anemic hypoxia include anemia, abnormal hemoglobin, or exposure to chemicals or drugs that disable O_2 or CO_2 binding to hemoglobin. In stagnant (ischemic) hypoxia, circulatory failure occurs, either through cardiac failure, obstructed blood vessels, congenital heart defect, or cardiovascular disease.

Toxic Substances

Like carbon monoxide, certain chemicals combine with hemoglobin to cause hypoxia; some form methemoglobin (metHg), which does not carry oxygen and thus causes hypoxia that may be symptomatic. Substances that can cause methemoglobin formation are common and include topical anesthetics, silver nitrate, sulfonamide antibiotics, cyanide, aniline compounds (found in inks, polishes, paints, and varnishes) and organic nitrates.

The accumulation in well water or ground water of nitrates from fertilizer runoff can cause oxygen stress or be fatal to infants who drink the contaminated water. Cases of "blue baby syndrome" (infant cyanosis or methemoglobinemia) due to nitrate (NO_3) contaminated drinking water were first reported in the 1940s.

Severe Anemia

A shortage of hemoglobin from anemia or hemorrhage decreases oxygen-carrying capacity, and therefore oxygen content, causing hypoxia. If chronic, some of the responses to anemia resemble those due to high altitude; if acute, the "struggle responses" appear. A shortage of circulating hemoglobin is a relatively common cause of everyday hypoxia. Interestingly, anemia does not cause pulmonary hypertension.

A young woman bled internally from a ruptured ectopic pregnancy. She had a cardiac arrest in the ambulance and was comatose and in shock, with a hematocrit of 13 percent in hospital. She remained comatose for a month, then began slow recovery.

TABLE 8
SIGNS AND SYMPTOMS OF METHEMOGLOBINEMIA

% MetHg	Effect
10–20	Mild cyanosis
30–40	Headache, fatigue, high pulse, weakness, dizziness
>35	Labored breathing, lethargy
50–60	Acidosis, arrhythmia, coma, seizure, low pulse, hypoxia
>70	Fatality

In a severe case of circulatory hypoxia, shock decreases blood flow, and when the brain is deprived of both nutrients and oxygen because of decreased blood flow (due in the above case to shock plus anemia), the damage is more severe than when either circulation or oxygen alone is reduced.

Heart Problems

When heart muscle is damaged because *arteriosclerosis* has reduced circulation to one or several parts of the heart muscle, it cannot pump enough oxygen-carrying blood to the body to meet demands. Rare congenital defects also jeopardize the heart as a pump. Distortion of one or more heart valves may cause reflux or obstruction, reducing blood supply to the body. These are common causes of lack of oxygen to cells and, depending on where the lack is more pronounced, cause signs of hypoxia. Ross McFarland, a dedicated student of all forms of hypoxia, compared the effects on mental functions due to altitude with those of aging. He has made a persuasive argument that most of the mental changes blamed on age were really due to narrowing of arteries to the brain, which decreased its oxygen supply.

Mutant Hemoglobins

When individuals with sickle trait become hypoxic, the abnormal cells are distorted into shapes that cannot take on as much oxygen as normally; this reduces the oxygen-carrying capacity of blood and decreases supply to the tissues. In addition, the distorted, burrlike cells often plug small capillaries, causing death of the tissues they supply. (Abnormal hemoglobins that impact oxygen-carrying capacity are discussed in Chapter 4, "Moving Blood: Circulation.")

HISTOTOXIC HYPOXIA

When cellular metabolic processes are impaired and tissues are unable to use oxygen, despite normal oxygen delivery, the situation is known as *histotoxic hypoxia*. Excessive oxygen demand due, for example, to strenuous exertion, high fever, or an overactive thyroid—in short, anything that increases tissue demand without an adequate compensatory increase in oxygen supply—may result in hypoxia severe enough to cause signs or symptoms. The delirium of a thyroid storm—a condition caused by the uncontrolled release of thyroid hormone and which results in a highly elevated metabolic rate—may be partly attributable to cerebral hypoxia. The defensive measures taken by the body are the "struggle" type. Even when the flow of oxygen is normal, cold (*hypothermia*) or low blood sugar (*hypoglycemia*) interferes with the higher brain functions and causes problems that are similar to, and synergistic with, those of hypoxia.

POISONS

A variety of poisons that interfere with the mitochondrial energy cycles cause tissue or cellular hypoxia. The best known of these is cyanide, which inhibits cells' use of oxygen. Hydrogen sulfide (H_2S, sewer gas) and several pesticides also inhibit essential metabolic processes. The role of these and many other synthetic (and some natural) substances in disturbing molecular metabolic processes is being studied extensively, but is beyond the scope of this book.

This chapter provides only a rough outline of the various causes of hypoxia at sea level, and it is far from complete. The purpose is simply to acquaint the reader with the possibility that a person can be very short of oxygen even at a low altitude, and the consequences can be as serious as they can be on a very high mountain.

What has not been addressed is the matter of how the signs and symptoms of hypoxia at altitude (hallucination, confusion, ataxia, and so forth) may appear during similar hypoxia at sea level, for the very simple reason that such descriptions do not appear often in clinical literature. When they do occur they are often attributed to the underlying disease rather than to lack of oxygen. Perhaps this outline will suggest to the practitioner—and to patients and families—that lack of oxygen might be suspected, searched for, and treated.

This chapter has not discussed whether or not "acclimatization" occurs during chronic hypoxia at sea level as it does over weeks or months at altitude. Many individuals slowly develop diseases or injuries that make them short of oxygen; other individuals are born with defects that make them short of oxygen for as long as they live. Very little hard data is available for such patients. This may be a rich area for further study; we would like to know how many of the changes in acclimatization at altitude actually appear during long periods of hypoxia at sea level. We need the hard data.

PART IV **THE MOUNTAINEER'S WORLD**

CHAPTER 13

ACCLIMATIZATION

In 1991, at age 78, I took my last foray into the great mountains. I walked to the base of Nanga Parbat at 14,000 feet on a small photographic expedition. It was a rather casual trip, and I took a rather casual attitude toward it— taking no medication and not thinking at all about the altitude. Not surprisingly, I developed high altitude pulmonary edema shortly after my arrival at 14,000 feet, and—disregarding all the advice I give to other people—stayed on for thirty-six hours to finish the job before staggering home. I was fortunate: I might very well have come down with a near-fatal case, and would have had to be carried down 40 or 50 miles to the road head.

This was my first experience with serious altitude sickness, because on all my previous high-altitude visits I had taken ample time to acclimatize during the long march in.

Acclimatization is the word mountaineers use to describe the changes that take place during a slow climb to gradually increasing altitude. It is the process that enables sea-level man to climb slowly over a period of several weeks to the summit of Everest, breathing only the ambient air around him. Were he taken directly to the summit without acclimatization, he would be unconscious in a few minutes, and most likely dead in less than a few hours. Acclimatization comprises remarkably delicate interlocking processes involving almost every part of the body.

On April 15, 1875, as Paul Bert was completing his studies proving that lack of oxygen caused mountain sickness, two of his young colleagues, Croce-Spinelli and Sivel, died during the ascent of their balloon *Zenith* to over 28,000 feet; the third balloonist, Tissandier, survived unscathed. His dramatic story is included in Bert's book:

> I come now to the fatal hour when we were about to be seized by the terrible influence of the atmospheric decompression. At 7,000 meters we are all standing in the basket; Sivel, numbed for a moment, has revived; Croce-Spinelli is motionless before me.... At this height, however, I was writing in my notebook almost mechanically.... But soon I was keeping absolutely motionless, without suspecting that perhaps I had already lost use of my movements. Toward 7,500 meters the numbness one experiences is extraordinary. The body and the mind

weaken little by little, gradually, unconsciously without one's knowledge.... I wanted to cry out, "We are at 8,000 meters [above 26,000 feet]." But my tongue was paralyzed. Suddenly I closed my eyes and fell inert, entirely losing consciousness. It was about 1:30.

At about 3:30 I opened my eyes again. I felt numb, weak, but my mind was active. The balloon was descending with terrifying speed.... My two companions were crouched in the basket, their heads covered by the travelling rugs. I assembled my strength and tried to raise them. Sivel's face was black, his eyes dull, his mouth open and full of blood. Croce's eyes were half shut and his mouth bloody.

CAN EVEREST BE CLIMBED?

These were not the first deaths at high altitude, and although widely noticed, they did not end interest in climbing Mount Everest. Twenty years later, surgeon Clinton Dent speculated:

Possibly even while these lines are being written, Mr. Conway and his mountaineering party in the Himalayas may have collected that grain of fact which proverbially outweighs the pound of theory.

To the writer the question has been for years a subject of interest from the mountaineering world as well as from the physiological point of view; on neither ground does [climbing Everest] appear an impossibility. To some extent a question of men, it is still more largely a question of money. Prejudice, perhaps, is father to the idea that the money which is always forthcoming to favor attempts to reach the North Pole may be still more advantageously employed in attempting to reach the top of Mount Everest. Selected men will have to work for a year or more with the one definite object before them. What they have to do is to ascend some 8,000 feet higher than any point that has hitherto been reached on foot. We may agree with Mr. Whymper that the effects on respiration will impose limits on the range of man, but it does not seem inconceivable that this limitation is beyond the highest point on Earth's crust. The attempt would be costly, laborious, long and possibly not free from risk. The same may be said of any extension of discovery. Let those who think that what can be done in the way of enterprise and discovery should be done consider the matter well. It is a tremendous undertaking, but a magnificent possibility.

In 1907 W. G. Fitzgerald, himself not a mountaineer, quoted observations made by those who were—Martin Conway, Fanny Bullock Workman, Douglas Freshfield, Edward Whymper, and others—and agreed with Dent. He quoted Angelo Mosso, a mountaineer and researcher in high altitude. Mosso had exercised Alpine troops at 14,000 feet and conducted experiments in a small decompression chamber in which a man could exercise while being taken to a simulated altitude of almost 30,000 feet! In 1898 Mosso wrote:

> If birds fly to a height of 29,000 feet, then man ought to be able to reach the same altitude at a slow and cautious rate of progress. I am convinced that a capable climber may attain the summit of Everest without serious sufferings.

Douglas Freshfield, one of the leading mountaineer-explorers of that time, was also cautiously optimistic:

> I see no reason why the modern mountain explorer should not attain Everest's 29,028 feet. Remember how gradually the rarity of air increases between 20,000 and 30,000 feet. I am sure too that a big expedition can attack Everest.

In 1920 Alexander Kellas, a mountaineering chemist, calculated from data collected by others:

> Mount Everest could be ascended by a man of excellent physical and mental constitution in first rate training, without adventitious aids if the difficulties of the mountain are not too great, and with the use of oxygen even if the mountain can be classed as difficult from the climbing point of view.

In 1953, with oxygen, and in 1975 without it, these predictions made at the start of the century were proven true.

Are Everest Summiters Different From Us?

Since Kellas wrote, more than a hundred men and women have stood on top of Everest breathing only the high, thin air about them. Are they somehow different from Croce-Spinelli and Sivel, who died at the same altitude in the balloon *Zenith*? Do those who summit very high mountains have some secret ingredient in blood or tissue, or do they react differently to lack of oxygen? What might they share with the thousands who suffer hypoxic illness at sea level? Or with the millions who are born, live, and die three miles high in the Andes or Tibet?

Based on what we know today, most extreme climbers differ very little from the rest of us. Whether genetically or through exposure to high altitude, some may have the advantage of a larger ventilatory capacity or may increase their ventilation to a higher degree in response to hypoxia (that is, they may have a more sensitive hypoxic ventilatory response, or HVR). Nevertheless, several who have summited Everest without bottled oxygen actually possess lower than normal hypoxic ventilatory responses. Furthermore, as a person becomes more acclimatized over the course of a long stay at altitude, his or her HVR tends to become blunted. Individuals with a brisk HVR also tend to show more periodic breathing at altitude. It is remarkable that after having acclimatized many times, climbers' bodies seem to *remember* how and do so more easily and completely.

The immediate reactions of sea-level humans to abrupt oxygen lack are the "struggle responses" (see Chapter 12, "Hypoxia in Everyday Life"), prompted soon after exposure to hypoxia, by which the body tries to keep the oxygen flow to cells as close to normal as possible. Alexander von Muralt appropriately called these struggle responses *accommodations*. Today we add the terms *acclimatization,* for changes that develop in weeks or months, and *adaptation,* for those that take generations.

In 2004, the world received news of yet one more phenomenal accomplishment in high-altitude climbing. On May 21, 2004, twenty-six-year-old Sherpa Pemba Dorje set a new world record by ascending the nearly 12,000 vertical feet from Mount Everest Base Camp to summit in eight hours, ten minutes. Dorjee had previously established a record at twelve hours, forty-five minutes a year earlier, only to see his effort bested three days later when Sherpa Lakpa Gyelu summited in ten hours, fifty-six minutes. Clearly climbers like Dorjee and Gyelu are well acclimatized. They are also extremely fit (see Chapter 17, "Limits to Work at Altitude") and may be adapted to high altitude. These remarkable accomplishments motivate us to learn more about the process of acclimatization.

STUDIES OF ACCLIMATIZATION
Pikes Peak

The first studies of acclimatization on a high mountain came about almost by chance, when Yandell Henderson, a young professor from Yale, met John Haldane at a medical meeting in Vienna in 1910. Haldane rather casually said he would like to find "a nice comfortable hotel on a high mountain" where he could continue his study of how oxygen passes from lungs into blood. Henderson suggested Pikes Peak and helped make arrangements for two leading physiologists—Edward Schneider and C. G. Douglas—to join Haldane and himself in Colorado. The four spent a month atop Pikes Peak, where they measured respiration and alveolar and arterial gases at rest and during and after exercise, and charted Cheyne-Stokes (periodic) breathing. And so began a century of studies on 14,000-foot Pikes Peak.

These four men shaped generations of students and scholars, and their happy communion, rather than their data, was probably the most lasting heritage of that summer. (Chapter 3, "Moving Air: Respiration," recounts the debate between Haldane and Joseph Barcroft over oxygen secretion, which Haldane insisted was one of the major contributors to acclimatization, even after Barcroft had effectively disproved it.)

An incidental product of the first Pikes Peak project came about because the mores of the time considered it "unsuitable" for a single lady to be un-chaperoned for weeks on the summit with the men. Mabel Fitzgerald was undaunted and, alone with her pack mules, took her gas analysis equipment with her and visited mining communities throughout Colorado. After several weeks she brought back the first—and still the most complete—alveolar air samples from men and women living at different elevations.

Later Studies of High Altitude

The next major study of acclimatization was conducted in 1935 by a large international expedition led by Bruce Dill. The party spent six weeks at 14,000 feet in Peru examining the physiochemical changes of blood in natives and in acclimatizing sojourners.

World War II halted mountain research but energized scores of studies of acute hypoxia, because aircraft could go higher than their crews, whose lives depended on oxygen when flying at altitudes that afforded tactical advantage. (Acute hypoxia causes severe effects immediately, and has little in common with acute mountain sickness, in which onset is more gradual.) Even a brief interruption of the pilot's oxygen supply could cause errors of judgment or even unconsciousness at combat altitude, so aircrew had to be taught to recognize the early, subtle effects of hypoxia. Before this training was available, many pilots perished—some unaware that their night vision at altitude was half that at sea level, others because they failed to recognize the early warnings of hypoxia. Some were too confident—"I've been to 20,000 feet many times and it never bothered me a bit" was one refrain—and some of the overconfident died.

> Our task as flight trainers was to demonstrate realistically to pilots what lack of oxygen would do by outfitting the decompression chamber with a model airplane equipped with a stick and rudder simulating actual aircraft controls. The pilot was asked to "fly" this little model after he had removed his oxygen mask at 25,000 feet, but was told to replace his mask immediately when he noticed anything at all wrong with his "flying." In my unit, which taught some 55,000 pilots and gunners, we asked one or two men from each group to do this demonstration, and I don't believe more than a few dozen were able to replace their masks, even when ordered to do so, before falling unconscious. It was a small demonstration but showed aircrew quite convincingly how hypoxia at altitude would affect their skills.

It would have been unfortunate if all the energy invested in altitude research had been squandered at war's end, and happily it was not. Many of those who would later contribute mightily to what we know about oxygen and humans became interested in altitude physiology in these military aviation training and research programs.

> My interests were in climbing and medicine rather than in flying, and I was able to persuade the U.S. Navy to let me organize a research study called "Operation Everest," even though it was more relevant to mountaineers than to aviators. This project and its sequel forty years later are described in Chapter 16, "Operation Everest I and II." Most of my colleagues went back

to their clinics and laboratories, but my special friend Dick Riley remained and shared the major part of the Everest study. As we anticipated, hypoxia would soon become less relevant to flying with the advent of pressurized aircraft, but mountaineering was about to enter a new era wherein altitude research would be very important.

The Himalayas Become Popular

In 1950 Nepal, closed to foreigners for centuries, opened some of its highest mountains to climbers, and the Golden Age of Himalayan climbing began. Within a few months the first 8,000-meter peak, Annapurna (26,700 feet), was climbed. Others soon followed. That same fall a small party (which included one of the authors, Charles Houston) was granted the first permission to visit Everest from the south side, access from the north being forbidden by the Chinese occupying Tibet. In 1951 and 1952 attempts were made on Everest and other high peaks in Nepal, and finally in 1953 Everest was first climbed by Edmund Hillary and Sherpa Tenzing Norgay, with supplementary oxygen.

In 1952 prominent British physiologist Griffith Pugh led a small party to Cho Oyu primarily to gain experience with oxygen equipment for the next attempt on Everest, which he would accompany the following year. Pugh and others brought back a wealth of data from these expeditions, some from as high as 25,000 feet. Pugh predicted that on the summit of Everest, without extra oxygen, a person would be close to his or her limit and able to do very little physical work: Staying alive would be difficult enough no matter how well acclimatized he or she might be. Since then, over a hundred men and women have reached Everest's top breathing only air. But, as Pugh predicted, they have been at the limits of their strength and will, and more than 180 have died, with and without oxygen.

The Silver Hut

Pugh returned to the Himalayas in 1961 as scientific leader of a project called "The Silver Hut." Some of the finest British and American mountaineers and physiologists participated. An insulated hut was erected at 19,000 feet and continuously occupied for five and a half months. (See Figure 30.) Some of the men stayed as long as nine weeks without descending, although others went down for short periods of rest and recuperation. Despite good food and comfortable living conditions, all of the party lost weight, and they concluded that 19,000 feet was too high for long-term living—a conclusion supported by the fact that no high-altitude natives live permanently above 17,500 feet. In one of his many studies, Pugh reported:

> After weeks at altitude, lack of oxygen was still driving respiration despite the lowered blood carbon dioxide, but the respiratory center had become more sensitive to carbon dioxide.... Newcomers were as physically fit or even fitter after a few weeks at altitude as those who

---

The Silver Hut

Prominent British physiologist Griffith Pugh went to the Himalayas in 1961 as scientific leader of a project called "The Silver Hut." A prefabricated insulated hut was erected at 19,000 feet in the Everest region, and was continuously occupied for five and a half months. Some of the people stayed as long as nine weeks without descending, though others went down for short periods.

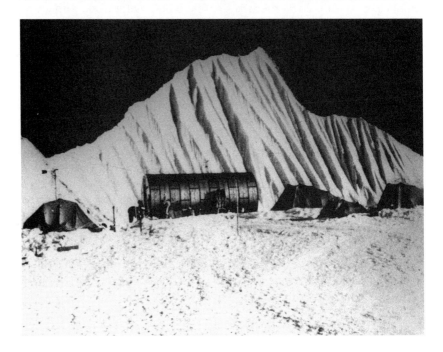

Figure 30. *Silver Hut*

had been there for months.... Physical work seemed to be limited by the fatigue of working, and respiratory muscles and the heart could only work at about two-thirds sea level capacity. Diffusion of oxygen from lung to blood was also a limiting factor at 19,000 feet....

Pugh implied that 19,000 or 20,000 feet was the highest altitude at which further acclimatization was possible. We now recognize that at or above this altitude, deterioration outstrips acclimatization.

Pugh's comment that the respiratory center becomes more sensitive to carbon dioxide is significant because it suggests that physical work by a fully acclimatized person might cause more shortness of breath than in the unacclimatized. This implies that the accumulation of carbon dioxide during work might drive breathing as hard as or harder than hypoxia. As an aside, it is interesting to note that breathlessness with exertion is rather prominent for a few days after returning from high altitude.

This was the first thorough study of acclimatization at very high altitude; it was a major contribution to altitude medicine.

The Sino-Indian Conflict

The importance of acclimatization was highlighted dramatically a year later when Chinese armies crossed their troubled border with India high in the northwestern and southeastern Himalayas. There was fighting at altitudes as high as 18,000 feet in very difficult conditions. The Chinese were well acclimatized after having lived at 15,000 feet in Tibet for many months; Indian troops, on the other hand, were hastily moved to altitude by truck or aircraft from the low Indian plains. As a result of their rapid ascent, Indian soldiers suffered more casualties from altitude illness than from enemy action, while the Chinese suffered no altitude problems other than cold.

The experience of the Indian Army on the high frontier yielded more information than had ever before been collected about mountain sicknesses, and led to publication of many landmark papers by I. Singh, N. D. Menon, and others. (See the Bibliography.)

Military men around the world should not have been surprised by what happened on that high faraway frontier. It was quite predictable: Other armies had suffered on high mountains many centuries ago.

The Arctic Institute's Mount Logan High Altitude Physiology Study

The Indian experience stimulated several studies of high-altitude physiology, some by the military, others supported by state or private sources. From 1967 to 1979 the Arctic Institute of North America, with support from the U.S. National Institutes of Health, the Canadian Armed Forces, and others, carried on research in a summer laboratory at 17,500 feet near the summit of Mount Logan, a massive mountain in the Canadian Yukon. The first studies attempted to define exactly what caused mountain sickness and how this could be prevented. But after a few years, and some rather frightening experiences, studies were designed to look at the process of acclimatization in subjects who spent several weeks at the high laboratory. In addition to the high altitude retinal hemorrhages seen on Logan (described in Chapter 9, "Vision and the Eye at Altitude"), many other important observations were made and collected in the book *High Altitude Physiology Study*. One study documented how Diamox eliminates periodic breathing during sleep at altitude. Another demonstrated that most subjects accumulated a small amount of fluid in the pulmonary interstitial space, while showing no evidence of high altitude pulmonary edema (HAPE).

Meanwhile, Himalayan climbing increased dramatically; speed climbing at dangerous altitudes became popular, and hordes of unsuspecting and inexperienced tourists, trekkers, and climbers were flown too rapidly to dangerous altitudes. Hundreds became sick and many died—not only visitors but experienced mountaineers as well.

Everest

In Nepal in 1973, John Dickinson and Peter Hackett (and later David Shlim) organized the Himalayan Rescue Association, which established a clinic below Everest Base Camp where volunteer doctors took care of the sick and collected a great deal of information about mountain sickness. Altitude physiology became even more popular and facilitated (or was used to justify) many big-mountain climbing expeditions.

A large and elaborate Italian expedition to Everest in 1973 not only managed to get seven men to the summit but also made extensive studies of work capacity and metabolism in thirty-six men during a long stay at 17,500 feet. The American Research Expedition to Everest led by John West in 1981 set up a well-equipped laboratory at 17,700 feet and a smaller one at 20,700 feet, where many exercise studies were done. Alveolar gas samples from one man were collected on the summit and matched with blood samples taken later and lower on the mountain. The findings of this major scientific effort can be briefly summarized as follows:

- Confirmed the Silver Hut estimate of the barometric pressure on the summit of Everest.
- Confirmed the Silver Hut estimate of maximum work capacity (VO_2 max) high on the mountain.
- Obtained alveolar gases on one subject on the summit.
- Calculated blood gases on the summit from blood drawn at 26,000 feet.
- Correlated hypoxic ventilatory response of climbers with their performance at altitude.
- Obtained hormonal, blood electrolyte, ventilatory, and circulatory data higher than ever before on a mountain.

These were important observations, made in the real world and subject to all the stresses of the mountain environment.

Denali

From 1982 to 1989, a combined rescue clinic and research laboratory was established by Peter Hackett and Bill Mills at 14,000 feet on Mount McKinley (also known as Denali, The Great One), a mountain that attracts almost 1,000 mountaineers each year. The clinic-laboratory was ideally sited to study and treat the dozens who required treatment for altitude illness. The project was generously supported by the U.S. Army and the National Park Service, and many climbers attempting Denali passed through the facility daily. Many healthy individuals volunteered as control subjects, and those badly affected by altitude provided a wealth of research data. The climbers covered a wide spread of age, both sexes, different experience levels, and different rates of climb, so the large amount of information collected was broadly representative of the population attempting a big mountain. The most important observations as reported in more than forty medical papers can be summarized as follows:

- Between 2 and 3 percent developed life-threatening high altitude pulmonary edema (HAPE).
- Fluid drawn from lungs showed more protein and evidence of inflammation in seven HAPE victims than in seven control subjects, indicating that leaking lung capillaries may contribute to HAPE.
- The hypoxic ventilatory response (HVR) was weak and the arterial oxygen saturation low in those who developed HAPE. Periodic breathing during sleep seemed related to a brisk HVR.
- Thirty percent of those studied had acute mountain sickness (AMS), with headache and sleep disturbance as major symptoms.
- Diamox relieved periodic breathing during sleep but did not increase cerebral blood flow. Diamox was shown to be helpful in *treating* as well as *preventing* AMS.

Doctors working on the Denali project rescued many sick and injured climbers and collected more important data on various aspects of altitude illness than any other mission before or since. Hackett was among the first to state unequivocally that AMS originates in disturbed brain functions.

Mountain laboratories are the "real world," where people are exposed to many stresses. Nevertheless, these mountain studies made it clear that one could not tell whether effects attributed to altitude might be due in part to cold, dehydration, exhaustion, inadequate food, or other environmental influences. There was still a need to study hypoxia in its pure form, in the more sheltered decompression chamber, bigger of course than the small cylinders used by Paul Bert a century earlier. An important and often overlooked advantage of chamber studies is the fact that the observers themselves are not affected by altitude. So in 1985 Operation Everest II, a repeat of the first one in 1946, was completed. (See Chapter 16, "Operation Everest I and II.")

THE PHYSIOLOGY OF ADJUSTMENT AND ACCLIMATIZATION

The simplest way to describe acclimatization is as a set of adjustments our bodies make when exposed to hypoxia. These changes occur in the respiratory, cardiovascular, renal (kidney), and endocrine systems. Because the respiratory system is so central to our performance at high altitude, let us begin there.

The Respiratory System

When we first ascend to high altitude, lower oxygen levels produce low blood oxygen (hypoxia) and stimulate the *carotid bodies,* small organs located on the wall of each carotid artery that sense the blood oxygen level and send a message to the brain when that level falls. The brain sends a message to the muscles of respiration causing an increase in the rate and depth of ventilation. This is known as the hypoxic ventilatory response (HVR). The more vigorous the adjustment to HVR, the greater the volume of oxygen to reach the cells. But hyperventilation comes at a cost—the loss of carbon dioxide as it is washed out of the lungs and blood.

Because it is a gas, and easily soluble in water and blood, carbon dioxide is the principal and most effective mediator of blood acidity. In solution it forms a weak acid, and therefore when more CO_2 than usual leaves blood and diffuses into alveoli, the blood becomes more alkaline. Normally, the acidity (pH) of blood lies between 7.35 and 7.45. The quickest way to correct alkaline blood is to decrease the loss of CO_2 by breathing less, but obviously this is not desirable at altitude. Next best is to excrete bicarbonate in urine, a process that takes longer and also causes water loss. This strategy is basic to acclimatization. It is how Diamox works to speed acclimatization and minimize mountain sickness.

Over the course of several weeks at high altitude, the carotid bodies become increasingly sensitive to hypoxia and, through the HVR, increase ventilation to even higher levels. As a result, blood oxygen levels are better maintained than they would be in the absence of HVR, but blood CO_2 falls still more. Clearly, the HVR helps a climber at high altitude compensate for the low atmospheric oxygen levels, and the increased sensitivity of the carotid bodies with time at altitude is part of acclimatization. The importance of the HVR to acclimatization to altitude is further underscored by the fact that climbers with a brisk HVR may be less likely to get HAPE than those with a more modest response.

The carotid bodies, and other body sensors that control ventilation, also react to CO_2 levels but inversely to their reaction to oxygen. Low blood CO_2 decreases ventilation, thus blunting the HVR. Furthermore, if a person remains at altitude for months or years, a paradoxical effect occurs. Their carotid bodies become larger but less sensitive. HVR eventually falls. Fortunately, by this time, changes may have occurred in other body systems (including the cardiovascular system) that compensate for the potential negative impact of this reduction in HVR.

Given the role of hypoxia in stimulating the HVR and the importance of the HVR in acclimatization, we might well ask if it is possible to adjust our exposure to hypoxia in such a way that we speed or enhance acclimatization. Climbers have attempted this by exposing themselves to hypoxia for relatively brief but repeated periods. This pattern, known as *intermittent hypoxia,* is well suited to expedition climbing in which climbers commonly spend many days ferrying loads to high camps and returning to base camp each night to sleep—a practice known as "carry high and sleep low."

Intermittent hypoxia seems to stimulate increases in the HVR, and does so faster than continuous hypoxia. Climbers ascending this way might have a peak HVR in five days rather than in the several weeks it would take with continuous hypoxia. Sleeping low on an expedition has the additional advantage of helping climbers minimize the sleep disturbance, dehydration, and inadequate diet that seem to be endemic to life at high camp. It is, therefore, not surprising that many high-altitude climbers, including guides who take clients to the highest peaks on the planet, use a "carry high and sleep low" approach to their ascents. Further support for the use of intermittent hypoxia to enhance acclimatization comes from the finding that climbers exposed to periods of hypoxia in a low-pressure chamber prior to an expedition have, on average, higher blood oxygen levels at altitude and may acclimatize more quickly. Although the evidence is persuasive, we still need more hard data to conclude that intermittent hypoxia alone enhances high-altitude performance.

The Cardiovascular System

The "struggle" or "fight or flight" response at altitude also impacts the cardiovascular system. Arteries constrict, increasing the resistance to blood flow and raising blood pressure. Increased blood pressure may be of particular importance in the pulmonary artery, where, if excessive, it can contribute to HAPE. The heart is also stimulated to beat faster. However, the amount of blood pumped with each heartbeat (the stroke volume) may actually decrease so that the amount of blood that the heart pumps each minute (the cardiac output) is little changed. Within hours of ascent to high altitude, we also experience a decrease in blood plasma volume, indicating that fluid has escaped the blood vessels and entered the interstitial space surrounding the cells. Both increased blood pressure and leaking capillaries may contribute to this plasma loss.

The loss of fluid from blood into tissue interstitia concentrates the blood so that more oxygen is carried in each milliliter of blood. However, it does not increase the blood's oxygen-carrying capacity, because the total number of circulating red blood cells has not increased, as it will when the bone marrow makes and releases more red cells. When that happens, both the blood's oxygen content and its carrying capacity increase, and acclimatization progresses well.

With time at high altitude, additional changes occur. Hypoxia increases erythropoietin (EPO) production by the kidney. Increased EPO, which can begin to occur following even a few hours of hypoxia, stimulates the bone marrow to produce and release red blood cells, increasing the number of red blood cells in a fixed volume of blood (red blood cell count) and the fraction of the total blood volume made up of cells rather than plasma (hematocrit). Raised red blood cell count and hematocrit are certainly part of acclimatization because they increase the ability of blood to carry oxygen and partially compensate for the reduced atmospheric oxygen levels at altitude. However, it takes a week or more for the full increase to occur. In addition to its affect on HVR, intermittent hypoxia also may be a strong stimulus of EPO release.

Over longer periods (months to years) at high altitude, some but not all of these cardiovascular changes reverse themselves. Blood pressure returns to normal, probably as a result of arterial dilation, as each tissue regulates its own blood flow (see Chapter 7, "The Body Up High: Cellular and Vascular Responses to Hypoxia") and sympathetic nervous system stimulation decreases. Unfortunately, blood pressure in the pulmonary artery may remain elevated, and this can eventually produce heart strain and even heart failure. (See Chapter 11, "Chronic and Subacute Mountain Illness.") The hematocrit also remains elevated for as long as we remain at altitude.

The Renal System

The kidneys are very busy organs, almost as hardworking as the heart. About a fifth of the blood pumped by the heart passes through the kidneys, which filter some 180 liters a day. Of this filtrate, 99 percent is reabsorbed, and one or two liters of urine excreted. Figure 31 provides a condensed view of the elaborate mechanism of this small human wastewater treatment plant

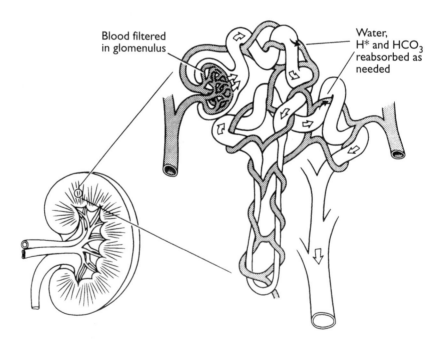

Blood filtered in glomenulus

Water, H* and HCO$_3$ reabsorbed as needed

Figure 31. *The kidneys*

> ### *The Kidneys*
>
> Arterial blood is pumped through a dense network of capillaries surrounding thousands of tiny filtration capsules (*glomeruli*), where fluid is filtered from the blood into the forming urine. As the urine moves through the kidney tubules, active transport removes selected substances (such as glucose and amino acids) from the urine and returns it to the blood. Other substances (such as hydrogen ions) are actively added to the urine. Much of the filtered water is returned to the blood as well. The net result is that most of the unwanted wastes and a relatively small volume of water are excreted in the urine while valuable substances are retained.

and suggests how important the kidneys are to acclimatization. However, in the words of Eric Swenson at the 1997 Hypoxia Symposium: "Despite much intensive field and laboratory investigation, the responses of the kidney and its role in acclimatization remain uncertain."

At least one of our two kidneys must function reasonably well for us to survive. Not only does the kidney regulate water balance, it must also carry away many waste products of metabolism and wear and tear on tissues. Also vital is the kidney's role in the maintenance of acid–base balance. The kidney has the ability to excrete both bicarbonate ions (base) and hydrogen ions (acid). When the blood becomes alkaline (increased pH, more basic), as it does when hypoxia stimulates an increase in the rate and depth of respiration at altitude, kidney function shifts in favor of bicarbonate ion excretion. Over the course of a few days at high altitude, this function of the kidney partially compensates for the alkaline blood (alkalosis) induced by overbreathing. A normal blood pH is vital for a range of physiological functions, from enzyme activity to cerebral blood flow. This action of the kidney to maintain blood pH is therefore a vital part of acclimatization. Thus we see that changes in breathing are the body's "quick fix" to regulate blood acidity, while the kidneys perform the same job over the long haul.

"Drink Lots of Water"

The kidneys need to excrete some water to eliminate bicarbonate and other waste substances. This suggests the need to drink more water in the mountains and has led to the assumption that a copious flow of urine at altitude would minimize mountain sickness and speed acclimatization. The basis for this advice came from a report of altitude diuresis by Frederick von Wendt, who measured his urine while climbing in the Alps in 1910. The term *Hohendiuresen* ("high diuresis," in German) was coined in 1944 after the observation on the Jungfraujoch that those new arrivals above 10,000 feet who passed the most urine tolerated altitude better than those who passed only a little. Right or wrong, this belief has become conventional wisdom and is taken as a good sign that acclimatization is progressing satisfactorily. It led logically enough to the use of diuretics to increase urine output. But again quoting Eric Swenson's comments at the 1997 Hypoxia Symposium:

> Despite physiological plausibility, careful examination of the older literature and now more recent studies suggest that the fancy that a lack of high-altitude diuresis precedes the development of AMS and is a critical determinant in the pathophysiology of AMS is not true.

Those who do not pass excess urine have been shown to secrete excessive *antidiuretic hormone* (ADH) and this has come to be considered, perhaps wrongly, a contributor to AMS.

Sojourners in the mountains have long been urged to drink extra water to replace that lost in exhaling and sweating. There is little question about the wisdom of taking on sufficient fluids, although it may not be true that more urine lost means less edema.

A word of caution: Drinking too much water also can cause problems: *A young woman called me from a mountain resort several years ago. She had been at 8,000 feet for a week and was feeling steadily worse. Her head ached and she felt bloated; indeed, she had gained ten pounds and her face, hands, and feet were badly swollen. She told me she had done just what her doctor ordered: "Drink plenty of water and take extra salt because you'll lose a lot in sweat." She had done this in spades! The surplus water and salt had caused massive edema, which disappeared rapidly when she stopped taking salt and cut down her water intake.*

Even without salt, excess water can cause problems. Head injuries and brain swelling from other causes like high altitude cerebral edema (HACE) may cause *hyponatremia* (low blood sodium), not from excess water or too little salt, but because the body secretes an abnormally large amount of ADH. Some schizophrenic patients with an obsession to drink water dilute their blood and lower serum sodium enough to cause collapse, coma, convulsions, and death. Sometimes marathoners drink more water than they need and do not replace lost sodium; they too risk collapse from hyponatremia.

The Endocrine System

A number of hormones are affected by high altitude. Antidiuretic hormone (ADH) is produced by an area of the brain known as the hypothalamus and released into the blood by the posterior pituitary gland at the base of the brain. It acts on the kidney to increase water reabsorption and decrease urine output. Although the details are not well understood, exposure to high altitude seems to decrease ADH release and, consequently, cause a reduction of water in the urine. We do know that fluid retention at altitude is associated with the development of high-altitude illness. Thus, a diuresis at altitude may be a necessary part of the acclimatization response. *Acetazolamide* (Diamox) has been used for years by climbers to enhance acclimatization and reduce mountain sickness. It acts primarily to increase bicarbonate excretion, but it is also, independently, a mild diuretic and thus also enhances acclimatization. Diamox also can improve sleep at altitude.

Because the metabolism of glucose produces more energy per oxygen molecule consumed than does the metabolism of other possible energy sources (such as fats), hormonal changes that increase the blood sugar or enhance glucose uptake into cells theoretically could contribute to acclimatization. High-altitude natives do appear to have higher blood levels of several hormones that can raise blood sugar, including growth hormone (from the anterior pituitary gland) and cortisol (from the adrenal gland). These individuals also have elevated levels of thyroid hormone, but it is not clear if stress or hypoxia or cold is the major cause. This elevation causes mild hyperthyroidism, which may contribute to weight loss after a long stay at altitude. We should also keep in mind that these hormonal changes have been documented predominantly in high-altitude natives as compared to lowland dwellers. Therefore, their role in the acclimatization of climbers who come to altitude from more modest elevations are less completely understood.

ACCLIMATIZATION AT THE CELLULAR LEVEL

Throughout this chapter, and indeed throughout this book, reference is made to a wide variety of body cell types, tissues, and organs responding to hypoxia. In many of these cases, the responses involve production of specific proteins by cells. So it is not unreasonable to ask just how a cell might sense hypoxia, and how hypoxia might stimulate protein production within cells. While we do not know all the details of how cells sense hypoxia, some of the broad outlines of this response mechanism are beginning to emerge.

All cell types important to the response to altitude seem to produce the protein known as *hypoxia inducible factor* (HIF). When oxygen is abundant in cells, cellular enzymes degrade HIF and render it inactive. But under the hypoxic conditions of high altitude, these enzymes are suppressed, and HIF retains its active form. HIF is a transcription factor. It binds to certain genes, setting in motion a chain of events that leads to the production of specific proteins. HIF induces the genes for a range of proteins that play a role in the cellular response to hypoxia including the genes for erythropoietin (EPO), vascular endothelial growth factor (VEGF), and endothelin. (For more information on the process by which genes direct protein production, and the functions of EPO, VEGF, and endothelin, see Chapter 7, "The Body Up High: Cellular and Vascular Responses to Hypoxia.") So while HIF is not the only factor involved, it is certainly an important common pathway in the response of many cell types to hypoxia and a vital link in our ability to acclimatize to the hypoxia of high altitude.

Because they are responsible for the motion needed to climb high, muscle cells must have a particular ability to respond to a sudden call for more oxygen. Ordinarily, as we start to exercise and the muscles require more oxygen, the heart speeds up and more blood is pumped to the muscles to meet this demand. An additional supply of oxygen is available in the muscles, loosely bound to myoglobin. During acclimatization, myoglobin increases substantially, and we might think of this substance as a storehouse or a facilitator of oxygen transfer, even though myoglobin may not be as fully oxygenated at altitude as it is at sea level. It is interesting that myoglobin has a left-shifted oxygen dissociation curve, admirably suited for release of a lot of oxygen rapidly when the local supply gets very low. Diving mammals have a large supply of myoglobin from which they draw oxygen during long submersion.

Each of the many functions that change in response to hypoxia is affected by the others, and together they produce a stable condition of acclimatization—if, but only if, (1) hypoxia is not too severe; (2) exposure is not too rapid; (3) the individual does not remain too long at the thin edge of survival, which is considered to be at about 23,000 feet; and (4) a negative predisposition, possibly genetic, does not interfere.

Life depends on an adequate flow of oxygen into each cell, where it is used by the mitochondria, the factories where every life function is energized. (See Chapter 5, "Cells: The Ultimate Users.") Although the number of mitochondria apparently does not increase during acclimatization, their size does, increasing extraction of oxygen from blood before it returns to the lungs.

Table 9 summarizes these major changes in oxygen acquisition, transport, and delivery that tend to bring the oxygen supply to the tissues closer to that available in the lungs.

TABLE 9
MAJOR CHANGES IN ACCLIMATIZATION

Increased breathing	Better exchange of air in alveoli
Increased cardiac output	Temporary; more blood is moved
Increased red cells	More oxygen carriers available
More tissue capillaries	Brings blood closer to cells
Increased myoglobin	More oxygen is locally available
Increased urine output	Temporary; concentrates blood

ACCLIMATIZATION IN PRACTICE

We must now look at some practical aspects of acclimatization: How long does it take? How long does it last? How can it be speeded up or enhanced? And—of special interest—is it helpful to acclimatize at high altitude for competitions held at sea level? To compete at high altitude, where should one train—and how? Training for competition is only peripherally related to mountaineering, and this topic is discussed in Chapter 17, "Limits to Work at Altitude." Only partial answers are available to such questions, and individual variation makes a great deal of difference.

We can say quite confidently that a month of gradual ascent is enough for most people to acclimatize well to 18,000 to 19,000 feet. We can also say, from a lot of experience, that at above 20,000 feet, deterioration outstrips acclimatization, and those who stay so high for many days do not improve with time. No people are known to have lived for more than a few months above 17,500 feet, and in addition to high altitude, other harsh conditions contribute to their failure to thrive.

Chapter 15, "Prevention and Treatment," examines appropriate rates of climb for the unacclimatized sojourner to moderate altitude. In general, taking a few days for the ascent will protect against altitude illness at up to 10,000 feet, and in less than a week most people feel as well as at sea level.

Acclimatizing to Climb the Highest Peaks

Many generations of mountaineers used siege tactics on the highest mountains, slowly building a pyramid of well-stocked camps to within striking distance of the summit. Climbers relied on the daily work of carrying loads up, and returning to a lower camp to sleep. During a long siege, or after a long period of bad weather has kept one in a high camp (a debilitating experience), descent to base camp for a rest in richer air is prudent. There are many advantages to this approach—but it takes more time and more equipment, and for the last few decades other approaches have been tried.

One of the newer methods is to spend more time at base camp, climbing higher every day or two on mountains nearby, gradually building acclimatization while enjoying the relative "luxury" of base camp. Then, when the climbers feel fit and the weather is good, they may go for the summit, perhaps from base camp or perhaps from a higher intermediate camp. Using this approach, some superclimbers have summited Everest in less than twenty-four hours; one has done it on K2.

Always at the mercy of weather, experienced climbers have developed several different programs for acclimatizing on the highest summits. David Breashears, who has summited Everest multiple times, recommends going up one to two thousand feet a few days after reaching base camp and then returning to base. He then climbs to Camp One for a night, and again descends to base. By then, if acclimatization is well under way, he and his team carry loads to Camp Two once or twice, and finally move up to sleep at Camp Three before going to the South Col in promising weather to summit the next day. Others have slightly different programs; all rely on a few nights at higher and higher camps for a week or ten days before attempting the summit—and this after several weeks at the 18,000-foot base.

Other veterans modify siege tactics by setting up a few camps, then retreating several thousand feet for a week or so of real rest. After this, some parties have been able to reach the top in only a few days—if the weather holds. On the highest mountains, weather is often the most decisive factor.

In any of these plans for going to high altitude over the course of days or even weeks, it might seem that retreat to low altitude and return to high altitude could make the climber vulnerable to reentry HAPE. (See Chapter 10, "HAPE: High Altitude Pulmonary Edema.") But apparently the altitude stay usually is not long enough; no such cases have been reported.

One extreme approach has not yet been tested: An expert climber, fully fit at sea level, might breathe oxygen night and day above 12,000 feet and, following a prepared track, climb at a reasonable rate of 1,500 feet an hour, reaching the top of Everest and returning in less than twenty hours. It would be risky: Should his or her oxygen fail, unconsciousness would be swift and death not far behind. From what we know about acclimatization, this fully oxygenated approach would make the climber only as breathless as at sea level, allowing him or her to start out well rested, well fed, and hydrated—but it would not seem to be a very joyful way to go.

For now, different individuals and groups continue to try various patterns of ascent, work, and rest.

Medication

Will medication or diet or breathing exercises speed acclimatization? Of these, the only one that makes a real difference is acetazolamide (Diamox). This and other means of prevention are discussed in Chapter 15, "Prevention and Treatment." One could call Diamox an "artificial acclimatizer," because it facilitates the excretion of bicarbonate and normalizes blood pH. Several expeditions have used Diamox every day, but their experiences differ, and there are too many variables to allow a definitive conclusion. Taking Diamox regularly during a major climb may be more helpful than harmful—if one insists on taking some kind of medicine. There may be a risk: Some who have taken Diamox regularly and stopped it abruptly while at high altitude have then developed acute altitude problems rather unexpectedly.

Respiratory stimulants do not seem to speed acclimatization. Hormones (steroids, human growth hormone, and others) and psychotropic drugs have not been adequately tested.

Changing Hemoglobin

When we try to decide what is an optimal level of hemoglobin, we are on uncertain ground. Crude efforts have been made to improve altitude tolerance by transfusing blood into the acclimatizing mountaineer. The results have been conflicting. Removing what might be called excess hemoglobin and replacing the blood with plasma has also been tried. Again, no clear result. Sound theory and a lot of anecdotal evidence suggest that a hematocrit of less than 56 percent to 58 percent is optimal, but we cannot conclude from this that removing blood is beneficial to the acclimatized climber.

We know how to convert adult-type hemoglobin to the fetal or fast form—but this is justifiable only in certain serious illnesses, and so far no method has been considered for the healthy mountaineer. Undoubtedly, tinkering with the ability of hemoglobin to pick up and release oxygen may help in some situations—but not today, not yet. A few studies of tolerance for hypoxia in individuals with mutant hemoglobin do not seem to have much relevance to mountaineering.

LOSING ACCLIMATIZATION

There is not much firm data about how long it takes for a person to lose acclimatization once acquired, but most of the changes—even the blood count—revert to normal within a week or two of returning to sea level. It is interesting that shortness of breath on exertion may last for a week at sea level after returning from several weeks at high altitude. This period of "de-acclimatization" has not been studied, but the persistent shortness of breath could be due to an increase in sensitivity of the respiratory center to carbon dioxide. In addition, the alkaline reserve (base excess) has been decreased, making the pH of blood more sensitive to small changes in carbon dioxide or to the lactic acid produced by exertion.

And what of the longtime high-altitude resident who travels to sea level? Will he or she have trouble deacclimatizing? The answer is firmly "no"—adjustment takes only a few days or a week. The mountaineer coming home from high in the Himalayas is euphoric and elated. Simple things like green grass, flowers, warmth, and space to move about delight him or her. Life is precious, filled with joys and surprises. But within weeks, the trivia of every day intrude: There is money to deal with; the daily round is dull and uninspiring compared to the high drama of a strenuous climb where a single purpose dominates. Life seems to have lost its savor; some climbers become depressed; divorces or broken relationships are common before one adjusts to the old routine. It is tempting to blame these emotional events on lasting effects of severe hypoxia. But men and women returning after great experiences at sea or long trips in the polar or desert regions have experienced similar emotions. It seems to us that they are due to shifting gears, rather than to hypoxia.

ACCLIMATIZATION FOR COMPETITIVE SPORTS

A vast amount of thought, effort, and money has been invested in the question of sports training. Will you compete better at sea level after acclimatizing to high altitude? If competing at high altitude, should you arrive weeks in advance and acclimatize? How will you fare if you go directly from sea level and at once compete at high altitude?

The enormous and saddening commercialization of most sports (including mountain climbing) has made the answers to these questions potentially worth billions of dollars but, not surprisingly, throwing money at the questions has resulted in more questions than answers. Because it is such a major issue, training is discussed in more detail in Chapter 17, "Limits to Work at Altitude." The bibliography lists some scientific papers addressing the subject.

Acclimatization to altitude is a wondrously complex process wherein many interwoven changes enable survival under extreme conditions. When we look at sea-level humans and observe how within seconds they become unconscious when deprived of oxygen, the wonder grows that we are able to get anywhere near the harsh, hostile, and spectacular summit of Everest. We wonder even more that whales and seals can dive without breathing for an hour, that turtles can hibernate for months under water, that the lungfish can go for years without breathing, that some forms of life exist completely without oxygen. As our understanding of acclimatization grows, we gain a fuller understanding of how these seemingly impossible feats can be achieved.

CHAPTER 14

GENETICS OF HIGH-ALTITUDE PERFORMANCE

In my adult lifetime I have seen four wars and served in one. I have survived unscathed a spiraling stock market that crashed thunderously, and lived through a worldwide depression. I have witnessed the arrival of television and the incredible wizardry of electronic communications around the world. Beyond everything else, I experienced the arrival of the nuclear age.

During my hospital training I saw the arrival of sulfanilamide, which presaged an array of drugs that permit us to control almost any infectious illness. On the heels of this revolution came steroids, which offered relief from or cure of other major ailments. Diagnostic and therapeutic tools have multiplied, and procedures we consider commonplace today were undreamed of a few decades ago. Medicine has progressed at unbelievable speed, but not without a few casualties.

In 1990, when scientists undertook the task of revealing the genetic code, few of us had much idea of what the implications might be. As I write, we can read the code, and are beginning—but only beginning—to recognize its profound possibilities for both good and evil.

To me this entry into the world of genetics, coupled with our fledgling ability to manipulate genes, may be one of the most significant advances in all of medicine, bringing with it both rewards and penalties that we are only beginning to grasp.

This chapter discusses a few of the known and possible effects that genetics may have not only in high-altitude medicine but on the entire field of oxygen utilization and hypoxia. We already know that different individuals use or reject different chemicals differently and that literally "one man's meat is another's poison." We know too that a few individuals are unable to tolerate high altitude—and by implication hypoxia—as well as others. We can now manipulate DNA in ways not thought of just a few years ago, and we are able to predict with some accuracy the likelihood of several congenital illnesses in utero.

This chapter can only be a very brief introduction to what is known as it is being written, and even more may be known by the time you read it. So extraordinary is the rapid introduction of new information that you can, with a few clicks on your computer, read about the latest developments in genetic engineering and how they may affect tolerance for hypoxia.

This is indeed a new world, and hopefully we can handle ourselves better in it than we have in the past.

In several parts of the world, many generations of altitude natives are thoroughly at home up to 17,500 feet (the elevation of the highest permanently inhabited villages) and can do hard physical work. As Joseph Barcroft wrote in the 1920s after visiting a mine in Peru at 14,000 feet:

> Every few minutes, like a bee out of some hive in cold weather, someone would appear from the mouth of the mine. He would be much out of breath, he would take frequent pauses on the way up, but the weight on his back would be a hundred pounds...he would sit for a while to rest and then down into the mine again he would go to bring up another load.

Natives of the high Andes, the highlands of Ethiopia, and the Tibetan plateau do seem to be different in some ways from people living at sea level. Many scientists have proposed that high-altitude natives have *adapted* (in the Darwinian sense) through inherited changes that make them better able to live and work where the new arrival from lower altitudes becomes sick. However, it is important to distinguish the genetic adaptation that occurs over many generations from the acclimatization that any person, regardless of ethnic background, experiences over days and weeks at altitude.

In the fifteenth century, Mirza Muhammad Haider described mountain sickness at around 15,000 feet in Tibet, noting, "This malady only attacks strangers; the people of Tibet know nothing of it, nor do their doctors know why it attacks strangers." However, he was not in a position to know how adaptation and acclimatization contributed to his observation.

The distinction between acclimatization and adaptation was the subject of a rather heated exchange in the middle of the twentieth century and continues more collegially today. In 1925, after working for many weeks at 14,000 feet in Peru, Joseph Barcroft (who knew as much about high altitude as anyone at the time) wrote:

> The acclimatized man is not the man who has attained to bodily and mental powers as great in Cerro de Pasco as he would have in Cambridge (whether that town be situated in Massachusetts or England). Such a man does not exist. All dwellers at altitude are persons of impaired physical and mental powers. The acclimatized man is he who is least impaired, or, in other words, he who has made the least demand upon his reserve.

Carlos Monge, Sr., a respected pioneer in altitude research, was outraged by Barcroft's assertion. We do not have access to his paper published at the time (in Spanish), so we can only imagine what he told Barcroft. But years later he was still angry and wrote:

> For our part, as early as 1928 we proved...that Professor Barcroft was himself suffering from mountain sickness without realizing it. His substantial error is easy to explain as resulting from an improper generalization on his part of what he himself felt and applying his reaction to Andean man in general.... Andean man must be physically distinct from sea level man, requiring much further research before one may define, let alone apply, the terms inferior and superior.

Monge was right: He recognized that Barcroft was comparing longtime residents who did not have the health and educational benefits he himself enjoyed, as a visitor who had partially acclimatized. But Barcroft was also right to a degree: Even the longtime resident above 14,000 feet is often not as physically or mentally able as his counterpart living at sea level.

In an attempt to understand possible adaptations in high-altitude natives that might make them more suited for life at altitude than lowlanders, early scientists who studied the response of the human body to high altitude often looked to differences in the respiratory and oxygen-carrying systems of the human body. In Paris, over fifty years before the Barcroft–Monge controversy, Paul Bert's colleague Dr. Denis Jourdanet anticipated Monge. He had spent twenty years studying Mexico and its people. Noting the stocky build typical of the highlander, he described "the vast chest [which] makes him comfortable in the midst of this thin air," an observation echoed years later by Barcroft in the Andes.

Jourdanet's writings caused quite a storm among entrepreneurs who were contemplating establishment of a French empire on the high plateaus of Mexico, and the French military surgeon L. Coindet was sent to investigate. He reported that natives had the same respiratory and pulse rates as the more recently arrived French, but acknowledged that natives could do more strenuous work for longer periods than could newcomers.

GENETIC ADAPTATION IN HIGH-ALTITUDE NATIVES

People live at high altitude in several places around the globe, including East Africa, the Himalayas, Central Asia, and the Andes. Some of these locations have been populated for at least several hundred generations—long enough for genetic adaptation to altitude to take place. So it is not unreasonable to propose that natives of high altitude may have gained a genetic advantage compared to low-altitude natives.

None of us can choose our ethnic heritage or place of birth, and so the question of adaptation in high-altitude natives might seem to be of academic interest only. However, there is much that we can learn from studies of high-altitude natives. For instance, if specific genetic adaptations to high altitude are found among these groups, we may gain insight into the mechanisms by which acute mountain sickness/high altitude cerebral edema (AMS/HACE) and high altitude pulmonary edema (HAPE) develop and learn how to avoid or treat these diseases.

Comparisons Among High-Altitude Native Groups

Studies of adaptation in high-altitude natives fall into two major categories: "within-group" studies and "between-group" studies. Between-group studies are easy to understand. They compare a set of physiological responses in one group to the same responses in another group. For instance, levels of ventilation, pulmonary artery blood pressure, or uterine blood flow of Andean natives might be compared to the levels found in Himalayan natives.

This may seem like an odd list of traits for scientists to study, but it really is not. The process of evolutionary adaptation selects only for traits that confer an advantage in successfully producing and raising offspring, and each of the traits listed above meets this criterion. Low hypoxic ventilatory response (HVR) is associated with HAPE, and high pulmonary artery blood pressure can strain the heart and produce heart disease. Low uterine blood flow in a mother during pregnancy can reduce her baby's birth weight and decrease its chance of survival.

Tibetan natives seem to have more favorable responses to altitude than do Andean natives. In addition, the birth weight of babies born to Tibetan natives decreases less sharply as the mother's altitude of residence increases than does the birth weight of babies born to Andean natives. This suggests that Tibetan natives, whose ancestors have probably lived at high altitude longer than the ancestors of Andean natives and therefore have had more generations to adapt, are indeed better adapted to high altitude.

The evidence supporting the hypothesis that the genetic adaptation to altitude among Tibetan natives is superior to that of Andean natives is far from conclusive, however. These two groups are also exposed to very different environments, and there is no foolproof method for distinguishing environmental effects from genetic differences. In addition, it is important to remember that as much as 95 percent of the native Andean population died during the Spanish conquest 400 years (about twenty generations) ago. This level of population destruction can entirely eliminate some genetic traits and radically alter the frequency of others. Thus, there is no way to know how the genetic makeup of the current Andean population compares to that of pre-conquest natives.

There are also studies that compare ethnic groups native to high altitude with groups that live at sea level. While these results are tantalizing, we need to keep in mind the great environmental differences between high-altitude and low-altitude areas and the complexity of acclimatization before we conclude that the differences we see are genetic. Some evidence suggests that humans born of generations of high-altitude residents may have more alveoli than those born at sea level. This adaptation would improve oxygen uptake by providing more area for diffusion and is more effective than simply developing a larger chest capable of moving more air in and out, an adaptation found in Andean natives but not in Tibetans.

Sherpas, who descend from generations of high-altitude residents, have a healthy response to oxygen lack (brisk HVR) and have slightly more hemoglobin than do sea-level natives. However, Sherpas are also generally physically fit and their maximum exercise capacity is high. They do not lose much weight at high altitude, and they seem to sleep more soundly. Andean natives have larger than normal carotid bodies, and this enables them to respond more briskly to hypoxic challenge.

Sherpas have only a little more hemoglobin than their sea-level cohorts, but Andean residents have a lot more. However, most Andean studies have been done on Aymara and Quechua natives, who live at higher altitudes than do the Sherpas. Tibetans are more like Sherpas, but there are some suggestions that Tibetans have a "fast-" as well as a "slow-"type hemoglobin—like their versatile servant the yak. Many Sherpas whose forebears lived on the high Tibetan plateau now live at somewhat lower altitude; their oxy–hemoglobin dissociation curves tend to be left-shifted, like the Himalayan bar-headed goose. This allows their hemoglobin to bind oxygen more readily as it passes through their lungs. Sherpas seem able to do more work at extreme altitude than can even well-acclimatized sea-level natives, but there are few well-controlled studies to support this.

When the chips are down, willpower, motivation, and spirit are arguably the major forces that drive the climber up the last exhausting feet on Everest, where he or she is moving almost automatically. But whether by better genetic heritage or more determination, one Sherpa, a man named Apa Sherpa, has summited Everest thirteen times. Several other Sherpas have done so four or five times, and so have some Caucasians.

Within-Group Studies

In contrast to between-groups studies, within-group studies examine a single group of high-altitude natives and ask if traits associated with high-altitude performance "run in families." Such studies have examined the ventilatory response to hypoxia (HVR), the oxygen saturation of the arterial blood, and hemoglobin concentration.

In some high-altitude populations, close relatives are more similar in their response to the hypoxia of altitude than are unrelated members of the same population. This suggests a genetic component to the control of these traits, at least for specific groups of people. However, these are complex traits that are almost certainly controlled simultaneously by many genes. To make matters even more confusing, the specific genes that control these traits are not known. Because of this, we cannot even conjecture how these genes might interact with the environment to produce their effects. Our current state of knowledge presents tantalizing suggestions that high-altitude performance may have a genetic component. But we have yet to discover the exact genes responsible, to determine what proteins they produce or how these proteins work, or to understand how these genes and proteins interact with the variable environments found at high altitude.

HOW GENES CONTROL BODY FUNCTIONS

We can begin to understand how genetic factors influence the body's ability to tolerate high-altitude environments by first describing what genes are and how they work. For our purposes, we can define a gene as the bit of DNA that carries the code for a single protein. There are about 30,000 genes in the human genome, and each of our body's cells contains the same genes. Genes are found on chromosomes in the nucleus of the cell.

We have known for fifty years that DNA is a two-stranded molecule that contains a linear array with thousands of repeats of only four bases. These bases are designated A, C, T, and G. DNA carries its genetic information through the ordering of these bases along the strands. When scientists first studied DNA, they found it difficult to believe that all the information needed to direct the function of all our cells could be stored in a mere four-letter code. Today we are familiar with the fact that computers can store vast amounts of data using only a binary (two-symbol) code, so the concept of storing of a huge amount of information in the four-letter code of DNA is easier to grasp.

The two paired strands of DNA carry complementary information. When a gene is stimulated, or *induced*, the information on its DNA is used to make a single-stranded RNA molecule that carries this same information. The RNA then leaves the nucleus of the cell and enters the cell cytoplasm, where it interacts with an intracellular structure known as a *ribosome*. (See Chapter 5, "Cells: The Ultimate Users.") It is on the ribosome that the RNA directs the production of a protein. (See Figure 32.)

Figure 32. DNA transcription and protein production

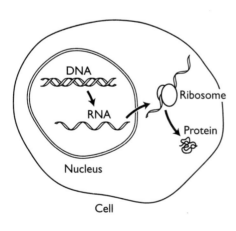

Proteins make up many of the important structural parts of cells. They also function as enzymes that speed biochemical reactions within cells. Because virtually all cell functions are based on biochemical reactions, proteins are responsible for pretty much every aspect of how cells work.

We have two copies of each gene, one inherited from each of our parents. Most genes come in several related forms called *alleles* that make slightly different versions of the same protein. Because these different versions of the proteins perform their jobs in a slightly different way, we are all different in appearance and function. As an example of allele function, consider the question of blood type. Blood type is determined by a single gene with three alleles—A, B, and O.

If we get an A allele from one parent and a B allele from the other, we are type AB. If we get an A allele from one parent and either an A or an O from the other, we are type A. If we get two O alleles, we are type O.

Are there alleles for specific genes that confer on the person lucky enough to inherit them some advantage in performance at high altitude? Attempts to answer this question have focused on several genes, including the gene that produces *angiotensin converting enzyme*, also known as ACE.

ACE Alleles and High-Altitude Performance

Our bodies maintain blood pressure through several intricate feedback loops, including one that involves ACE. Specialized cells in the kidney are able to sense when blood pressure falls. These cells release an enzyme called *renin* that sets in motion a chain of biochemical reactions ending with the production of *angiotensin II* by the capillaries of various organs, most notably the lung. Angiotensin II is a vasoconstrictor and also acts on the adrenal gland to cause the release of the steroid hormone *aldosterone*. Aldosterone acts back on the kidney to conserve salt and body fluid. Thus, angiotensin

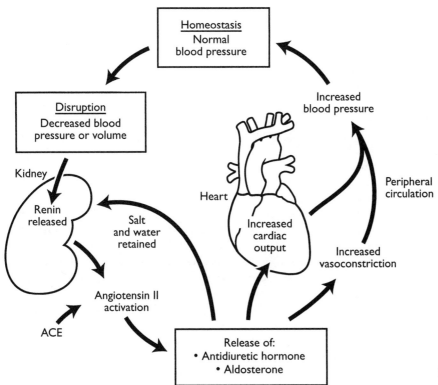

Figure 33. *ACE and high-altitude performance*

Biofeedback: Blood Pressure Regulation

A drop in blood pressure is sensed by the kidney, which releases renin. The release of renin sets in motion a chain of events that leads to the production of angiotensin II. Angiotensin II causes the blood vessels to constrict and directs the adrenal glands to release aldosterone. Aldosterone acts on the kidney, causing it to retain salt and water. The combination of vasoconstriction and fluid retention raises the blood pressure.

II raises the blood pressure in two ways—by direct vasoconstriction and by fluid retention. ACE enters the picture because it is the enzyme responsible for the production of angiotensin II, as illustrated in Figure 33.

The gene for ACE has two alleles, one with an extra bit of DNA inserted called the insertion, or I, allele and one without this additional DNA called the deletion, or D, allele. The D allele seems to be associated with elevated blood levels of ACE, as well as with a higher risk for diseases associated with elevated blood pressure, including coronary heart disease and abnormal thickening of the heart muscle. By contrast, the I allele seems to turn up frequently in elite endurance athletes and successful high-altitude climbers. Scientists also have studied the ACE genes of high-altitude natives to determine if these groups are more likely than lowland dwellers to have the I allele. The results of these studies are equivocal.

If the I allele of the ACE gene does imply an advantage for exercise in general, and for exercise at altitude in particular, how might it work? This is tough to answer for several reasons. First, the extra bit of DNA found in the I allele is in a part of the gene that does not directly carry information for protein production. Thus, the ACE protein made by the I and D alleles of the ACE gene should be identical. The two alleles could still produce different *amounts* of ACE, however, and this does seem to be the case. People with the I allele have lower ACE levels than do those with the D allele.

The simplest explanation of how extra ACE causes problems might be that it increases angiotensin II production, and the extra angiotensin II raises blood pressure. This could limit athletic performance and produce diseases associated with hypertension. One problem with applying this thinking to high altitude is that there is some evidence that, among high-altitude natives in Central Asia, those with two copies of the I allele actually have higher blood pressure in their pulmonary arteries and are more likely to suffer from the negative effects of this pulmonary hypertension than are those with two copies of the D allele.

Therefore it is likely that any advantage conferred by the I allele of the ACE gene comes from some other mechanism. Some studies suggest that those with the I allele may benefit from improved blood oxygen saturation, enhanced cardiopulmonary fitness, and more efficient muscle metabolism compared to those with the D allele. Others have proposed that the I allele may offer benefits in muscle building during training. Because angiotensin II and aldosterone have a range of effects on the body in addition to their impact on blood pressure, it is not unreasonable to propose that ACE could have numerous and complex effects. The most we can say at this time is that, if the I allele of the ACE gene provides those who have it with an advantage in endurance sports and at high altitude, the exact mechanism for this effect remains unknown.

Other Genes and High-Altitude Performance

Several other specific genes also have been tested as possible contributors to performance at high altitude. One of these is the gene for *tyrosine hydroxylase* (TH). To get a better idea of why researchers might look to TH to explain why some people perform better than others at high altitude, recall first how our bodies sense and respond to hypoxia.

Changing levels of blood oxygen are sensed by small organs called the *carotid bodies,* which lie on the walls of the carotid arteries—the major arteries carrying blood to the brain. The carotid bodies use *dopamine* as a neurotransmitter to produce an electrical signal that travels to the brain. The brain then signals the muscles of respiration to work harder and faster. This response, known as the hypoxic ventilatory response (HVR), brings more oxygen into the body.

Because TH is a vital enzyme in the production of dopamine, an abnormal TH gene could limit a climber's ability to make dopamine and respond to hypoxia through the HVR. There is also some evidence that climbers at high altitude who get HAPE do not have as brisk an HVR as other climbers. It is quite logical for scientists to ask whether the TH genes of those who get HAPE differ from those who do not. However, to this date at least, no such differences have been found.

A similar story can be told for the *myoglobin* gene. Myoglobin is a protein similar to hemoglobin. Myoglobin, found in the sort of muscle that contributes to endurance exercise, acts as an oxygen storage depot and can, in theory, contribute to a climber's ability to perform at high altitude. Scientists have looked for specific alleles of the myoglobin gene that might help explain why some people perform so much better than others at high altitude, but scientists have yet to find them.

Are there any genes that *do* impact performance at high altitude? There are at least two candidates. One is the gene for endothelial nitric oxide synthase (eNOS), the enzyme responsible for production of nitric oxide (NO), a potent but ephemeral vasodilator. (For more on eNOS, NO, and HAPE, see Chapter 7, "The Body Up High: Cellular and Vascular Responses to Hypoxia.") If the gene for eNOS is abnormal, NO levels may be low and blood vessels in the lung may constrict, which could lead to HAPE. Indeed, scientists have found two specific abnormalities of the eNOS gene that are more common in climbers who develop HAPE than in those who do not.

Cell surface proteins called *human leukocyte antigens* (HLAs), which play a major role in the immune response, have also been implicated in susceptibility to HAPE. Two alleles of the genes for these HLA proteins also seem to be present more often in climbers who get HAPE than in those who do not. While it may be difficult to see how alterations in genes for immune system proteins could play a role in HAPE, there may be a link. Stimulation of immune system proteins can cause inflammation, and inflamed blood vessels can constrict and leak, potentially opening the way for HAPE. One of the HLA alleles seems to cause particular elevation in the pulmonary artery pressure of those with HAPE who carry it. This HLA allele also seems to be associated with high pulmonary artery pressure in several diseases.

Have we found the genetic key to understanding susceptibility to HAPE? Before we rush out to have our eNOS and HLA genes checked, a word of caution is in order. The connection between specific alleles of these genes and HAPE has thus far been studied only in a relatively small number of Japanese climbers. Because the population of Japan is somewhat more genetically isolated than other ethnic groups, these studies need to be repeated in larger and broader groups of people before we can draw any hard conclusions.

Is performance at high altitude influenced by genetics? The answer is probably yes, to some extent. Yet the exact genes responsible for these effects remain in doubt. Even if these genes are found, how will this knowledge alter our approach to high-altitude climbing? A person who knew that he or she was genetically predisposed to high-altitude disease might choose not to go high or might be particularly careful in acclimatization. The susceptible person might use all available medications to prevent high-altitude disease and descend upon any sign of sickness. Most of these ideas are good general precautions for all climbers. It is certainly possible that there will come a time when gene therapy will be so safe and commonplace that climbers simply will have defective genes replaced. That day is far in the future. Nonetheless, some of the advances in genetics *will* have an impact on how we react to hypoxia, whether it be at altitude or sea level.

In the final analysis, unless you climb with your identical twin you will have a different genetic makeup than your partner's. This may help you in some circumstances but produce added challenges in others. As is always the case in climbing, the key to dealing with genetic differences is to use your strengths, compensate for your weaknesses, and choose climbing partners whose strengths complement yours.

CHAPTER

PREVENTION AND TREATMENT

*Over the ten seasons of the Mount Logan High Altitude Physiology Study,
we looked at many different aspects of altitude sickness, notably high altitude retinal hemorrhages (HARH). Only on two occasions did we try to
study the effects of diet on wellness or illness.*

*In the first study, at 17,500 feet, to try to achieve a uniform diet
among the participants, we asked the subjects, Canadian Airborne soldiers,
to eat U.S. Army Meals Ready to Eat (MRE) and to record their altitude
symptoms on a standard form. Our study ran into great difficulty because
the soldiers insisted on trading foods they disliked for foods they liked!
Many of them did not cooperate. We arranged to store the used food boxes
and later brought them down to base lab to quantify the leftover food, and
we were able to get a reasonably good estimate of what that select group
had eaten. Toward the end of the summer, when the project had ended, the
boxes containing half-eaten meals piled up and were shipped back to Ham-
ilton by air. Due to some snafu, this pile of boxes arrived three months later
in Dr. John Sutton's laboratory, heralded by a distinctive smell that filled
the entire laboratory. The boxes, which had become rotten and moldy, were
quickly disposed of, abruptly ending this experiment.*

*In another Mount Logan trial, we persuaded half of a group of volun-
teers (not soldiers this time) to eat a pure carbohydrate diet. We compared
their symptoms with those of other volunteers who were on an unrestricted
diet. Alas, the experimental subjects could not tolerate the restrictive diet,
and after two days they rebelled, quickly marking the end of another futile
experiment.*

More than a hundred years ago, the first people to travel in the high Himalayas took days or weeks of hard walking to gain altitude, and thus attained
enough acclimatization to prevent mountain sickness. Since then, particularly in the last seventy-five years, we have found that the slow ascent is
crucial, and by far the best protection against mountain sickness.

Obviously, the best way to avoid mountain sickness is to stay home and
not venture above 5,000 feet. But if you go to the high mountains, there
are several good ways to stay well. It doesn't take much. Many climbers can
avoid the worst effects of mountain sickness simply by ascending slowly,

recognizing their individual susceptibilities, and taking some relatively in-nocuous medications if needed.

To understand prevention, you must first know the potential problems of high altitude and why they exist. Even a little understanding of air and the atmosphere, even a vague idea of how the heart and lungs do their work, is a good start. Earlier chapters explained how lack of oxygen affects the body and how to recognize when minor discomforts become dangerous. This chapter discusses what you can do to avoid some of the problems and, should that fail, describes possible treatments.

The first and best preventive measure is to take your time—go up slowly. How slowly? Very few people notice the effects of altitude at 5,000 feet. We used to advise climbing only 1,000 feet a day above this altitude—but in the real world, few are willing or able to take that much time. We all seem to be in a hurry these days.

PREVENTION: HOW SLOW IS SLOW ENOUGH?

Except for those who have had and fear they will again have mountain sickness, most people can go from sea level to 7,000 feet in one day and feel little discomfort. The higher you climb and the faster you ascend, the greater your chances of getting mountain sickness. Approximately one person in five has some symptoms of acute mountain sickness (AMS) at 7,000 to 9,000 feet elevation, but twice that many develop symptoms at 10,000 feet. Most healthy people can ascend rapidly to 5,000 feet without experiencing symp-toms of AMS, and then proceed to 9,000 or 10,000 feet the next day without significant difficulties. Above this altitude, the pace of ascent should be slowed to 1,000 feet a day, and above 14,000 feet the rate of ascent should be slower still. As discussed in the chapter on acclimatization, the altitude at which you sleep is also a factor in the severity of AMS symptoms. Sleeping low can help you avoid AMS. A demanding climb requires more oxygen for physical and mental effort, and both of these strain physiologic resources. However, the better your acclimatization, the higher you can climb in a day.

If you are planning to climb or ski or hike above 9,000 feet, it might be wise to spend a few days at a lower elevation first. There is much evi-dence that altitude sicknesses are uncommon at 8,000 feet but more likely at 9,000 feet. Although there are no firm data, anecdotal evidence suggests that there is more difference of physiological relevance between these two altitudes than one would expect from a mere 1,000 feet. Why this might be so, anyone can guess! But if you do plan to stop over, stay for more than thirty-six hours: Less time does not seem to have much effect, according to Honigman's study (see Chapter 8, "The Spectrum of High-Altitude Illness: AMS/HACE").

If you are going higher—say, to peaks of 14,000 to 15,000 feet like Mount Rainier—you will do better by halting for two nights on the way up and setting a pace that accommodates the slowest member of the party. If your climbing plans require a faster pace, then it is reasonable to turn to some of the preventive medications suggested later in this chapter. Almost half of those who try to summit Rainier in one or two days get sick on the way, and many are forced to turn back.

Higher mountains require more time. You can drive or fly to the foot of Denali, the volcanoes in Central and South America, the smaller peaks of the Andes and Himalayas, and even to some high peaks in Africa. It is tempting to start climbing right away. On very popular mountains like Kilimanjaro, tour conductors and guides too often rush the party higher and faster than is prudent. As a result, many get sick, some seriously, and are disappointed. Now and then someone dies from avoidable altitude illness.

Denali is a special case. Being closer to the pole than other major mountains, it is physiologically several thousand feet higher than its measured altitude of 20,300 feet, a fact that few climbers make allowance for. Those who rush Denali are likely to get sick, perhaps very sick, and some die. Others are so impaired by hypoxia that they make bad decisions, move awkwardly, and are likely to fall, often to their deaths. Only half of those who attempt Denali make it, and of those who fail, many become sick or injured. Denali is always cold, often as cold as any mountain anywhere; this adds hypothermia to the stress of hypoxia, making it even more dangerous. Denali is in a class with the major Himalayan giants and should be approached as such.

Why Go Slow?

How does going slowly help the unacclimatized? The obvious reason is that it gives the body accustomed to sea level time to set in play the many physiological changes needed to function with less oxygen. Some of these changes begin very soon after you start up; others develop over the course of several weeks.

Conventional wisdom advises mountaineers to "carry high and sleep low," and this is smart. Why? Because during sleep at high altitude, breathing is less efficient and often erratic, so one's arterial oxygen saturation periodically swings downward from the waking level. During sleep, most people breathe less often and less deeply even at sea level, lowering the blood oxygen slightly. This means that, in terms of oxygen delivery, you go up a little higher in altitude during sleep.

This book focuses on the body's immediate and delayed responses to hypoxia. When these are given time to mature, they are lifesaving. But if you do not give your body time to adjust to altitude, you are likely to experience mountain sickness. And don't forget that conditions that cause lack of oxygen are not rare at sea level, where many of the same functions respond to the need for more oxygen, often in similar ways.

It is important to listen to your body. In circumstances in which you are in danger, your body will signal what it needs—whether that is more oxygen, water, warmth, or fuel. These needs are synergistic; that is, lack of any one of them increases the effect of the others. When your body screams, "Help!" or "Stop!" you'd better pay attention.

> *A friend of mine was climbing Kilimanjaro (19,340 feet) with a distinguished group of college presidents and other leaders. Their guide had led them up gradually, but even so, some were feeling the altitude. A few thousand feet below the summit, several of the party sat down to rest while the others continued on, slowly. After a while my friend said to the others, "I feel awful. I don't know about you, but I think if we stay here we might all die. I think we should go down, now," and they did. His description in his diary of how he felt is typical of early high altitude cerebral edema (HACE), and the group made the right decision to get down, as they all agreed later. They were wise.*

In extreme conditions it is sometimes not possible be prudent. Know your absolute limit and quit before it is too late. The tragedies on Everest in 1996 and K2 in 1986 are examples in which people's judgment was so blunted that they stretched themselves too far and paid with their lives. In these sad cases, as in many others at different times and on other mountains, climbers ignored and then did not hear the warnings screamed at them by their bodies. They passed the point of no return—and died. Their judgment was blunted, their perception blurred by the combination of lack of oxygen, cold, hunger, thirst, and lack of sleep. On Everest in 1996, four individuals did realize the extremity of their situation, turned back below the summit, and made it down safely.

Is Everest that much more dangerous and difficult than the other Himalayan giants that are a few hundred feet lower? On these the available oxygen is only 1 or 2 torr greater—does that make such a big difference? No, it does not.

Mountain tragedies attract attention, and in 1996 a whole series of events cascaded, many of which could or should have been avoided. By contrast, on May 10, 1993, in perfect weather, forty people reached the summit; during the unusually mild spring of 1992, fifty-eight people summited. No, altitude alone is not the major killer, but it certainly exacerbates all the other stressors.

Adjustment and Acclimatization

Why can't you speed up the adjustments? Isn't there some way you can hurry them along? Can you "train up" for the summit? Good questions—to which the answer is a qualified "no." Chapter 13, "Acclimatization," discussed various ways of acclimatizing for the highest mountains. Different veterans choose different methods, but they all have one thing in common—time.

Recall the immediate adjustments to hypoxia known as the "struggle responses": deeper breathing, greater output from the heart, more concentrated blood. These are temporary measures that cannot be sustained for long; they keep you functioning while the slower changes of acclimatization develop.

Obviously, avoiding strenuous effort for the first few days after a rapid ascent to moderate altitude is sound advice because of the additional demands that heavy work places on breathing and the pumping of blood. Wait until the adjustments have had a few days to develop into acclimatization before tearing off on a strenuous ski or climbing day.

Individual Susceptibility

There are some obvious individual attributes that may render a climber more or less likely to develop mountain sickness. For reasons that are not completely understood, people over fifty years of age are slightly less likely to suffer from altitude sickness than are younger climbers. Some studies suggest that obese climbers are at greater risk than those who are thinner. Women may be less likely than men to acquire high altitude pulmonary edema (HAPE), but do not seem to be protected from other forms of mountain sickness (AMS/HACE, for example).

Most of the variability in whether or not a person gets altitude sickness seems to reside in his or her individual physiology. Cold (which causes arterial constriction) and exercise (which increases blood flow through the lungs) can increase the risk of HAPE. For those with previous experience at altitude, however, there is one possible clue to individual risk. People who have had high-altitude sickness once are likely to experience it again. So, if you have suffered from mountain sickness before, you should take particular care. Those particularly susceptible to altitude sickness should consider the prevention measures discussed below. All climbers should listen to their bodies and pay attention to the messages!

Reversing the Hypoxia of Altitude—The Most Obvious Treatment

If the hypoxia that results from going high is the cause of altitude sickness, the most direct treatment is to raise the blood oxygen level. The most obvious way to do this is to descend. Even a relatively modest descent (1,500 to 3,000 feet) may be enough to produce significant improvement in mild AMS symptoms, although climbers who have developed frank HACE or HAPE may need to descend further. If a climber develops more than mild AMS (and certainly if he or she develops HAPE or HACE), immediate descent or evacuation is mandatory.

If a climber develops more than mild AMS and immediate descent is not possible, he or she should receive supplemental oxygen to raise the blood oxygen level. This treatment is particularly vital in HAPE because the lung fluid symptomatic of this disorder can slow the diffusion of oxygen from lungs to blood, further reducing the blood oxygen level and contributing to the progression from AMS to full-blown HACE. In situations where supplemental oxygen is not available, a portable hyperbaric chamber, or *Gamow* bag (see page 225), can simulate descent and raise the blood oxygen level. The importance of descent and vigorous treatment for mountain sickness is underscored by one study that reported a mortality rate of 50 percent for Himalayan climbers who developed HAPE in a setting where descent was not possible and no treatment was available.

Preventive Medicine

Because many of those who go to the mountains are impatient, have little time to spare, or want to get up there quickly, use of preventive medication is enticing. We are accustomed to taking a pill for anything and everything—why not one to speed up adjustment to altitude? Why not, indeed!

Acetazolamide (Diamox)

One medication enables a climber to breathe more often or deeper without paying the price of an altered blood acidity. It has been proven an effective preventive over many decades, and its benefit is based on solid theory and controlled experiments as well as experience. Think of *acetazolamide*, widely known as Diamox, as an artificial acclimatizer. It blocks or slows the action of *carbonic anhydrase*, an enzyme that regulates the conversion of carbon dioxide to bicarbonate. When a climber takes acetazolamide, he or she excretes more bicarbonate (base) in the urine. This acidifies the blood and partially counteracts the loss of carbon dioxide and acid produced by the hypoxic ventilatory response (HVR). The end result of taking acetazolamide is a brisker HVR and higher blood oxygen levels. (See Chapter 13, "Acclimatization," for more detail on the impact of the HVR on blood acid levels.)

Because it helps to normalize the pH of blood, thus modifying the impact of pH on the respiratory center, Diamox also decreases the swings in respiration known as Cheyne-Stokes, or periodic, breathing during sleep. Some periodic breathing occurs normally in many people during sleep at sea level, but is exaggerated at altitude and in other cases of hypoxia. By smoothing out the fluctuations in arterial oxygen saturation, Diamox decreases the morning headache and the "wobbles" due to AMS. Currently there is some argument about just how Diamox decreases AMS, but the strong association between more normal breathing and lower incidence of AMS in almost all people taking Diamox is quite persuasive evidence.

For some (but not all) people, Diamox increases urine production and so interrupts sleep; because of this, some climbers do not favor its use. In fact it was originally developed as a diuretic, but prevention of AMS requires a small enough dose that the diuretic effect is slight. It is also used to treat glaucoma, as discussed in Chapter 9, "Vision and the Eye at Altitude."

For sixty years climbers have taken acetazolamide both to prevent and to treat AMS. Years ago, the recommended dosage was 250 mg three times a day, starting several days before the ascent. This dosage increased urination, especially at night, and caused some unpleasant symptoms. Now physicians generally recommend 125 mg once a day, at bedtime. This amount is effective for most people, causes few symptoms, and does not increase urine flow at night. If the lower dose does not prevent symptoms, one can increase the dose to 250 mg twice a day, starting on the day of ascent. It is important to tailor the dose to a person's experience or wishes, and over time an ideal dose can be found for each individual. Other authorities and many articles and books still suggest the larger dose. Because Diamox is an enzyme inhibitor and acts rapidly, you may not need to take it several days before starting your climb, as is sometimes advised. Delayed-action pills provide a sustained slow release, and some climbers prefer this. With the regular form, however, the dose can be adjusted rapidly if needed.

Some critics of Diamox say it is better to rely on natural acclimatization rather than on pills—and there is little quarrel with this. Others don't like the numbness and tingling in the fingers or lips, and the bad taste it gives to beer and other carbonated beverages. But these symptoms are absent or slight with the smaller dose, and probably indicate that one has more than enough of the medication on board. A rare individual who is oversensitive to sunlight may develop a rash while taking Diamox (as is true of many sulfa drugs). A few individuals feel nauseated or sick while taking Diamox, but this is unusual with the smaller dose. The few who are sensitive to sulfa or to sunlight should not take Diamox.

All things considered, the aphorism "if you can't take time, take Diamox" is good advice. But if you do take Diamox, start with a small dose and drink plenty of water. There is some good—but also a great amount of bad—advice on the Internet about Diamox use for climbing, so be wary of counsel from sources you do not have reason to trust. Unfortunately not all doctors are familiar with the proper dose of this very useful medicine—or, in fact, knowledgeable about altitude in general. Not many doctors will take time to explain why these suggestions are important. You, the climber or tourist, must take the initiative to learn—and teach. One doctor told his patient to keep her windows closed in the mountains to decrease lack of oxygen! A recent book about the 1996 Everest tragedy states categorically that Diamox is not a preventive but should be used only for treatment; this is completely false.

Dexamethasone

Another currently used preventive is *dexamethasone*, a steroid. Although its exact mechanism of action is unknown, this steroid blocks inflammation and vascular endothelial growth factor (VEGF) formation (see Chapter 7, "The Body Up High: Cellular and Vascular Responses to Hypoxia") and thus may decrease fluid and protein leakage from brain capillaries at high altitude. As a result, it may decrease brain swelling. Dexamethasone can be lifesaving in moderate to severe cases of AMS and in HACE, but offers no benefit in HAPE. Some climbers have used dexamethasone to prevent AMS, with success. However, the side effects of steroids (mood changes and elevated blood sugar, to name only two) and the availability of alternative prevention strategies (slow ascent and acetazolamide) make dexamethasone a poor choice for prevention of mountain sickness. Dexamethasone taken for a long time has also been reported to cause osteoporosis and gastric bleeding, but this is not a problem if used for a few days at altitude. The optimal dose for prevention is 2 to 4 mg twice a day.

Syringes loaded with dexamethasone were carried by many Everest climbers in 1996, and used by one or two in the emergency. The rationale was that it would give an added burst of energy, or decrease the hypoxic impact on the brain, but both of these are improbable because this steroid takes time to be effective, especially in the brain.

Both acetazolamide and dexamethasone require a doctor's prescription, but only Diamox has been certified by the FDA for preventing mountain sickness.

Other Medications

Nifedipine, a calcium channel blocker, relaxes the muscular layer of small arteries throughout the body and lowers blood pressure. This pulmonary artery dilator reverses hypoxia-induced constriction of the pulmonary arteries (hypoxic pulmonary vasoconstriction, or HPV), decreases pulmonary artery pressure, and reduces fluid movement out of the pulmonary capillaries, which makes it a valuable *treatment* for HAPE. However, it is generally necessary only when the climber cannot be given supplemental oxygen. It has been wrongly used to *prevent* AMS—which it does not do. Some recommend nifedipine to *prevent* HAPE (which it does), but because it may also lower systemic blood pressure, it should be used only by those who have had HAPE a few times and are considered HAPE-susceptible. These individuals are a recognized group (HAPE-S) and should be advised to take nifedipine if going above 8,000 to 9,000 feet. For dosage recommendations, see the section on treatment (page 221).

Beta-agonists, new to the field of high-altitude medicine, mimic some of the "fight or flight" responses. They act on a channel in the cells lining the alveoli (air sacs of the lung) that allows sodium to move from the alveoli into the cell lining. From there, sodium is pumped into the interstitial space by the sodium-potassium pump and is picked up by the blood vessels. Because water follows sodium, beta-agonists increase the clearance of water out of the alveoli and prevent pulmonary edema. (For more on the movement of sodium and water out of alveoli, see Chapter 7, "The Body Up High: Cellular and Vascular Responses to Hypoxia.") Inhaling the beta-agonist *salmeterol* may prevent HAPE, and some experts have suggested that this drug could be an effective treatment as well.

Nonsteroidal anti-inflammatory medications (NSAIDs), including aspirin and ibuprofen, also can be useful for the treatment of headache from AMS. However, this is a treatment of the symptom rather than a cure of the underlying problem.

Nitric oxide (NO—a gas), while clumsy to use, is an effective treatment for HAPE. It should not be used for prevention, however. *Nitroglycerine* tablets beneath the tongue have been unwisely used for treatment of HAPE, and certainly cannot be recommended for prevention or treatment.

Another preventive medication, *ammonium chloride* (to acidify the blood), was carefully studied and recommended many decades ago but has not been revisited for a long time. Newer coating materials may make the tablets less irritating to the stomach and yet allow them to dissolve in the small intestine. Ammonium chloride is worth another look. Rolaids have been touted by a few individuals, but have neither a scientific nor experiential justification.

There is a lot of interest in *alternative medication* to prevent AMS. Of these so-called natural drugs, the most popular is *Ginkgo biloba*. Extensive study has shown that ginkgo has, at best, only marginal benefit. As a preventive for AMS it is much less effective than acetazolamide. Visitors to La Paz and other high-altitude Andean cities are sometimes offered a variety of "altitude cocktails." These are various mixtures; one common ingredient is a small trace of *cocaine*, which acts as a euphoriant but has little if any effect on hypoxia. These cocktails are not worth the money, and they can render users insensitive to the very real challenges their bodies are facing. This is not advisable.

Other Means of Prevention

The possible value of brief repeated exposure to simulated altitude has been well publicized recently. Popular sports clubs and some fashionable hotels in the United States and in Europe offer low-oxygen "acclimatization" rooms where one can rest or exercise at a simulated high altitude in preparation for a climbing or ski trip to a mountain resort. Enticing though this method sounds, it remains unproven.

Japanese mountaineers and others have prepared for an assault on Everest by sleeping in decompression chambers at progressively higher simulated altitudes, but their climbing records do not show impressive benefits. With so many variables, it would be very difficult to arrange a statistically significant controlled study.

An ambitious French study called "Everest Turbo" ran a program to pre-acclimatize five elite mountaineers for an attempt on Everest. The procedure called for a week on Mont Blanc up to 15,000 feet, then many hours during the next four days going a little higher each day in a decompression chamber; they went up to 28,000 feet simulated altitude on the fourth day. Many tests were done every day. About a week later, after flying to Nepal, they were at 16,000 feet on Everest. Unfortunately, despite very rapid climbing, the weather turned them back at 24,000 feet.

The findings of this project suggest that continuous and then intermittent exposure to increasing altitude triggers acclimatization without the deterioration often encountered on a high mountain. A significant observation was that the subjects experienced dramatically fewer symptoms of AMS each day during the four days of intermittent exposure to increasing and very high altitudes. The study was an "experience" and not a practical effort to acclimatize.

A highly secret program to improve competitive edge by intermittent exposure to altitude was developed in 1969 for Olympic candidates in East Germany. The Kienbaum project is described in Chapter 17, "Limits to Work at Altitude."

All of these intermittent exposures to progressively higher altitudes are similar to the successful tactics used in "Alpinestyle" climbing, which are discussed in Chapter 13, "Acclimatization."

Interval Hypoxic Training

Interesting studies supported by the Russian Academy of Medical Sciences have been conducted in Moscow since 1989 at the Clinical Research Laboratory of the Hypoxia Medical Academy (HMA). This laboratory is testing the hypothesis that repeated brief exposures to lack of oxygen are useful for treating a variety of illnesses, and also in training for athletic performance. This concept would fit Selye's General Adaptation Syndrome, which was also described independently in Russia several decades ago.

Selye argued that any stress—injury, illness, or a hostile environment—provokes a general response by the endocrine system, which then causes adaptation leading to either recovery or failure. His specific evidence fills a very large book but can be simply defined in Figure 34.

The HMA's interval hypoxic training (IHT) consists of "courses" of cyclic repetition of brief normobaric hypoxic episodes and subsequent re-oxygenation. The intensity and duration of each "session" and the number of "sessions" in a "course" are customized for specific diseases and individuals. The air–oxygen mixture is exactly measured and administered by a calibrated machine, with oxygen provided through a membrane generator. A variety of illnesses are

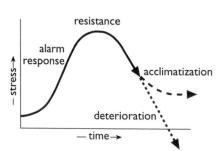

Figure 34. *Selye's General Adaptation Syndrome*

Selye's General Adaptation Syndrome

From 1936 to 1980, Dr. Hans Selye published 1,700 papers and thirty-nine books defining how organisms respond to stresses of different kinds. He concluded that response to any threat follows a general pattern of alarm, resistance, and outcome. Fortunately, in everyday life humans generally react by adjusting or accommodating, after which the physiological changes return to normal. If adjustment fails, deterioration results in either chronic illness or death.

Hypoxia is a classic example of a stressor in Selye's General Adaptation Syndrome. Hypoxia stimulates prompt alarm responses and resistance—the "struggle" responses. If the altitude is not too high, or the hypoxia too severe, the body acclimatizes by slowly replacing the "struggle" responses with those that are more sustainable. These changes enable humans to live permanently as high as 17,500 feet, or to live with illnesses that cause the same degree of hypoxia at sea level. Above 17,500 feet (or equivalent), deterioration sets in.

---

treated in different "courses" of varying length.

Results have been published in Russian in the Russian press, and in a quarterly journal in English published by the HMA. Few of the reports have appeared in peer-reviewed journals, which may explain the skepticism with which some American scientists regard the materials—but which few have read. Many of HMA's studies appear to have been carefully done, well controlled, and statistically significant, although exact procedures are not always well described.

Dr. E. N. Takchuk, director of the HMA, explains why she believes the treatments are effective:

Mechanisms of IHT include both central mechanisms of neuro-humoral regulation and local regulatory mechanisms. This is the reason for the increase in efficacy of the oxygen-transporting and oxygen-utilizing systems at all levels of the organism, similar to the physiological acclimatization as a result of prolonged altitude exposure....

IHT effectively decreased the response of pulmonary ventilation and heart rate to a physical load (the effect similar to that observed in altitude exposure).... At a load of 150 watts, the double product (heart rate multiplied by systolic blood pressure), an indirect measure of myocardial oxygen consumption, was significantly lower ($p<0.04$) in the group of volunteers (sports students) after the IHT course as compared with placebo group. Similar results were obtained in patients with coronary heart disease (stable angina of effort). At a load of 50 watts, the decrease of the double product was accompanied by the increase of physical load tolerance ($p<0.05$). [When the load was further increased, the benefit attributed to IHT was increased (p<0.01).] The above results suggest the outlook for the therapeutic use of IHT.

IHT might be considered for use in altitude preacclimatization.... The placebo controlled study was carried out...on young healthy volunteers...at the altitude of 3,000 meters (10,000 feet) in the decompression chamber.... [The course of IHT] was shown to retain significantly higher arterial blood oxygen saturation (p<0.05) than placebo controls.

[There was] a statistically significant 1.7-fold increase in erythropoietin level in blood...from the fourth IHT session, with the level remaining high during the IHT course.

The HMA has used IHT to decrease the rise in epinephrine and glucose in pregnant women before and immediately after Caesarean section delivery. Good results have been claimed in treatment of rheumatoid arthritis, chronic bronchitis, and asthma, and in preparation for general surgery. IHT is also used in training for competitive sports, allegedly decreasing the product of heart rate times blood pressure (the *double product*, a rough measure of fitness) during a set level of performance.

One element common to the wide variety of illnesses reportedly benefited by IHT appears to be stress, which IHT is said to decrease "through neuro–humoral and local regulatory mechanisms." This is not unreasonable, in keeping with Selye's General Adaptation Syndrome. The procedure is interesting and possibly an important alternative approach to stress, and perhaps a helpful means of acclimatizing to high altitude. Another possible explanation is that IHT may work by stimulating increased rate and depth of respiration and by increasing red blood cell production. While keeping an open mind, it is nevertheless appropriate to reserve judgment until more detailed information is widely available, and until similar results are obtained by others using the same procedures.

PREVENTIVE STRATEGIES FOR WORK AT HIGH ALTITUDE

Mines have been operated at 10,000 to 14,000 feet in the Andes for many centuries. Some mining companies have been developing new approaches because valuable minerals are now being mined at altitudes over 20,000 feet. One program calls for high-altitude miners to work every day and to go down several thousand feet to sleep, with an occasional homestay at low altitude, even though daily travel time takes away from work time, and transportation is expensive. Some of the miners get mild AMS, and a few are said to have experienced re-entry HAPE from this yo-yo life.

A new proposal is now being tested at the mine site by providing sleeping quarters near the mine in which, overnight, a steady flow of oxygen sustains an oxygen partial pressure equivalent to that at 10,000 to 12,000 feet. This may prove to be a more effective and efficient way of adjusting people for prolonged high-altitude work.

A few resort areas at 10,000 feet have considered making similar rooms available, where tourists who are feeling the altitude can sit and read, exercise, or even sleep in a higher oxygen partial pressure. None have been made available so far, possibly because of safety restrictions, but the idea appears to have merit.

In competitive athletics, one attempt to gain a competitive edge is to live at altitude and to train there in an oxygen-enriched room, which would enable training at peak intensity, while acclimatizing during the night. This technique, which is almost the mirror image of the "carry high and sleep low" strategy, may be efficient in time and money but, like other training programs, has not been adequately tested—and because of the many variables is difficult to test well. This and other training strategies are discussed in Chapter 17, "Limits to Work at Altitude."

Diet and Vitamins

Can you prevent mountain sickness and adjust more rapidly to altitude if you add vitamins, minerals, and other supplements to your diet? This depends on your usual diet—which, under some conditions, may not be adequate. For those subsisting mostly on expedition supplies for a few weeks, added vitamins may be a good idea. Dozens of diets have been recommended for big expeditions, but appetites are capricious and fade at high altitude. Absorption of food from the intestinal tract is thought (but not proven) to be impaired at very high altitude, bowel action is often a problem, and in the end the carefully planned diet usually comes down to food that the individual finds most palatable and easily digested.

If you do take vitamins, nutritionists advise a balanced formula rather than large doses of one or two. Despite a good bit of publicity, no research indicates that vitamin E, or any other vitamin, improves tolerance for altitude. Folic acid (folate) may be shown to be important at high altitude because it sharply reduces homocysteine in the blood. (A high level of homocysteine is associated with a higher risk of heart disease, stroke, and other vascular diseases.) But this has yet to be explored.

The popularity of vitamins ebbs and flows, depending on the intensity with which they are promoted commercially. Many people hunger for a panacea or elixir of health, and are willing to pay without looking critically at the promised benefits.

Adding an iron supplement is important if iron stores in the body are low—but you have to test your blood to know if this is the case for you. Because many women do have low iron reserves and some are actually iron-deficient, added iron is reasonable for young women going to altitude for a long time. The benefits of supplements of other minerals like selenium, calcium, and trace substances never have been carefully evaluated. Here too there are shifting vogues and fashions.

There is a good theoretical basis for believing that a diet high in carbohydrate with virtually no fat or protein decreases the chances of mountain illnesses. In practice, though, a pure carbohydrate diet becomes distasteful after a day or two. Recent studies of a diet that is 70 percent carbohydrate have shown no benefit in preventing mountain sicknesses.

Generally accepted is a game plan for eating frequent small, high-carbohydrate snacks during the working day, and adding protein at night. A few special high-carbohydrate products have been touted, but so far no well-controlled study at altitude has been reported.

For years climbers have been urged to drink extra water, and there is a good basis for this. In an earlier chapter it was suggested that on high mountains you should consume less alcohol because "one drink does the work of two" at altitude. This is an unproven recommendation, awaiting a good controlled study, which might be a rather attractive project. The rationale is that the effects of hypoxia and alcohol on the brain and its functions are similar—and additive. Alcohol is one of the few substances that passes rapidly through the blood-brain barrier into the brain.

Fitness

Finally, there is the vexing question of physical fitness. Does the fit and trim athlete tolerate high altitude better than the couch potato? The short answer is "not exactly." In Chapter 17, "Limits to Work at Altitude," this is discussed in a little more detail. The cheering fact is that the trained athlete and the experienced mountaineer climb more efficiently, with less exertion, and therefore use and need less oxygen than the neophyte to make the same climb.

It is not a waste of time to train before any climb that will place you at high altitude. The more fit you are, the less of your total physical capacity you need to use on any given day, and the more reserve you have for hardships higher on the mountain. How rigorously to train is difficult to say. Most athletes rely on sports-specific training regimes, but climbing is such a "total body" exercise that these may be difficult to define for climbing. Logically, one would expect that increasing muscle fitness of arms and legs would be most helpful. If you are a bit overweight, should you trim down, eat a bit less, toughen up, run more? That probably is a good idea—but in the olden days one great climber deliberately gained a dozen pounds before going to a major peak so he would have some fat to lose. Some arctic expeditioners say they are ready to begin their trips when they are "fit and fat," but this is obviously an individual preference.

From all the studies that have been done in laboratories and from actual experience on mountains, only two strategies have been proven to prevent or minimize mountain sicknesses: slow rate of ascent and use of acetazolamide. Others remain to be substantiated.

TREATMENT OF MOUNTAIN SICKNESSES

Obviously, the treatment for lack of oxygen from any cause is to get more oxygen to the cells. In clinical illness or injury, it is sometimes difficult to change the basic problem, but breathing extra oxygen usually helps. In the mountains treatment is often simple—get down to thicker air, with a degree of urgency that depends on the problem.

Acute Mountain Sickness

Most symptoms of simple acute mountain sickness (AMS) fade away in twenty-four to forty-eight hours and do not require any treatment except the conservative approach described earlier in this chapter. If the mild symptoms are bothersome, 125 mg or 250 mg of *Diamox* or 4 mg of *dexamethasone* every six hours will help; if one is already taking either of these, extra doses can be added. Breathing supplementary oxygen during the night will likely improve sleep if insomnia is a problem, and will make one feel better in the morning. Periodic breathing, often a cause of insomnia, is relieved by low-flow oxygen and almost eliminated by a small bedtime dose of Diamox.

Nausea or vomiting, troublesome symptoms of AMS, can be helped by one of the many anti-emetic medicines available. *Compazine,* an old standby, is still used. *Zofran,* a treatment for motion sickness, has proven to be quite effective in decreasing nausea and vomiting in AMS (although it does not seem to have any effect on other symptoms of the disease). As soon as vomiting stops, it is important to replace fluids (as well as in case of diarrhea, which is not common in AMS and more likely due to something else) with small sips of tea, slightly salted water, or diluted juice. If an intravenous solution and set is available, fluids might be given by vein. If the victim is very dehydrated, water can, with some difficulty, be given by rectum, and dexamethasone can be added to the water in an urgent case.

If the headache of AMS is quite bad, *ibuprofen* usually is a little more effective than *aspirin*; breathing supplemental oxygen for a few minutes wipes out the headache quickly—but it tends to return after a while. Various medications used to treat or prevent migraines have been tried for altitude headache, but none has proven to be effective.

High Altitude Cerebral Edema

If the headache of AMS worsens or early warnings like confusion or a stumbling walk (ataxia) appear, medical advice is important, because these symptoms mean that the problem has moved toward the high altitude cerebral edema (HACE) end of the AMS/HACE spectrum. More dexamethasone by mouth may help, but it is more effective and faster if given by injection or intravenously. A careful medical examination is important to determine if immediate descent is imperative. Of course, on a big mountain or away from medical care, that may be out of the question, and one can only carefully watch developments and treat them with one's best judgment. Discretion should dictate descent before things get out of hand. Even a descent by the sick party with assistance is far easier than an evacuation. Breathing oxygen will buy time, but do not mess around with HACE: Evacuating a semiconscious patient with HACE is very serious business. Helping a semiconscious but walking patient is a lot better than trying to carry him or her a day later! The pressurizable Gamow bag is discussed later in this chapter. It is a good way to buy time when the victim is far from help and evacuation will be long and difficult, but it does not always work. Once the diagnosis is clear, it is best to get down!

> During the early days of the Mount Logan project, a young paratrooper was flown from 2,500 to 17,500 feet. He was in charge of a small squad, which might explain why he did not mention his headache as it grew worse. By day's end he was obviously confused, and sixteen hours after arrival he became comatose. The radio was nonfunctional for several crucial hours, delaying rescue. During midnight evacuation by air I thought he would die. But by the time we reached low altitude, his alarming periodic breathing had become normal, and my partner and I thought it best to hold him at our base laboratory and give him large doses of dexamethasone intravenously. He regained consciousness eight hours later and made a rapid and complete recovery.

In retrospect, several things are worth mentioning. First, in those days we took a big risk by flying people directly from 2,500 to 17,500 feet in ninety minutes. Even in 1968 there was enough experience to show the likelihood of serious altitude illness. Second, lack of a way to get down except by air was also dangerous, and in this case, a temporarily inactive radio delayed evacuation for several hours, which could have been disastrous to the victim. Third, although he was given oxygen at the high laboratory, he did not improve. This is an alarming sign, as others have since learned on high mountains. Finally, it might seem a mistake that the victim was not flown to a fully equipped hospital, but the rationale was that the best experts were on hand.

High Altitude Pulmonary Edema

If the normal and expected shortness of breath of high altitude gets worse, or if a cough appears, perhaps with some frothy, pink, or bloody sputum, the problem is probably high altitude pulmonary edema (HAPE). Even an inexperienced person can often hear rattles and wheezes and crackles in the chest of a HAPE victim that do not disappear after a cough, strong evidence of HAPE. This can progress rapidly from a serious to a lethal situation.

In HAPE, *nifedipine* (50 to 100 mg) by mouth usually improves breathing and decreases the cough in less than an hour, and is faster and more effective than oxygen. Nifedipine rapidly lowers pulmonary artery pressure. It may also lower systemic blood pressure and cause dizziness or faintness, so the smaller dose should be tried first. If the improvement wears off, as judged by worsening of cough, cyanosis, or dyspnea, the dose can be repeated every hour or two—or given intravenously.

But descent should not be delayed. Getting down a few thousand feet almost always improves the situation, often dramatically. Strong diuretics such as *Lasix (furosemide)* are potentially dangerous and are not always effective; they should not be used except in extreme circumstances.

In 1969 while we were working on the Mount Logan study, a young climber in another party became weak and short of breath at 14,000 feet and was half-carried down to 9,000 feet, where both his lungs were found to be filled with fluid and HAPE was obvious. High-flow oxygen did not improve his rapidly worsening condition, so he was given several doses of Lasix. He did not diurese, and in a few hours became shocky and then unconscious. I flew through a gathering storm in a small helicopter and brought him down. To add fuel from a reserve gas can, we landed on a moraine at 4,000 feet. The patient roused enough to leave the aircraft and pass a very large amount of urine. When we landed at 2,500 feet, he was alert and able to walk around and even joke, and although his pulmonary rales took several days to disappear, he recovered rapidly and completely.

This young man would have died had he not been brought down, and it seems likely that the diuretic had worsened his condition until descent may have enhanced its effect. Herb Hultgren has described HAPE patients who were ambulatory until loss of fluid by diuretic caused shock due to a sharp fall in blood volume and complicated rescue.

The most effective treatment for HAPE depends on release of nitric oxide (NO) in the lung, which lowers pulmonary artery pressure. Nifedipine, a calcium channel blocker that is effective in lowering pulmonary artery pressure (PAP) and relieving HAPE, also may cause significant lowering of the systemic blood pressure. Other activators of NO are not as effective. Recently, Viagra in a dose of 25 mg every three to four hours has proven to be effective in treating HAPE (and does not produce the other major effect of sexual performance enhancement induced by larger doses). A new, long-acting NO activator called Cialis has appeared, and although it has not been fully tested in the treatment or prevention of HAPE it does show promise. Should drugs like Viagra and Cialis be used to prevent HAPE by those who are going to the mountains and know they are susceptible to this disorder?

While more research is needed before answering this question definitively, existing studies of diseases like idiopathic pulmonary hypertension, in which patients have high pulmonary artery pressure at sea level, may be helpful.

Morphine has been used to treat HAPE because it slows the rapid respirations seen in HAPE victims. However, this drug is potentially dangerous in HAPE because it may suppress breathing, even though it does relieve the pulmonary hypertension and decrease alveolar fluid. Strong diuretics and morphine are treatments of last resort.

A small masklike device is sometimes helpful in treatment (as in prevention) by increasing the pressure of exhalation, which increases the alveolar gas pressures slightly, holds the alveoli open, and enhances gas exchange at the pulmonary membrane. This allows the wearer to inspire easily, but requires him or her to breathe out against a spring-loaded valve. This simple device has been quite helpful at night for patients with moderate chronic obstructive pulmonary disease (COPD), helping them to sleep, as does low-flow oxygen, but it is not clear yet whether either the mask or nighttime oxygen changes the long-term course of COPD. It does seem to benefit a few HAPE patients.

This device is similar in principle and action to something called "grunt breathing," advocated by some mountaineers. This technique originated during World War II as an emergency breathing method for airmen who lost their oxygen supply at a dangerous altitude, and early tests appeared to show it was effective. However, further studies showed that the emergency (pressure) breathing procedure (EBP) was no better than simple overbreathing without the grunt!

> *In my altitude training unit, we proved that deliberate, careful hyperventilation, or overbreathing, increased the arterial oxygen saturation as much or more than EBP. The subjects performing the deliberate overbreathing could maintain consciousness while doing assigned tasks (without oxygen) for an hour during several test flights in a B-24 bomber aircraft at 25,000 feet. In fact, the extra effort of "grunt breathing" uses more oxygen than simple overbreathing. In a then-confidential report, brief training in controlled overbreathing was recommended as an emergency survival method at altitude.*

A word of caution: Any voluntary increase in respiration must be carefully done to avoid excess, because it washes out carbon dioxide and causes anxiety, tremor, tingling in face and fingers, and soon severe muscular arm cramps and even unconsciousness from alkalosis. Try it—but be careful. Nor are these measures the best prevention or treatment, and they should not delay more effective measures (as has happened in one or two instances).

Simply exhaling against pursed lips may also increase alveolar pressure slightly, and without grunting. In fact many asthmatics have known for years that this is a good way to open airways and to breathe more easily. There are no controlled studies to show how much, if any, this technique increases arterial oxygen saturation.

The Pressurizable Bag

On a mountain, there are three ways to get more oxygen into the lungs: (1) going down to thicker air, (2) breathing supplementary oxygen, and (3) increasing the atmospheric pressure around the victim. This last can be done in some sort of pressurized bag or room in which the patient is placed and the opening sealed while an air pump increases the pressure.

The best-known device in the United States is the cylindrical Gamow bag, made of tough canvas or plastic with a clear window, a tight-locking zipper, and safety tapes around the cylinder. Pressure is increased in the bag through a tube from a pump of some kind, with a pressure relief valve to prevent overpressurizing. Some form of absorbent for carbon dioxide is necessary inside the bag, because the pump cannot move enough air to get rid of the carbon dioxide exhaled by the patient as fast as it is produced. Different sized and shaped bags or "tents" are available, for one patient or a patient and attendant.

The sick person is placed inside the bag lying down, and communicates with helpers by voice; occasionally a small radio is used. A pulse oximeter to measure arterial oxygen saturation is helpful, but basically the patient's appearance and clinical condition determine the course of events. The bag is inflated and maintained at about two pounds pressure above the outside atmosphere; this "takes the patient down" several thousand feet, which is sometimes enough to relieve the problem for several hours. But if HACE or HAPE is severe, the bag gives only brief benefit; descent is mandatory.

Using the bag plus dexamethasone is slightly more beneficial than using either alone, and should be tried early in severe cases, but again, do not delay descent. In the mountains, there is no question that the bag has saved lives in difficult circumstances far from definitive care. In some cases the bag has enabled a victim to recover enough to totter down to safety or rescue.

In several instances it has improved the individual enough to go on climbing higher. This is not an appropriate use because symptoms are likely to return in a few hours. In one case the second attack that followed when the climber went up the next day was fatal. The bag is not worth using where oxygen and skilled care are quickly available, as in mountain resorts.

Most models are difficult or impossible to use during a carry-out, but they do protect the critically ill patient in camp. Although some victims have been in a bag for many hours, most become restless as they improve and do not tolerate the bag for more than a few hours. It is also difficult to monitor vital signs or to give medication without releasing pressure for a brief time, which may undo some of the benefit.

The pressurizable bag is a special instrument that is valuable in limited circumstances but should never be seen as a substitute for descent to more complete treatment. Unfortunately, this is not adequately recognized; guidelines are under consideration to make a pressurizable bag a requirement on big expeditions to high mountains (and even on treks), not so much because of need, but for fear of litigation if a bag is not available when and if needed. It is unfortunate that in the effort to cover all bases and protect people from every hazard, fear of lawsuits has made life so complicated—and not only in the mountains!

Clearly, acute altitude illness is a serious medical condition that can develop rapidly and threaten the life of a climber. Unfortunately, altitude sickness all too often develops in circumstances where descent, the most obvious and effective treatment, is difficult or impossible. This places a premium on preventing AMS/HACE and HAPE. Climbers should be aware not just of the symptoms of these diseases, but of their own limitations, and act accordingly. Newer, more effective treatments are being developed all the time. While these are welcome, they will never replace the need for caution and common sense.

CHAPTER

OPERATION EVEREST I AND II

In the spring of 1941 it seemed likely that the United States would be involved in the war that was engulfing much of Europe and Asia. I wanted to be involved. In late spring I applied for a commission in the Medical Corps of the United States Navy. I was secretly engaged to the lady who would be my head nurse during my residency, and when we both finished on July 2 we were quietly married. In August I received my commission, and we returned home. Thanks to an introduction from Dr. Ross McFarland, an expert in aviation medicine, we arranged to meet with Captain J. C. Adams, the U.S. Navy's chief flight surgeon. We drove down to Washington and spent an hour with him. He asked about my experience at high altitude, which was considerably more than that of most American doctors at that time. At the end of a very pleasant interview he summoned his aide and dictated orders for me to be sent to Pensacola, Florida, to enter training as a flight surgeon, and from there I would go to one of the newly established altitude training units.

Aircraft of the day were able to go higher than a pilot could fly without supplementary oxygen, and even with supplementary oxygen there was some risk. The oxygen equipment was primitive, and pilots had very little idea of how to use it, or of what could happen if they ran out of oxygen at high altitude. Older pilots boasted that they could fly to 18,000 or 20,000 feet without using oxygen at all, although they were certainly impaired if they stayed up long enough.

After graduating with my wings as a flight surgeon, and knowing a little more about high-altitude physiology than when I started, my wife and I drove north, stopping in Virginia on December 7, where that afternoon we heard about the attack on Pearl Harbor. I immediately reported for duty in Norfolk, Virginia, where I stayed for three or four months working in the dispensary, and then went to the altitude training camp in Jacksonville. The training protocols in 1941 were primitive. The Navy, and I believe the Army as well, used exposure in a high-altitude decompression chamber to separate fighter pilots, who flew higher, from the bomber pilots, who would fly lower. It was, as we soon discovered, a ridiculous screening process. Beyond that, our task was to teach pilots and aircrew how to use the equipment and what to do when the equipment failed. I had studied a great deal more about high altitude than my immediate superior, a regular Navy lieutenant. We soon disagreed on certain things, and I was outraged when I found out that he was sending inaccurate reports to Washington about the altitude chamber. One thing led to another, I was reprimanded for discourtesy to an officer, confined to quarters for four days, and promoted to lieutenant commander. Orders came to transfer me to Miami, where I was stationed at the fighter base. My command was the altitude-training unit, with a small crew of hospital corpsmen and staff officers. We developed and promoted our own flight training program, and, somewhat chastened by having been disciplined by the admiral, I was much better behaved. After a few episodes in which equipment in the decompression chamber failed and one of the passengers collapsed, it became apparent to me that there was little gain in telling aircrew to use their oxygen. It would be a more powerful lesson if we taught them what to do when the oxygen equipment failed. Therefore, without authorization, I began a procedure of asking one of the pilots in the decompression chamber to remove his oxygen mask at 20,000 feet, telling him to replace the mask when he felt anything unusual. We pressed urgently that he put on his mask before he lost consciousness. In the next few years as we used this demonstration on three or four of the pilots or aircrew in each decompression chamber run, I cannot recall more than a dozen men replacing their oxygen equipment before passing out. It was a very dramatic and persuasive demonstration. I reported this through channels to Captain Adams in Washington, and shortly afterwards received a letter stating in rather gentle terms that I was not complying with the directives, that there were risks attached, and that if I continued to do the procedure it would be at my own risk! I read between the lines that he wanted me to continue, and we did so. Following a long period of clinical research we demonstrated that voluntary hyperventilation could prolong consciousness when oxygen failed. This was dramatically demonstrated when I borrowed two B-24 bombers and took an entire crew to 25,000 feet, where we flew for about one hour. One pilot and one member of the flight crew who volunteered to hyperventilate removed their masks and demonstrated that they could fly for forty-five minutes, and that the gunner was able to operate his gun for roughly the same amount of time. Those who had not been instructed usually passed out within two minutes.

At the end of the war I was sent back to Pensacola, and there the great altitude chambers lay empty and unused. It was there it occurred to me that we had a perfect opportunity to test whether or not a man could survive in the thin air at the summit of Mount Everest, weaning him slowly over a period of several weeks in the chamber. That idea became Operation Everest and, forty years later, a repeat study called Operation Everest II.

When the height of Mount Everest was measured in 1856, it excited little interest among mountaineers. This disinterest remained for forty years, because many believed that spending a night above 20,000 feet would be fatal. Besides, Tibet was firmly closed to foreigners. But as the nineteenth century ended, a handful of explorers had begun to climb higher and sleep higher, and the highest summits beckoned. Leading mountaineers wondered: Could Everest be climbed?

After Paul Bert showed that lack of oxygen caused altitude sickness, which could be treated or prevented by breathing oxygen, his colleagues Croce-Spinelli and Sivel died in a hot air balloon when they ran out of oxygen while ascending almost as high as the summit of Everest. (See the account in Chapter 13, "Acclimatization.") To many, this put Everest—without oxygen—beyond reach. Others were more optimistic.

Surgeon–mountaineer Clinton Dent thought the climb possible, but barely so. In 1918 chemist–climber Alexander Kellas, projecting from data at lower elevations, agreed. Climaxing the 1924 attempt on Everest, Lieutenant Colonel Edward Norton, one of the more experienced Himalayan climbers, reached 28,300 feet without supplementary oxygen, only 800 feet below the summit, where the oxygen pressure in air is only 2 to 3 torr higher than on the summit. This was a record that would stand for fifty years. In 1953 Edmund Hillary and Sherpa Tenzing Norgay reached the top breathing supplementary oxygen. Since 1975, more than one hundred people have summited Everest breathing only the air around them, and now there is nowhere higher to climb. But many have died from the combined stresses of high mountains.

Lack of oxygen is not the only problem on high mountains, and by 1940 climbers began to ask a new question: How much does the almost unavoidable cold, exhaustion, thirst, fear, and hunger affect performance and even survival on the highest peaks? How could the effect of these additional stresses be measured?

This chapter describes two studies of acclimatization in which Charles Houston was a key player. Because the data were unique at the time, and may be of interest to scientists reading this book, some details are included. For the nonscientific reader, this may be hard going, although descriptions are given in nonmedical terms. The following is Charles Houston's firsthand account.

OPERATION EVEREST I, 1946

I proposed to the Navy a project, to be called Operation Everest (OE), in which my team would study acclimatization to hypoxia in a warm, comfortable setting. We hypothesized that our findings would be relevant to illnesses causing hypoxia at sea level. Of greater importance to the military, the study would also compare the maximum altitude achievable by unacclimatized men breathing oxygen with the altitude that could be reached by well-acclimatized men also breathing oxygen. Such acclimatization could have provided air combat superiority in those days. For mountaineers, we would see if acclimatized men could reach 29,000 feet breathing only the ambient air.

The Navy approved the proposal for Operation Everest five months after it was requested. Four healthy young men volunteered as subjects to live in a cramped decompression chamber for thirty-five days, during which time the chamber would be gradually decompressed. Recruiting scientists was more difficult because many thought the project either dangerous or foolish.

Our plans called for "climbing" to 8,000 to 9,000 feet in one or two days and thereafter decompressing the chamber at a rate equivalent to climbing 2,000 to 3,000 feet a day. When we felt acclimatization was adequate, we would have the subjects taken to 29,000 feet during a long eight-hour "climb." Detailed protocols were prepared for measuring the more important changes we expected and would be able to measure inside the chamber.

A laboratory with the best equipment available at the time was staffed by several experts, and the Navy loaned us a nutritionist. The chamber was staffed by a crew of thirty enlisted men and petty officers, standing four-hour watches in pairs around the clock. My partner Dick Riley and I were assisted by student flight surgeons; I lived in a room next to the chamber for the duration.

After the volunteer subjects had been examined and all equipment thoroughly checked, the massive steel door of the chamber was closed on June 28, 1946, and after three days at sea level for control studies, the subjects "took off."

During the next thirty-five days, the chamber was kept warm and humid and continuously ventilated, carbon dioxide was absorbed, and the oxygen level in the chamber air was monitored. The barometric pressure in the chamber was measured by aircraft altimeters, calibrated with a mercury barometer to the International Civil Aviation Organization (ICAO) altitude–pressure curve.

Arterial blood and alveolar air samples were taken repeatedly, and pulmonary ventilation was measured at rest and during and after exercise up to 20,000 feet. Electrocardiograms were recorded every few days and chest X rays taken at seven altitudes. We did not try to do very many studies but rather to do well those we did undertake. The subjects were well fed and encouraged to take fluids, but neither fluid intake nor output was measured. Three of the four subjects smoked cigarettes. Two exercised every day on a stationary cycle or climbing bars, but the others worked out only sporadically.

During the slow ascent, the subjects said they felt well but with occasional mild headaches, periodic breathing during sleep, and easy fatigue. As seen by observers sitting at sea level, the subjects appeared to be increasingly impaired although they "felt just fine," as the chamber was slowly "climbed."

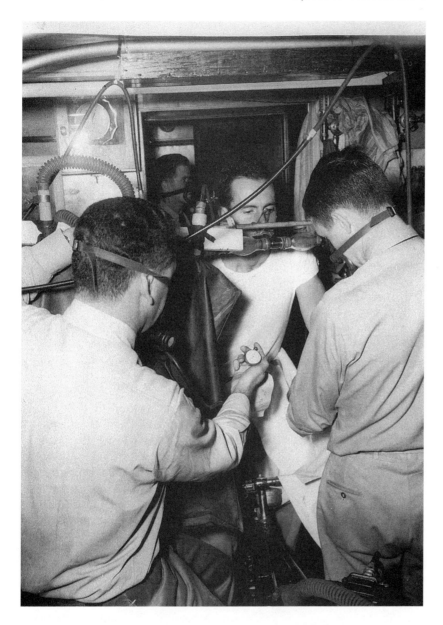

Figure 35. *Operation
Everest I decompression
chamber*

*We worried that, without the hypoxic drive to breathe, they might stop
breathing if some emergency required that the chamber be taken abruptly
to sea level. We also were concerned that their hearts might dilate, as had
been reported by Dr. Somervell on the early Everest climbs.*

*After four days at 22,000 feet, the chamber was "taken up" at the rate
of 1,000 feet an hour. Each subject rode the stationary cycle briefly every*

hour. At 26,700 feet one man requested oxygen, and a second did so 1,000 feet higher. The other two continued, and after eight hours reached 29,025 feet according to the aircraft altimeter. Both were alert and cycled for a short time, but appeared to be close to their limit. After twenty minutes we brought the chamber down to 20,000 feet.

These two men had shown that the hypoxia on top of Everest would not rapidly kill acclimatized men. But the eight hours for the final ascent from 22,000 feet had been too fast, and it was obvious that our men could not have done the hours of heavy work needed for the actual climb. Nor were they fully acclimatized.

On the following day the two subjects were taken slowly to 50,525 feet breathing oxygen, watched from outside the chamber by sea-level observers who could not tolerate that high an altitude, even breathing 100 percent oxygen. Both subjects were alert, weak, and yet able to function moderately well. Because sea-level pilots are seriously impaired at 42,000 feet even breathing 100 percent oxygen, we concluded that acclimatization had clearly raised the altitude ceiling of our partially acclimatized subjects. Of great interest at that time, the accomplishment was soon moot because all aircraft would be pressurized to provide a low cabin altitude.

The information collected during OE I was unique because it was the first time humans had been observed, by scientists at sea level, as they acclimatized to increasing altitude. Absent the powerful stresses on a high mountain, these subjects experienced only the hypoxia of decreased barometric pressure, although it is true they were confined and unable to exercise very much.

Some of the observations can be summarized in a few sentences; the full data are given in one of my published papers describing OE I and II. Pulmonary ventilation increased steadily with altitude as expected. Hemoglobin, hematocrit, and arterial oxygen capacity increased steadily. Arterial carbon dioxide fell and pH rose. When we plotted blood oxygen saturation against oxygen pressure on the oxy–hemoglobin dissociation curve for the appropriate pH, there appeared to be a shift to the right. Resting pulse rate

TABLE 10
ALVEOLAR GASES (MEASUREMENTS IN TORR)
(Supplemental oxygen was not used.)

	Oxygen	Carbon Dioxide
Four subjects at 26,000 ft	26, 26, 30, 31	17, 16, 14, 14
Two subjects at 28,200 ft	23, 24	15, 13
Two subjects at 29,030 ft	23, 21	13, 14
Same subjects second time	24, 22	13, 14
Normal sea-level values	100	40

increased and cardiac output increased two to three times the sea-level value. Electrocardiograms and X rays showed no evidence of cardiac enlargement or strain. Of some interest are the alveolar–arterial oxygen gradients, which decreased with increasing altitude almost to zero at 20,000 feet, the highest point where we drew arterial blood. All A–a gradients increased sharply with exercise at high altitude.

As expected, alveolar oxygen pressures decreased with altitude, but were partially sustained at the expense of a fall in carbon dioxide, due to the increasing ventilation. Not shown here is the decrease in work capacity with altitude; although improved by breathing oxygen, it did not reach sea-level capacity.

From this study—a "pure culture" of hypoxia without the confounding effects of the mountain environment—we showed that people could live and do light work for a short time at the height of Mount Everest. In fact, the "physiological altitude" at the "summit" in the chamber was about 1,000 feet higher than it would be on the actual mountain, because above 23,000 feet the ICAO calibrated altimeter (which we used) gave measurements several torr lower than those actually measured years later on top of Everest.

We could not measure the extent of acclimatization, but a volunteer brought to 22,500 feet from sea level collapsed in one minute and twenty seconds while riding the stationary cycle after his oxygen mask was removed. In contrast, one of the acclimatized subjects cycled for twenty minutes until bored.

As the altitude increased, the subjects slowly became less interested in various activities and less inclined to exercise. They had occasional headaches but not the full picture of mountain sickness. None complained of the sore throat or cough so common on high mountains. Appetites declined and they all lost weight. All had periodic breathing, and above 22,000 feet their cyanosis and general appearance during sleep was worrisome enough for us to monitor their pulse rates electronically, and even to keep a flight surgeon in the chamber for a few nights. Having myself spent many days above 24,000 feet, I appreciated how these subjects felt, but was worried by how badly they appeared to us unaffected sea-level observers. In Chapter 10, "HAPE: High Altitude Pulmonary Edema," it was shown how Haldane appeared to those who were watching him and Kellas from outside the decompression chamber; the subjects in OE I were slightly less affected.

Of special interest to military aviation in that era, we showed that this degree of acclimatization could significantly raise the "ceiling" for pilots breathing oxygen.

We were greatly relieved to see that the subjects were breathing normally when they descended in a few hours to sea level and showed no ill effects from their exposure. The frequent X rays had shown no sign whatsoever of cardiac enlargement.

OPERATION EVEREST II, 1985

Air warfare in World War II stimulated interest in altitude research, and more studies of high altitude on mountains were done in the next twenty years: Among the many studies were the Silver Hut expedition near Everest (1960–61), the High Altitude Physiology Studies (HAPS) on Mount Logan (1967–75), and the American Research Expedition (AMREE) to Mount Everest (1981). (See Chapter 13, "Acclimatization," for details on these studies.) These and many others added greatly to our understanding of acclimatization—in the harsh mountain environment.

By 1980 it seemed appropriate to repeat Operation Everest with a more ambitious agenda, in a larger decompression chamber, again in a controlled environment. There we could use modern techniques to study hypobaric hypoxia in a setting in which many sophisticated studies could be done safely and conveniently.

It took five years to recruit scientists and subjects and to find money, but eventually the Army Research and Development Command agreed to cover the anticipated expense. The Army Research Institute of Environmental Medicine (ARIEM) in Natick, Massachusetts, provided a large decompression chamber and staff for six weeks. In September 1985, eight male subjects and two alternates completed baseline studies at ARIEM and were approved for the project. Much as we wished to include women subjects, the numbers would be too small, and female hormonal cycles might confound the data and blur our conclusions.

We wanted the rate of ascent to be slower than in OE I, hoping for more complete acclimatization, but a number of factors led to an ascent profile only a little less rapid.

Like the 1946 study, OE II was planned to be a "pure culture" of hypobaric hypoxia, without the cold, privation, and physical and mental stress unavoidable on a very high mountain. Ample water, appetizing meals, and ready access to stationary cycle and treadmill exercise resembled a sea-level setting. The chamber was kept warm and humid; entertainments were provided. Although the studies were demanding on both subjects and scientists, the subjects had time for rest and recreation. Most of them exercised regularly and they were watched day and night through ports in the chamber.

The Oxygen Cascade in Acclimatization

OE II focused on how changes in the oxygen cascade (see Chapter 3, "Moving Air: Respiration," and Chapter 13, "Acclimatization") affected acclimatization. Pulmonary ventilation and diffusion characteristics were measured by standard techniques.

We assessed heart function by cardiac catheterization (passing a thin catheter through a vein into the right side of the heart and then into the artery carrying blood to the lungs) done on each subject at three different altitudes, at rest and during and after exertion, and included pulmonary and systemic arterial pressures; mixed venous oxygen was also measured directly. Electrocardiograms and chest echocardiography were done at regular intervals.

Maximal exercise capacity and sustained exercise capability were measured on different days; muscle biopsies were taken during each test of sustained exertion. Vital signs and simple pulmonary function tests, as well as alveolar samples, were obtained every day on all subjects, with occasional simultaneous arterial blood gases. Fluid and caloric intake and output were measured each day.

Above 22,000 feet, most subjects complained of sore throat, which we had not seen in OE I below this altitude. This is particularly interesting because sore throat is a severe problem on very high mountains and has been blamed on the cold, dry air. But because our chamber air was warm and wet, we suggest that a direct effect of hypoxia may be part of the cause.

We realized, as had been true in OE I, that the subjects were not fully acclimatized, but most of the data we collected were new and showed how the process of acclimatization was evolving.

All the data gathered in the 1985 experiment have been published in a collection of medical papers under the title *Operation Everest II*, and have also been assembled in one volume by the Army Institute of Environmental Medicine. The principal findings can be summarized as follows:

1. The largest improvement in bringing oxygen to the body was the increased ventilation (i.e., moving air from the atmosphere into the alveoli), by increasing both rate and volume of respiration.
2. All subjects developed a consistent and sometimes remarkable ventilation/perfusion mismatch (areas of the lung that got the most oxygen did not always get the most blood flow, and vice versa) at the higher altitudes, and this was aggravated by exercise, paralleling the rise in pulmonary artery pressure. We believe this was due to accumulation of interstitial fluid in the lungs more rapidly than the lymphatics could remove it. No subject (or scientist) developed full-blown HAPE.
3. The heart functioned well and was not the limiting factor at extreme altitude, as shown by maintenance of cardiac output for a given oxygen uptake. Breathing supplemental oxygen did not increase stroke volume for a given filling pressure.
4. Electrocardiographic changes were compatible with the increase in pulmonary artery pressure. Even maximal exercise at extreme altitude did not cause the heart muscle to falter. This is a reassuring finding.
5. Pulmonary artery pressure increased with altitude; at very high altitude it was lowered by breathing 100 percent oxygen, which did

not, however, decrease the calculated pulmonary resistance. This rather puzzling observation was persistent and carefully checked.

6. Alveolar and arterial gases and arterial blood pH were obtained at an altitude equivalent to the summit of Everest, and showed higher oxygen and carbon dioxide and lower pH than were found in one subject on the summit during AMREE; that climber later said that he had been breathing ninety times a minute when he took the sample! This would have caused his very low alveolar carbon dioxide and low pH, indicative of extreme respiratory alkalosis.

7. Maximal exercise capacity decreased steeply at the highest altitudes, as others had found at lower elevations. This suggests that the degree of hypoxia inevitable on the summit of Everest may make that spot close to the highest achievable by even the best-acclimatized human. Some birds go higher, and many animals survive more severe hypoxia using different strategies.

8. As in OE I, all the subjects lost weight despite appetizing, balanced meals, for which they gradually lost appetite. The weight loss could not be explained by balancing energy output against intake, which suggests some malabsorption.

Both OE I and OE II are of interest to mountaineers because, among other things, they showed that our rate of climb was too fast to achieve optimal acclimatization. This may not be especially relevant for some of today's elite mountaineers, who consider siege tactics (slow, steady ascent) "out" and speed climbing "in," but others can profit from the examples.

Optimal Rate of Climb

Looking at the ascent profiles and symptoms experienced in these two studies, we can cautiously suggest that a healthy young person can go, during the course of three days, to 12,000 feet and not experience more than minor symptoms. Above this, climbing 1,000 or 1,500 feet a day, with a rest every third day, seems appropriate. Above 22,000 feet, our data confirm the belief that one does not acclimatize. The rate of climb above this should be dictated by individual tolerance.

The finding that the lung, not the heart, is the limiting factor at high altitude is reassuring to older persons, but cautionary for those with minor lung problems.

IMPORTANCE OF OPERATION EVEREST STUDIES

For research scientists, OE I and OE II established standards for the effects of hypoxia without the other stresses of a mountain environment, against which data on the real mountain can be assessed. The data make it possible to separate changes due to hypoxia from those due to cold, dehydration, and other mountain impacts.

Relevance to Everyday Hypoxia

But why are these two complicated studies important to those who have little interest or concern with mountains? OE I and OE II give us a background against which to appraise individuals who are hypoxic at sea level because of acute or chronic illness, injury, or disability. The data enable us to estimate which abnormalities are due to hypoxia alone and which might be caused by other aspects of the underlying illness or injury. We can approach diagnosis and treatment in many cases more precisely and often more effectively.

Snoring and periodic breathing should be regarded not only as a nuisance, but also as a problem that, if not corrected, can lead over time to serious consequences. Mental or personality deviations in patients with severe heart or lung disease may be recognized as partly due to hypoxia—and remedied—rather than being due solely to senility or emotional illness. We can be much better informed before we advise people with one or another illness about the benefits and risks of going to the mountains.

In short, these are not simply interesting but unimportant pieces of knowledge. To paraphrase Joseph Barcroft, lessons from high altitude can help us to better understand ourselves at sea level.

LIMITS TO WORK AT ALTITUDE

Like many teenagers, I was fascinated by the first attempts at Mount Everest in the late 1920s, particularly after my first alpine experience in 1925. The stories were romantic and exciting, adventures in a faraway, completely strange world. I had tasted the romance of mountaineering, but I had no idea what was involved until after my first two Himalayan expeditions, in 1936 and 1938, when I was gripped by a desire to go there myself. The story of the "discovery" of Everest, true or not, fascinated me: A junior clerk burst into the office of the Surveyor General of India in 1884 exclaiming, "Sahib, I have discovered the highest mountain in the world." Once his calculations were confirmed, a few mountaineers became interested in this strange, high mountain, which had never been seen except from a distance. It was remote, sealed off from the south by secretive Nepal, and on the north by an equally difficult country, Tibet, to which only the British had access.

The first serious attempts on the mountain, in fact among the earliest to first reach the mountain, did surprisingly well, considering that almost nothing was known about work at high altitude. The first question was whether the thinness of the atmosphere, at 29,000 feet, would be fatal. Second, would it be possible to work or even move around? In 1924 Colonel Norton reached the astonishing height of 28,300 feet. The question of whether a man breathing only air could survive 700 feet higher, on top of Everest, had not yet been answered.

At the end of World War II the decompression chambers were idle and offered a tempting opportunity to determine whether or not the very thin air on top of Everest would be fatal even to an acclimatized man. Operation Everest I and II, experiments conducted in 1946 and 1985 and described in Chapter 16 of this book, both proved that an acclimatized person could survive in that thin air. But the question remained, could he work?

In 1953 Sir Edmund Hillary and Sherpa Tenzing Norgay climbed Everest, breathing supplementary oxygen with much better equipment than had been available before. Within a dozen years several others had reached the summit breathing only air, but they were very close to their limits. The second question had thus been answered: a well-acclimatized person *could* climb to the top of Everest and climb safely down. But what were the limiting factors that would prevent most men and women from doing the same?

In 1978 Reinhold Messner and Peter Habeler made the summit breathing only air. Since then, over one hundred others have done the same.

There remained other questions. Would some people be limited by muscular fatigue, others by inability to pump enough blood, still others by inadequate circulation of blood? Would some fail because their willpower or judgment or skill faltered due to lack of oxygen to the brain? So still the question remains: What *are* the factors that limit work at high altitude? Maximum work capacity (VO_2 max) has been shown to decrease steadily with increasing altitude—and, obviously, on the summit of Everest very little work can be done.

My own experience is somewhat limited: In 1938 on K2 I sat down at 26,000 feet and thought. I was very tired, but not exhausted. I was quite rational and clear in my thinking. I was still interested in reaching the summit only 2,000 feet above, but my willpower and dynamic thrust had slowed down. At that time, knowing that we had completed the task we came to do—namely, to find the route up the mountain—I was quite happy to go down. Thus in my mind a failure of desire prevented me from going on. My companion went a little higher, but was equally satisfied to retreat. We had done the job we came to do.

In the last half-century dozens have summited Mount Everest without oxygen. Others have climbed high—faltered, failed, and retreated; a few have faltered and died. There are few hard data to explain why they failed and why they died.

In the decompression chamber in Operation Everest II (OE II), two subjects were removed to lower "altitudes" because of the effects of hypoxia. The six others reached the "summit," however, stayed there for half an hour without difficulty, and were able to work. OE II, like OE I, was a "pure" study of hypoxia, without the complicating effects of cold, hunger, dehydration, and many other impacts that the mountain has on humans. The data show that in the final push, inability to move enough air in and out of the lungs was the limiting factor.

In OE II, each subject's heart and circulation performed well, and were not limiting factors. Although the exercise on a stationary bicycle required to attain VO_2 max was tiring, it was not muscle fatigue in the legs that ended their effort. On Everest, it does not seem to be the fatigue of climbing that limits effort, for most of those who summit breathing air seem to plod on "like a sick man in a dream," as Mallory wrote. Cold, lack of sleep, dehydration, and hunger do play a role, and may cause the fainthearted to retreat before their breathing limit has been reached. All we can say is that, absent the mountain effects, lack of oxygen limits work by limiting the ability to move air.

Can anyone climb Everest? Today it is safe to say that a healthy, strong, determined person aged seventeen to seventy with technical climbing skills and experience, given good weather, competent guides, and a large supply of cash, can probably reach the summit, breathing oxygen. However, only a few with all the above, plus an unfailing determination, can do so breathing only the air about them.

Nevertheless, each individual has a limit imposed perhaps by other factors as well: We may not be able to define these precisely, in a complex organism like the human, but in the last analysis a weakening of willpower, failure of the determination to press on at all costs, may be the ultimate limitation.

WORK AT ALTITUDE

Only a few thousand people have any interest in climbing the highest mountains on Earth, and even fewer wish to do so without breathing supplementary oxygen. Far more important, therefore, is the question of how high human beings can work efficiently and economically. How high can people live permanently without ill effects?

The mining operations described by Joseph Barcroft in the high Andes had been going on for centuries. Today mining operations are far different, with much of the work being done by huge machines. However, machines must be operated by people; people must drive the trucks, set the dynamite charges, and do the myriad other activities that make mines work. These people could be working anywhere between 20,000 and 22,000 feet. Fifty years ago the life expectancy for these workers was short, and their labor inefficient. Improved working conditions eventually made life better, but even so it was necessary for the workers to go down to a lower altitude at least every few days to recuperate for a day before coming back up. Soon the procedure was modified to give workers one week of work at altitude and one week of rest at a much lower altitude. Various strategies were used, but basically they consisted of recuperating at lower altitude to work at high altitude. Medication was not helpful, and the improvement in efficiency was small. A far more healthy, economical, and effective strategy, described in Chapter 15, "Prevention and Treatment," involves having miners sleep in dormitories in which the air is oxygen-enriched during sleeping hours, allowing the laborers to work productively during the day at high altitude.

This strategy is quite similar that used by the Everest climber who, sleeping with low-flow oxygen, will be a much more efficient climber the next day. The oxygen is not stored; what happens is that the body recuperates from the anaerobic load placed on it during daytime hours of heavy work.

Of course, the secret to most of these altitude operations includes acclimatization, and Chapter 13 discusses how acclimatization occurs, how it affects people at altitude, and how it may possibly have bearing on the survival and health of people who are hypoxic at sea level.

With regard to permanent residence at altitude, there is little evidence of permanent habitation above 17,500 feet. For many centuries Tibetans have lived at altitudes up to 17,500 feet on the high Tibetan plateau, and in the Andes settlements have existed for centuries, but always below 17,500 feet. That seems to be the limit. But why? It cannot be because of the climate, because millions of people live under even harsher conditions, and those millions also struggle for food, fuel, and shelter. We know that several hundred years ago the Incas climbed to and worked at 20,000 to 22,000 feet. They built temples and shrines and were able to do hard physical work for short periods of time. But they did not live there.

The factors that enable some populations to live that high have been described in Chapter 14, "Genetics of High-Altitude Performance," and are adaptations acquired over many generations. The adaptations have included an increased ability to move air, a more efficient circulatory system, and other, less critical functions. It seems likely that the inability to do heavy work for more than a few weeks has set 17,500 feet as the limit for residence.

The Chinese (Han) have lived in parts of Tibet for only a few hundred years, and those who have arrived more recently do not fare well at altitude, and are subject to more problems from the thin atmosphere than are the Tibetans. Perhaps it will take a few more centuries for them to adapt completely—if they stay there that long! Two other factors have been influential in limiting permanent residence at altitude. First, fertility rates are lower at altitude, and so are birth weights, both of which correlate to increased infant mortality. Second, the incidence of certain congenital defects is more common at higher altitude.

LIMITS TO PERFORMANCE AT HIGH ALTITUDE
Metabolism

Getting to the summit of any high mountain requires expending a lot of energy. Scientists define the metabolic rate as the amount of energy (measured in *calories*) that we expend in a day. Each of us has a *basal metabolic rate*, the number of calories that we use at rest just to maintain basic life functions. We also have a *total metabolic rate*, which includes both the basal metabolic rate and the additional calories we use to power other activities, most notably physical activities.

Dividing the total metabolic rate by the basal metabolic rate gives the *physical activity level,* or PAL. The PAL that we can maintain for many days without losing weight gives a good measure of the amount of energy that we can put into physical activity over the long run. (Day-to-day weight loss may be your goal if you are planning a surfing vacation and want to look good in last year's bathing suit, but it is not something that you can afford on a high-altitude expedition.) Couch potatoes have an average PAL of about 1.5—that is, they can sustain a total metabolic rate only 50 percent larger than their basal rate without losing weight. This is, in a sense, good news because it implies that performing even a modest amount of exercise on a regular basis can help an overweight couch potato slim down.

Clearly, a climber who contemplates a high-altitude expedition would like to maximize his or her PAL. But how do you do this? Physical training certainly increases PAL. Strong recreational athletes can maintain an average PAL of 2.0 or more, a substantial improvement over the PAL for couch potatoes. Elite endurance athletes do even better. They sustain an average PAL of about 4.0 without weight loss, but very few exceed a PAL of 5.0. So there does seem to be a limit to the impact of training on PAL. Diet also impacts PAL. Eating a high-calorie, high-carbohydrate diet increases the PAL that trained athletes can sustain over days of intense exercise. But, again, there are limits. People can only eat, digest, and absorb so many calories.

Unfortunately, high altitude impacts PAL as well, and not in a positive way. High-altitude climbers generally have a fitness level similar to that of elite endurance athletes. However, when at high altitude, climbers sustain PALs of around 2.5, far below the levels reached by athletes at sea level. Certainly, climbers can, and do, expend more energy than this for a few days or more. But climbers expending this much energy lose weight, something that they cannot afford to do for very long.

Why do climbers lose weight at high altitude and what can they do to minimize this loss? The very nature of a high-altitude expedition predisposes a climber to weight loss. Calorie expenditure is high, both from physical activity and from exposure to the cold. Food is unpalatable, difficult to prepare, often of poor nutritional quality, and occasionally completely unavailable. The hypoxia of high altitude may also contribute directly to weight loss. Digesting and absorbing nutrients takes energy. As discussed in Chapter 5, "Cells: The Ultimate Users," optimum energy production in our cells requires oxygen, something that is in short supply at high altitude.

Being at high altitude also reduces appetite. Chapter 7, "The Body Up High: Cellular and Vascular Responses to Hypoxia," described how elevated levels of the satiety hormone leptin might contribute to poor appetite and weight loss at high altitude. Other hormones may play a similar role. *Cholecystokinin* (CCK) is a hormone released from the small intestine after a meal. Normally, CCK stimulates the liver, gall bladder, and pancreas to insure that there are sufficient digestive enzymes in the small intestine. It also signals the brain to produce a feeling of satiety. Like leptin, CCK is elevated at high altitude, possibly contributing to poor appetite. Interleukin, a substance that we have mentioned as a possible trigger for angiogenesis (see Chapter 7), is also elevated at high altitude and may cause weight loss.

What should a climber do at high altitude to maximize his or her PAL and minimize appetite and weight loss? Right now, our understanding of the hormonal control of these factors is not sophisticated enough to offer much help. Clearly, pre-expedition training, careful acclimatization, and consuming a high-calorie diet when available are all good ideas. But, at best, these steps will limit PAL reduction and weight loss, not prevent it.

Skeletal Muscle

We have seen how going high can cause weight loss. At moderate altitude, most of this loss is generally from fat, particularly in climbers from Western countries who, on average, begin their ascent with a higher percentage of body fat than do local residents. However, most climbers who go very high and stay long enough at high altitude, experience a loss of skeletal muscle mass as well.

How, exactly, do skeletal muscles respond to the stress of altitude? Skeletal muscles are made up of long slender cells called *muscle fibers* that contain multiple nuclei and run the entire length of the muscle. Over time at high altitude, muscle fibers get smaller in diameter. They also lose mitochondria and the enzymes responsible for the initial steps of glucose breakdown, or *glycolysis*. Because the mitochondria and the enzymes of glycolysis play vital roles in the process by which cells extract energy from nutrients, their loss reduces the ability of cells to use oxygen and perform aerobic work. These changes can limit our ability to perform optimally at high altitude. (For a more complete discussion of the functions of the mitochondria and the enzymes of glycolysis, see Chapter 5, "Cells: The Ultimate Users.")

At present we know of no way to completely eliminate the negative impact of high altitude on skeletal muscle. There may, however, be a way to reduce the effect. Training in hypoxia, for example, training at moderate altitude prior to a high-altitude expedition, seems to stimulate the gene for a protein known as *hypoxia inducible factor*, or HIF. The protein HIF, in turn, stimulates the genes for a range of proteins that help muscle performance at high altitude, including the genes for the enzymes of glycolysis, erythropoietin (EPO, the hormone that increases red blood cell production; see Chapter 7, "The Body Up High: Cellular and Vascular Responses to Hypoxia"), and myoglobin (a protein similar in chemical structure to hemoglobin that stores oxygen within cells; see Chapter 14, "Genetics of High-Altitude Performance").

Respiration and Circulation

Increased activity of the lungs at high altitude is matched by increased activity of the heart. The heart beats faster and more forcefully in an attempt to move more blood and oxygen to body tissues. This is a beneficial response, but it does have limitations. The harder the heart beats, the faster the blood moves through the capillaries of the lung, the pulmonary capillaries (see Chapter 3, "Moving Air: Respiration"), where the blood receives oxygen from the alveoli. If the heart beats forcefully enough, it can actually move blood through the pulmonary capillaries so rapidly that the blood cannot pick up even the reduced level of oxygen available in the alveoli at high altitude.

The Brain

Some climbers report that, while they may have had the physical strength to continue at high altitude, they lacked the will to do so. There are many factors that might contribute to loss of will in these conditions. Some speculate that brain function may be one of the important factors that limit our ability to perform at high altitude.

We do know that several aspects of brain function are compromised at high altitude. When tested, climbers at high altitude show decreased motor skills and cognitive ability. They think and perform more slowly, make more mistakes, and have poorer judgment at altitude than at sea level, and they may also hallucinate. These changes could certainly limit performance at altitude, and it is tempting to simply blame hypoxia. However, only the most severe levels of hypoxia produce brain injury unless blood flow is reduced as well. Is brain blood flow low at high altitude? We do know that while hypoxia dilates the arteries that carry blood to the brain (the cerebral arteries), the reduced carbon dioxide blood levels caused by overbreathing may reduce this blood flow somewhat back toward lower values.

Regardless of the mechanism by which high altitude impacts brain function, this effect should be considered as a possible limit to high-altitude performance. We should also note that some high-altitude climbers seem to have residual cognitive or personality problems that persist after they return to sea level. On the other hand, many climbers have ventured to the summits of the highest mountains and then gone on to have outstanding careers in medicine, the experimental sciences, and the arts.

Infection

Infection is not an inevitable part of high-altitude climbing the way hypoxia is, nor are there any infectious organisms found only at high altitude. However, infections of various types have ended enough climbing trips that they are worthy of mention in any discussion of factors that can limit our performance at high altitude.

The immune system is somewhat compromised at altitude (as it is from hypoxia due to other causes) and may impose a limit to work at altitude. Few bacteria live at altitude, but arriving climbers may bring a new supply to infect those already on the mountain. Most important are those bacteria that cause respiratory infections, because they may increase susceptibility to HAPE. Skin infections are also a risk because of poor hygiene and trauma from climbing, cold, and simple scratching. Only occasionally will an infection limit work at altitude, but it can be devastating.

As we have seen, a range of factors can limit performance at high altitude. There is no magic formula for avoiding these problems, but good common sense should prevail. In general, if we want to climb our best at high altitude, we should train hard (possibly at moderate altitude) and acclimatize carefully. We should also take care of ourselves during the expedition through proper diet, good hygiene, and early treatment of any developing infections.

TRAINING FOR ATHLETIC COMPETITION

There has been much talk, and hundreds of articles, about whether an athlete can improve sea-level performance by training at altitude, but few solid conclusions. So intense are competitive athletics today that even the smallest edge is important.

An athlete cannot train to his or her utmost limit at high altitude because, even as low as 5,000 feet, maximal work capacity is less than at sea level.

There might be some advantage from a small increase in hemoglobin, which can deliver more oxygen per unit of blood pumped. This increase comes with acclimatization to moderate altitude, but is partly offset by the slightly decreased alkaline reserve, which results from the small increase in blood pH. This means that the additional carbon dioxide and lactic acid generated by strenuous exercise will have more effect on blood pH and thus on respiration than when alkaline reserve is normal, and the well-acclimatized individual is likely to ventilate more than a sea-level rival during the same exertion.

In the past, to avoid the decrease in alkaline reserve that occurs upon acclimatization, elite athletes instead trained at sea level and took transfusions of blood (usually their own blood taken earlier). This practice of blood doping, however, is now banned in most sports. Injections of erythropoietin (EPO) stimulate formation of more hemoglobin and red blood cells, but this too is banned. Too much hemoglobin makes blood sluggish and harder for the heart to pump, an effect that can offset the slight advantage gained by an increase in hemoglobin. The bottom line seems to be that adding hemoglobin is not worth the risks.

One might find an answer by comparing how Denver-based professional teams compare with those from lower altitude. Our Olympic swimmers and skiers have trained at 5,000 feet or higher, but no proven benefits have been forthcoming. On the other hand, Boulder, Colorado (6,000 feet), is a center for world-class cyclists, who are convinced that training there gives them an edge. Some runners and prospective expedition mountaineers have trained while breathing low oxygen mixtures for a few hours at sea level each day. This is roughly the same as spending time at simulated altitude in a decompression chamber, but in this country, at least, that tactic has not proven of value. Several other countries have tried variations on these programs—anything to get that extra edge.

Kienbaum, East Germany, 1969

An interesting acclimatization program was carried on for more than a decade at a hidden facility in the village of Kienbaum in East Germany. The secret was so well kept that even the Russians who controlled East Germany during the Cold War were unaware of it. The program ran from 1969 until after the reunification of Germany, for the sole purpose of training East German athletes for international competition. The operation was based on the conviction that training at altitude improved competitive ability at sea level (which is not widely accepted).

The Kienbaum training center occupied several hundred acres of outdoor track and field courses, dormitories, and mess halls, and is at 500 feet altitude. The altitude training building was a large domed decompression chamber about the size of a basketball court buried deep beneath a low, innocent-looking mound of grass-covered earth. The interior of the chamber had two levels—the upper one with a circular running track and treadmills and a lower level with two large water tanks in which the flow could be controlled for rowing, canoeing, or swimming. The two chambers operated together and could be taken to a simulated altitude of 12,500 feet, with temperature controllable from +15 to +25° Centigrade.

In 1990 I was invited to visit the Kienbaum training facility and given a complete tour and somewhat limited briefing. I was told that the training protocols were adjusted to the sport and to each individual, but usually thirty to thirty-six athletes would work out in the chambers for two to six hours a day at 6,000 to 10,000 feet simulated altitude. They lived and exercised the rest of the day outside the chamber, essentially at sea level. This is just the reverse of today's more widely accepted plan for living high and training low.

Some scientific studies were probably done at Kienbaum but not disclosed to me then or later, and when I pressed, they answered, "Look at our world records compared with other nations." As the world knows, East Germans consistently took more medals than athletes from most other nations. Although the East Germans are said to have used hormones and other medications, it seems likely that the Kienbaum program did contribute to their success. It is important to note that although they trained at altitude, they also trained and lived most of the time at sea level. So far as I could tell, they believed that the increased hemoglobin was the principal benefit.

With the end of the Cold War, Kienbaum ceased operations. Now it is used as a general training facility. Its existence is a testimony to the great expense and effort international competition spawned, even in countries that had limited resources. The lengths to which the East Germans went to keep programs secret from the occupying Russians also has intriguing implications.

Live High, Train Low or Live High, Train High?

Ben Levine, who has done a great deal of work with elite athletes, says it is important to separate "altitude training" into two parts: (1) acclimatization, which depends on the altitude where the athlete lives for at least twelve hours every day, and (2) training, which is a function of the altitude where the athlete actually works out.

Acclimatization stimulates red blood cell and hemoglobin production and thus increases oxygen-carrying capacity. Other changes of acclimatization are more subtle and contribute less strongly. In a well-controlled study of thirty-nine distance runners who lived at 8,000 feet for four weeks, Levine found an increase of 9 percent in hemoglobin and an increase of 5 percent in maximal oxygen uptake over their low-altitude tests, regardless of where they trained. However, not all retained superior capacity at sea level. When the group lived at 8,000 feet but trained at 4,200 feet, performance in distance running at 4,200 feet was better than for those who lived and trained at lower altitude. An influential factor was the increase in EPO, and thus of hemoglobin formation. This study involved distance runners, who compete in events where endurance is more important than speed.

The role of altitude in training for other competitive sports is more difficult to evaluate. Studies do seem to support the idea that, for endurance events, living at high altitude and training at low altitude may improve performance at low altitude. For sports requiring both endurance and bursts of intense effort (such as football or soccer), the data are not so clear. For events demanding short, intense bursts of effort, like sprints, competitors do not benefit by living or training at altitude because they do not need additional oxygen-carrying capacity.

Levine concluded from several well-controlled studies that combining high altitude acclimatization with low-altitude interval/intense training in well-trained competitive runners results in significant improvements in sea-level 5,000-meter times above and beyond those achieved by an equivalent sea-level or high-altitude control.

Chuck Fulco of the Army Research Institute of Environmental Medicine reviewed hundreds of medical articles describing work at increasing altitude. From these he analyzed the effects of training, the changes that took place after both short and long stays at different elevations, and the effect of altitude on different types of exertion (rapid, short-duration effort compared to longer endurance work). Figure 36 shows the decline with increasing altitude in maximal work capacity (VO$_2$ max) as a percentage of sea-level capacity.

Fulco reached the following conclusions: Training and/or living at altitude can improve altitude exercise performance in athletic events...lasting more than about two minutes.... Controlled studies do not support

Figure 36. Fulco's VO$_2$ max graph

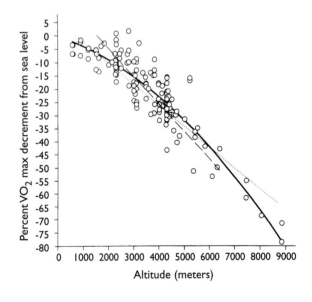

a beneficial effect of altitude training on subsequent sea level performance.... Living at altitude but training at a lower altitude permits the theoretical advantage of both acclimatization and training without reducing exercise intensity. This paradigm appears promising but is still open to question since altitude natives training at altitude with oxygen supplementation (in effect "living high, training low") did not improve maximal work capacity more than altitude natives training at altitude without oxygen supplementation.

Although the answers to many important questions about training and altitude are still vague, from the hard data now available we can draw a few conclusions that are widely accepted today, although not without disagreement:

- Beginning at above 5,000 feet, the maximum work one can do decreases by about 3 percent per 1,000 feet of altitude and improves only slightly after longer residence at altitude. Endurance or submaximal work shows a similar pattern, decreasing when one initially ascends to high altitude and increasing only slightly over time.
- Training at altitude cannot be quite as intense as at sea level, and the competitive edge is therefore slightly dulled. Thus training above 5,000 feet is of doubtful value for sea-level competition.
- Advantage does come from increased EPO and increased hemoglobin (and thus oxygen-carrying capacity), but this is partially offset by the decrease in buffering power that comes with acclimatization and perhaps also by the increased viscosity of blood.
- Athletes training for short, intense events do not benefit from training at altitude; those planning to compete in endurance events at altitude will probably benefit by training for weeks at that altitude.
- Some altitude natives do surpass their cohorts in sea-level competition, but others do not, and the explanation is more likely their lifelong dedication to running rather than their level of acclimatization.

One can conclude that if you want to get the edge at sea level, sleep high and train low—except for sprints, for which it does not matter.

WOMEN CLIMBERS

According to Francis Gribble's *The Early Mountaineers*, when a woman joined one of the first parties of climbers to visit the Dauphine Alps, a local chamois hunter declared: "The men are gold-seekers and the woman is a witch they have brought with them to show where the gold is hidden."

Today, of course, the place of women in mountaineering has been firmly established, and dozens have climbed the highest and most difficult peaks around the world, tolerating altitude, cold, and stress as well as men. Women have shown their skill in the Alps for more than a century, although not for several decades did they forgive Alfred Mummery, one of the leading climbers in the Victorian age, for his unintended slur (cited in Gribble): "All mountains seem to go through three stages: an inaccessible peak, the most dangerous climb in the Alps, and an easy day for a lady."

Even though women have climbed the highest mountains and eighty (as of early 2004) have summited Everest, until recently there has been little systematic study of their responses to hypoxia. Possibly this was because women's cyclic hormone variations might be expected to complicate already complicated responses to hypoxia. Perhaps some male chauvinism persisted even after female climbers proved they would gladly participate in such studies. Whatever the reasons, until the last few years data about the effects of female hormones at altitude were patchy and incomplete. Now there is a surge of interest, with research grants flowing readily from the U.S. government and military.

Influence of Menstrual Cycle on Mountain Sickness

For some women the menstrual cycle alters the salt and water balance and often causes edema, which might be expected to increase susceptibility to acute mountain sickness (AMS). Yet there is little agreement among the few studies on this topic. Lorna Moore has been leading a team that is examining the hormones *estradiol* (dominant in the follicular, or pre-ovulatory, stage of the cycle), *luteinizing hormone* (LH, which surges eighteen hours before ovulation), and *progesterone* (dominant in the luteal, or post-ovulatory, phase), the combined effects of which are complex. (See Figure 37.)

At any altitude, a woman's ventilation increases slightly during the luteal phase of the menstrual cycle due to the rise of both estradiol (estrogen) and progesterone. One might expect this to decrease the incidence of

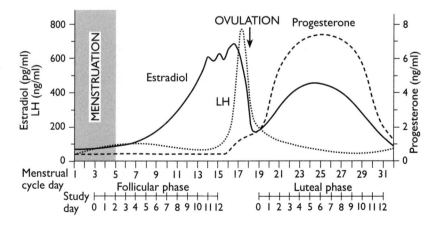

Figure 37. *Menstrual cycle*

AMS. Administration of progesterone to either men or women does in fact increase ventilation and decrease AMS slightly. But no statistical study has been published to confirm any relation of AMS or high altitude pulmonary edema (HAPE) to the menstrual cycle. While five studies have shown that the incidence of AMS is slightly less frequent in women than in men and that the incidence of HAPE is five times greater in men, none of these studies was able to correlate menstrual cycle to incidence. Nor has the occurrence of altitude illness in women taking contraceptive pills (that contain progesterone) been established, although several groups continue to study this.

Both plasma aldosterone and atrial natriuretic protein fluctuate during the menstrual cycle, but these affect ventilation and fluid retention in opposite directions and need more study.

The hypoxic ventilatory response (HVR) tends to be slightly lower in women, but when the data are corrected for body size, the HVR turns out to be slightly higher than men's.

Women may burn food somewhat differently than do men, but the limited data suggest that women have about the same energy requirements as men and, given the same fuel, can accomplish the same amount of work, although perhaps at a somewhat slower pace. Women's maximum work capacity (VO_2 max) is less than men's, but women can train up as well as men. Like men, those women who start with a higher maximum oxygen uptake at sea level may be better off at altitude, where both men and women function at a percentage of sea-level capacity that decreases proportionately as altitude increases. A few studies show that women's pulse rate and blood pressure, and thus the "double product" or approximate load on the heart, at altitude is as variable as men's. Women may acclimatize faster than men, and they do not lose as much weight during an altitude stay.

Pregnancy

When the Spanish *conquistadores* occupied the territory of the Incas in the sixteenth century, the Catholic priests who lived and traveled widely in the region commented on the high fertility of the natives and blamed the high infant mortality on cold. Spanish women became pregnant at a normal rate, but for decades all pregnancies ended in miscarriage or stillbirth. Not for fifty-three years did the first child of Spanish ancestry survive birth at altitude. Whether this was due to the altitude is unclear; there were many other adverse factors. But soon the Spaniards—and later many newcomers to altitude—would go down to sea level during the last trimester of pregnancy and remain there for a time following birth.

Today libido and fertility are reported to be normal in altitude residents, but in both residents and newcomers, complications of pregnancy, such as toxemia, uterine hemorrhage, premature delivery, miscarriages, and stillbirths, are more common at altitude. Newborns have a lower birth weight and gain weight more slowly. In children conceived and born at altitude, the small artery between the aorta and pulmonary artery (which is open while in the womb) may fail to close after the child is born. This condition, called *ductus arteriosus*, which allows some blood to bypass the lungs of the fetus, must be corrected surgically if the artery remains open a few months after birth. This defect is five times as common in infants at altitude as in infants of similar ancestry at sea level. A few other congenital defects are slightly more common at altitude.

Can a pregnant woman go to altitude without harming herself or the child she is carrying? In 1988 the late climber Alison Hargreaves summited Switzerland's 13,000-foot Eiger five months into her pregnancy without incident. One might expect that the fetus of a woman going from sea level to altitude in the first three or four weeks of pregnancy might be damaged by hypoxia. This does not seem to happen, but the higher incidence of miscarriage during this stage of pregnancy may mask it. Many authorities suggest that the pregnant woman go to lower altitude—as many do—during the last trimester of pregnancy to avoid complications, including congenital defects, although these would have developed earlier.

It has been suggested that placental circulation is such that a fetus lives in an oxygen environment equivalent to that on top of Everest, but the presence of fetal hemoglobin (see Chapter 4, "Moving Blood: Circulation") and a greatly increased red blood cell mass, as well as increased circulation, result in an oxygen-carrying capacity and oxygen content closer to normal. Nature has provided protection for the growing fetus against hypoxia. However, given the increased occurrence of fetal growth restriction and other complications, this protection is not complete.

Most authorities agree that a pregnant woman can safely go to moderate altitude—say, 8,000 feet—without fear for the fetus, although some put the ceiling lower. Few would consider it safe or appropriate to climb high in the Andes or Himalayas after the first trimester—but some have done so.

Other Hormonal Differences

Men have hormonal fluctuations in testosterone release, although this is neither as marked nor as regular as in the female cycle. The effect of the male cycle on altitude tolerance has not been adequately studied, but increased testosterone has been linked to sleep apnea. Testosterone secretion decreases during long exposure to altitude, with aging, and in chronic obstructive pulmonary disease (COPD).

Other hormones common to women and men, such as human growth hormone, change at altitude and fluctuate with time, but in the same general direction in each sex. Circadian rhythms almost certainly affect acclimatization and hypoxia tolerance each day because most of the powerful hormones in the adrenal glands normally are secreted at around 4 or 5 A.M., toward the end of sleep. The adrenal steroid hormones (aldosterone and cortisol, for example) affect salt and water balance, among other things, and have not been studied adequately at altitude. One can only speculate what effect circadian rhythms might have during climbs at night or during several continuous days, especially when climbers are stressed.

More common among women is a hidden iron deficiency, which becomes more significant as the body is required to make more red blood cells in acclimatization. Women recover their sea-level blood volume faster than men, but seem to be slower in forming red cells during acclimatization; whether this is due to low iron stores or some other factor is unknown. But if a woman is deficient and takes supplementary iron, her response to hypoxia improves.

Most women tend to have less muscle mass than men, but they can double their strength through training, often without a large change in bulk. Although women are almost as strong as men in trunk and legs, arm strength, even with training, is usually less than that of men. Endurance for exercise is decreased at high altitude. However, as Chuck Fulco has shown, for small muscle groups where strength is not limiting, women are protected from the decreased endurance that occurs in men because women seem to have a greater capacity for muscle oxidative phosphorylation. At least for some isolated muscle groups, women may have less impairment due to hypoxia than men.

Women who engage in prolonged strenuous physical activity—be it ballet, marathon training, or long mountain expeditions—tend to have scanty menses (*oligomenorrhea*) or even stop menstruating altogether (*amenorrhea*). Menstrual dysfunction is not due to altitude, but has been hypothesized to be caused by insufficient caloric intake with subsequent decrease in basal metabolic rate, resulting in hypothalamic dysfunction. Normal cycles may resume after strenuous training ceases.

AGING

Thirty-five years ago Ross McFarland, a pioneer in many aspects of oxygen and altitude medicine, suggested that the effects on the brain of hypoxia and aging were similar. He based his hypothesis on the following: (1) immediate recall, span of concentration, and reflex time are impaired with age and altitude; (2) sensitivity of vision in dim light decreases with age just as it does with altitude; (3) acuity of hearing decreases with age as with altitude. He added that "calculations are unreliable, judgment faulty, and emotional responses unpredictable" both with age and at altitude. Acknowledging great individual variation, one may be impressed by this concept.

Aging changes everything, and rarely for the better: imperceptibly at first, then slowly, but soon the slope becomes steeper. Fortunately, as with hypoxia, we do not notice much change. We believe we are as young as we feel, not as old as we act. Still, to paraphrase what a patient once told Walter Alvarez: "Age keeps taking little bites of me."

Exertion and Breathing

With age, muscular strength and endurance decrease, which is only slowed for a time by vigorous training. Maximal work capacity decreases along with maximal breathing capacity. Reflexes are slowed, increasing the time of response to any stimulus, even if only slightly.

The maximum achievable heart rate (MAHR) declines with age, but for many people both systolic and diastolic blood pressure slowly increase. Pulmonary artery pressure increases slightly with age, and peripheral circulation, including that to the brain, is decreased. The hypoxic ventilatory response (HVR) is blunted, and normal values of pulmonary function tests must be adjusted for age.

As McFarland suggested, many similar changes are likely to appear with aging, and it should not be surprising to find that the responses to altitude of most old folks are additive to those due to age. Most elders climb more slowly and carefully, most grow less ambitious as they find the spirit as willing as ever but the flesh weaker. There are many exceptions: hundred-year-old men and women who walk up Mount Fuji (12,395 feet), many even older who climb fourteen-thousanders with pleasure if not ease, and the rare veteran climber who summits Everest though over sixty. (In 2003, Yuichiro Miura, climbing with his son, became the oldest person, at age seventy, to summit Everest.) And hundreds of thousands of elders throng to mountain resorts at 8,000 to 10,000 feet, or trek in the Andes or Himalayas.

It is reassuring that several good studies have shown that at moderate altitudes, the incidence of AMS decreases linearly with age: Young folks are more likely to be sick, for whatever reason—speed, overactivity, or exuberance—than their elders.

Because older individuals have higher pulmonary artery pressure, which increases with hypoxia, one might expect them to develop HAPE more frequently. But not so: The incidence is higher in children under ten, and lower in older adults than in younger adults. HAPE is far more frequent in males than in females, though AMS is roughly equally distributed. However, pulmonary function at altitude, already lower in older people, is more sharply decreased after strenuous exertion at altitude, suggesting more interstitial edema than usual. This could, of course, be an early warning of HAPE.

FITNESS

Most of us aspire to be physically fit; we feel better, sleep better, think better when fit, or so we believe. Fitness and good health go hand in hand, and around the world people spend vast sums of money and great chunks of time exercising. In many countries health spas are part of the culture and include fitness programs along with beautification, mineral waters, medicated baths, and "fat farms." Many European industries give employees paid leave to attend health spas where fitness is stressed. Apparently they believe it pays.

Fitness, achieved by whatever level and form of exercise is appropriate to age and environment, is difficult to measure. Maximum work capacity (VO_2 max) decreases about 1 percent per year after the forties, but this decline can be slowed or arrested, possibly even reversed, by regular exercise. But VO_2 max does not measure endurance or ability to do prolonged moderate work. Is this important? It depends on what you want to do.

All our reflexes slow almost imperceptibly with age, but this can be compensated for, though not improved, by practice and regular exercise. Bone loss in men begins around age fifty. For women, bone loss occurs at an earlier age and often at a faster rate. The rate of bone loss increases slowly in many people; this can also be halted, and lost bone, like muscle, can even be rebuilt to some extent with regular exercise. Many functions worsen with age, but in some cases the decline can be slowed by staying fit.

Few would disagree that getting and keeping fit is a good way of life. Does it delay aging and death? Does it improve mental processes, creativity, sexuality? What do the hard data show? Perhaps most of us would say "yes, amen" to all of these and others, and the scattered information, some of it well controlled, tends to support the belief.

Does fitness at any age decrease mountain sickness? Can one climb higher, more easily and safely, and be less likely to develop AMS, HACE, or HAPE? Regrettably, there are few or no hard data to answer these questions conclusively. Physical fitness does not equate to better altitude tolerance at any age.

But wait a moment! The fit athlete at any altitude moves and works more easily, uses less oxygen per unit of work done in a fixed time, and is generally more oxygen- and fuel-efficient. This certainly suggests, if it does not prove, that a fit climber might do better in the low-oxygen atmosphere of high mountains. Logically and theoretically this is true. It is equally true that the experienced and skillful climber moves more easily and with less oxygen and fuel consumption than the amateur, but this does not necessarily mean that one is less fit than the other.

And, obviously, by being able to climb more rapidly, the fit and experienced climber will be in harm's way for a shorter time.

In short, staying fit is good medicine for living, but it may not protect you from mountain sickness.

CHAPTER

THE MOUNTAIN WAY

In 1938 I was part of a group that walked 350 miles from Kashmir to K2. We had the best mountain equipment available, a forty-day supply of food, and a tiny medical kit. (Bear in mind that this was before antibiotics and steroids!) We had no radio (and of course no cell phone) and no bottled oxygen. Local porters carried our equipment, but otherwise we were on our own. With luck we might send letters home, by dispatching a mail runner, but we could not and did not expect to be rescued in the event of trouble. We were well aware of the risks on the mountain, including potential illnesses.

Being aware of our isolation and independence, we were careful and did not push our limits. We had a glorious three months. That was how things were back then. The few groups that went into remote areas were self-sustaining and never expected rescue.

Since then, of course, there have been major changes. Today most major expeditions carry radios and cell phones and do not hesitate to call home, send news flashes, or ask for rescue. A few years ago, a doctor in remote Tibet telephoned Harley Street in London for advice about a difficult obstetrical problem. I myself have received several calls for advice from Everest Base Camp.

As a consequence of readily available communication, climbers take more chances, and because high risk may bring fame and fortune, climbers do push the limits. Not surprisingly, the number of injuries and deaths has increased considerably.

At the same time, we are hearing more stories of strange illnesses that may be due to high altitude. These anecdotes must be scrutinized carefully and, if possible, tested under controlled conditions. Nonetheless, these stories do give us a small window into physiology at altitude, which may become clearer with time. In my own case, in 1991 I participated in a small, casual expedition to Nanga Parbat. We walked for about a week to 14,000 feet, and within a day I developed high altitude pulmonary edema (HAPE). I had been too casual, not thinking of the altitude and taking no medication. I stayed at 14,000 feet for thirty-six hours to finish the job I was there to do before staggering down. I completely ignored the advice I'd given others, and if I had gotten worse, I would have been carried down 60 or so miles to the road head. Don't do the same yourself!

Mountains, whether large or small, offer large rewards to those who go to them. They can be awesome and beautiful, hostile and terrifying, peaceful or dangerous. Previous chapters in this book described some early visitors to the mountains, what they found, what they experienced, and what they thought. Other chapters discussed exploration of the atmosphere that surrounds us and how we came to understand the vital substance—oxygen—upon which most (but not all) life depends. Close attention was paid to how we acquire oxygen, move it throughout the body, and use it to fuel every activity. Mountains, especially very high ones, offer great hazards. This book is most concerned with those caused by lack of oxygen, and the most common forms of "mountain sickness" have been described as well as how they are recognized, prevented, or treated. This chapter examines the less common and less threatening forms of illness due to high-altitude hypoxia. It also makes suggestions about who can safely go to the mountains and who cannot.

The signs, symptoms, and dangers of high-altitude hypoxia are often mimicked by two other stresses encountered on higher mountains—hypothermia and hypoglycemia. All three can be insidious and capable of overcoming the unwary before he or she notices anything wrong. These stressors affect the higher centers of the brain first, dulling perception, impairing judgment and decision, and all too often progressing to unconsciousness and death if not treated. Their danger is magnified by the sleep deprivation, exhaustion, and emotional stress so often experienced on the great mountains. They are synergistic: The combination of hypoxia, hypothermia, and hypoglycemia can be deadly to the exhausted traveler who has not slept or taken food or fluids.

The sad stories of climbing deaths related at the beginning of this book are examples of how on very high mountains several elements can combine to cripple or kill. Most of those involved in the tragedy on Everest in 1996 had been strangers only a few weeks before and did not have the strong bonds between them and the sense of brotherhood that are essential in extreme situations. Some qualified for such a climb more because of wealth than experience. On K2 in 1986, some climbers had changed from one expedition to another, only a few shared a common language, and most were strangers to others. Fixed ropes on both Everest and K2 allowed climbers to move alone over much of the route, not roped to a climbing partner, often at night. Gone was the "Fellowship of the Rope."

The episode leading up to the heart-rending deaths of the Russian women on Pic Lenin in 1974 is a story of grace under pressure from cold and privation. These climbers chose to stay together, rather than to save themselves. It was an example of the best tradition of mountaineering. Their decision to go on to the summit (despite the increasing storm) and bivouac had been an error of judgment. Perhaps nothing could have prevented some or all of the deaths, but poor decisions, perhaps due to hypoxia, certainly contributed.

PROBLEMS ENCOUNTERED IN THE MOUNTAIN WORLD

From 1921 through 1996, 391 expeditions consisting of about 4,400 climbers attempted Everest; 679 climbers summited and 148 died. Between 1997 and 2002, more than 800 climbers reached the summit of Everest; over the same period, 27 died on that mountain. These numbers are the best now available, but they differ depending on who is writing and often do not include all the Sherpas. Most of the deaths have been during descent. Several of the Sherpas who had made the top three or more times survived the events of 1996.

On Everest in 1996, all involved during that ghastly episode were well acclimatized over the weeks they had spent reaching base camp and climbing higher. By the time they reached high camp, at 26,000 feet, their bodies had already adjusted as well as humans can—but they had stayed so long above 20,000 feet that "deterioration" had begun.

Since 1903, some 20,000 people have attempted Denali (Mount McKinley, 20,300 feet) and half have succeeded, while close to 100 have died from the same causes that killed climbers on Everest, K2, Nanga Parbat, and Pic Lenin. On Denali (which means the "Great One" in the ancient Athapascan Indian language) altitude illnesses have frequently caused death. Denali has the most severe weather of any great mountain. Few places ever get colder: "The cold chilled my soul," said one veteran. Storms strike with little warning, as they do on Everest, but often last much longer, tempting the impatient climber to start out before the snow and weather have settled. "Allow one month for McKinley," advises Brad Washburn, director of the Boston Museum of Science, distinguished photographer and mapmaker, who knows more about Mount Washington and Denali than anyone. "You cannot rush McKinley; some who have tried have died."

The mountain environment can be harsh even on much smaller mountains like 6,400-foot Mount Washington, the highest mountain east of the Rockies, where hypoxia is no problem but the weather is every bit as severe as on Everest. Sudden violent winds—at times gusting to 150 miles per hour—sweep across Washington's barren summit at any season, and temperatures plummet. The inexperienced hiker may start out at the base of the mountain on a balmy summer day and climb up toward the summit, unaware of the darkening clouds, and find himself or herself in a storm, blinded by fog or snow, disoriented, inadequately dressed for the surprising weather, and without extra food or drink. Over the last hundred years some thirty-five people have died on this low and apparently safe mountain.

Lack of Oxygen

The impact of lack of oxygen on the brain at high altitude has been the root cause of the great catastrophes like those on Everest in 1996 and K2 in 1986. Many less dramatic tragedies have been directly due to hypoxia because it weakens judgment, fosters indecision or bad decisions, fractures morality, and impairs the very skills most needed in climbing.

Because they are usually acclimatized during the approach, climbers on high mountains do not often have symptoms of HAPE or acute mountain sickness/high altitude cerebral edema (AMS/HACE). Even so, some healthy climbers—who should know better—die of HAPE and HACE each year on the highest mountains. Falls, rock and ice avalanches, and frostbite are more frequent, but altitude hypoxia is just as deadly.

Recently, trekkers in the Himalayas have been reported to have about the same incidence of mountain sickness as tourists in the Rockies. This began when, in place of the two- to three-week approach march, trekkers were flown to 11,000 feet and began the trek from there. Better education and better planning have reduced mountain sicknesses—but illnesses and deaths among tourists are still a problem, especially in the Everest region, which draws some 25,000 visitors a year. In 1950 we were only six.

Breathing bottled oxygen increases the partial pressure of inhaled oxygen (see Chapter 3, "Moving Air: Respiration"), in effect "taking the climber down" several thousand feet. In 1996 most of those who went for the summit on Everest were using supplementary oxygen during the final climb; for many, their oxygen supplies ran out at various times during the descent. The altitude had a greater impact on those who had used oxygen and then ran out.

One of the guides who died had been ill for a day or two; some suggest that he may have had HAPE and/or HACE but persisted in trying to reach the summit to take care of his clients. Too late, he turned back and died with one of them. It is difficult to doubt that his judgment and ability to make hard decisions were flawed by hypoxia. Another guide (Anatoli Boukreev), who had argued he would be safer without oxygen, after summiting with his group still had strength and will to attempt rescue three times during that awful night. Because he is known to be a very strong and experienced climber, no conclusions can be reached from his decision to forgo oxygen, but his argument against supplementary oxygen has some validity.

Many of the survivors have described a feeling of dissociation from their bodies and from each other, and the replacement of pain with total fatigue. Even their reasons for being there near the summit became hazy, replaced by an animal instinct to go on, to survive.

Hypothermia

Hypothermia mimics hypoxia in some respects. As the body chills, the brain falters, judgment and perception are blurred, and the victim does not realize what is happening. Mental confusion and hallucinations soon follow. Reflexes slow, muscles seem stiff, and movements are awkward and clumsy. The combination of cold and altitude is very powerful; together, the impact of each is perhaps doubled.

At a core body temperature of 95° Fahrenheit (rectal), hypothermia is serious; at 89° death is probable unless heroic treatment is provided; few victims survive a body temperature of 85°. Wind increases the rate of cooling by the square of wind velocity; the windchill is much colder than the actual air temperature and more dangerous because it cools one faster.

Even the best down- or fiber-filled clothing in a windproof breathable shell cannot protect completely against windchill for long. Bear in mind that air is only half as heavy at high altitude, and the windchill much less; therefore, the force of the wind is similarly decreased. Muscular exertion is the major heat producer, and if the victim stops moving and shivering, hypothermia will begin.

This is what happens on high mountains: The exhausted climber stops "to rest," sits or lies down, and usually will not rise again. But one of the 1996 Everest survivors did lie down for many hours and did survive. A companion never roused. Another spoke on the radio for many hours, slowly losing consciousness, and finally was silent. The Russian women on Pic Lenin in 1974 died slowly during three awful days. One by one those remaining described their plight. Their immense fortitude and courage to the end could not mitigate the impact of cold and altitude.

Hypothermia is said to be the foremost killer in outdoor winter sports. Twenty percent of the deaths on Denali are due to cold and exhaustion, as are most of those on Mount Washington. Even at low altitude or sea level, tens of thousands of people, mostly the poor and elderly sitting alone in unheated rooms, become hypothermic even when the outside temperature is not extremely cold. It is said that 25,000 elderly die annually in the United States from hypothermia, often misdiagnosed. The danger of hypothermia is that it is so subtle, so insidious that the victim is unaware of the slow slide toward unconsciousness. On high mountains, hypothermia and hypoxia together pack a double whammy.

After the exhausted rescuers had left two climbers on Everest in 1996, believing them too near death to attempt the desperate carry-out, one of them roused next morning. He believes he had been hypothermic, and of course he was. But few people survive deep hypothermia when they lie down for very long; it is more likely that he slept, exhausted. When the sun rose, he somehow gathered will and strength to stagger several hundred yards down to camp, where he collapsed. The other exhausted climbers expected him to die and did little more for him than provide warm coverings and some hot drinks. Next day he recovered enough strength to be helped down the mountain, terribly frostbitten but alive. His story powerfully shows the truth of the maxim "the hypothermic patient is not dead until warm and dead."

Hypoglycemia

Strenuous exertion combined with little or no food drains the reserves of fuel, notably carbohydrate. Some of the signs of the resulting low blood sugar resemble those of hypoxia and hypothermia: Confusion, bizarre behavior, clumsy gait and hand motions, or even paranoid hallucinations are not uncommon, especially in diabetics. Most of us are familiar with the shaky feeling, perhaps with cold sweats, we experience after skipping a meal or two; we are aware that just before lunch often is not the best time for a complicated discussion or decision. When cold is causing the body to burn more fuel (mostly glucose), hypoglycemia complicates life for the climber at any altitude. In the rush of excitement on a summit day, too many "can't eat" or won't, and pay for it later. "Brain waves" recorded by electroencephalogram (EEG) during hypoglycemia resemble those recorded during hypoxia.

The important thing to remember is that the symptoms of the stressors hypoxia, hypothermia, and hypoglycemia are subtle and insidious, and each reinforces the effects of the other.

> Two climbers were observed through binoculars from base camp as they proceeded from their tent at 23,000 feet across a steep slope, one by one. Soon the second man, moving slowly, stopped and sat down, but the leader continued on. After a time the second man stumbled to his feet, walked a few paces, and lay down in the snow motionless. The leader turned back past the apparently sleeping man, and went back to their tent. Rescuers the next morning found the leader in his tent, unconscious and badly frostbitten, but his companion was dead in the snow. Both were inappropriately dressed for the extreme cold, they had not allowed time to acclimatize, and seemed to have eaten little before starting out that day.

Although it may not be a major hazard, hypoglycemia adds to the odds against one on a high mountain; many of those on Everest in May 1996 had not eaten for many hours, and this contributed to their danger.

Dehydration

Dehydration is common on mountains because so much water is lost in overbreathing and in sweat (which is often imperceptible because it evaporates instantly in the dry air). The climber must drink water to keep the blood from becoming too thick and sluggish, allowing the red blood cells to pile up like plates, decreasing the surface for picking up or releasing oxygen, and thus adding to tissue hypoxia. The kidneys require water to form urine to eliminate bicarbonate (part of the acclimatization process described in Chapter 13) as well as to excrete waste products.

On high mountains the air is cold and almost completely dry. As inhaled air passes through the nose or mouth, it is warmed and humidified, sucking both heat and water from the body, and these are not recovered during exhalation. On the highest mountains, where breathing is so greatly increased, this heat and water loss cannot be sustained for long. Dehydration exaggerates the impacts of hypothermia and hypoxia.

Sleep Deprivation

Recent studies have shown that when a night's sleep is repeatedly interrupted, even for only a few seconds, the mental processes are impaired the next day, at any altitude. The fragmented sleep that most climbers experience at the highest camps adds to the likelihood of confusion, poor judgment, and bad decisions the next day.

One of the survivors on Everest in 1996, Jon Krakauer, described his experience as he reached the summit:

> I hadn't slept in fifty-seven hours. The only food I'd been able to force down over the preceding three days was a bowl of soup and a handful of peanut M&Ms...so little oxygen was reaching my brain that my mental capacity was that of a slow child...I was incapable of feeling much of anything except being cold and tired.

Each of these environmental impacts adds to the effect of the others and the combination produces the "sick man walking in a dream," as George Mallory described a climber high on Everest. (Mallory, with Andrew Irvine, was last seen near the summit of Everest in 1924, but whether they made the summit is unknown.) Several of the survivors in 1996 eloquently described their sense of isolation and loss of normal perception.

HEALTH CONDITIONS THAT MAY CAUSE PROBLEMS AT ALTITUDE

Bearing in mind these environmental risks, are there some individuals who should not go to altitude? The mountain world is attracting more and more people, and not only to small mountains but to big ones. Getting to the mountains has become easier and faster in most parts of the world, and millions of men, women, and children of all ages are going to potentially dangerous altitudes.

Almost anyone can go to 5,000 feet without noticing any effects. Above 8,000 feet, one of every five visitors is likely to have symptoms due to altitude, and what happens above this depends on the rate of climb and altitude reached, as discussed in Chapter 8, "The Spectrum of High-Altitude Illness: AMS/HACE."

But what about individuals with some illness or disability? How should doctors advise a pregnant woman, a man in his sixties with heart disease, or someone with diabetes, epilepsy, or asthma? Hundreds of people are asking their doctors these questions, as thousands who never would have dreamed of it a few decades ago are going up into the mountains.

A sixty-two-year-old woman wishes to take a six-day trip in the Andes, going as high as 12,000 feet after a rather rapid ascent. She had asthma as a child and smoked heavily until recently. Years ago she had an eosinophilic granuloma (an unusual malignant tumor) in her lungs and in her brain. The lungs healed slowly; the granuloma was removed from the brain surgically. She had several seizures after the operation and has taken the anticonvulsant dilantin ever since. A year ago she had a breast cancer removed and was given a course of radiotherapy. She has no symptoms, is moderately active in sports, and is not excessively short of breath. Her arterial oxygen saturation is 96 percent. Chest X ray shows little scarring, EKG is normal, but her pulmonary function tests show greatly reduced maximal breathing capacity with no improvement after medication.

S is a fifty-one-year-old mother of three who has rapidly progressive Lou Gehrig's disease (amyotrophic lateral sclerosis). She wishes to visit her family's home at 9,000 feet while she still is able. Her arterial oxygen saturation is below 85 percent at sea level. Her neurology specialists advise her not to go, but if she insists, they urge that she not go outside!

The first woman has several strikes against her. Her asthma did not leave any damage, but years of smoking did. The tumor in her lungs probably left some scarring, and x-ray treatment after her breast cancer was removed may also have caused fibrosis of lung tissue, even though carefully monitored. She decided not to go on the altitude part of the trip.

As for S, low arterial oxygen saturation suggests that her ability to breathe is limited because her respiratory muscles are compromised. This means she would lose one of the best defenses against hypoxia even as low as 9,000 feet and might have a serious problem. The advice not to go outdoors is silly. If she breathed supplementary oxygen during the flight and drive to the resort, and all the time while there, she should not be at greater risk than at sea level.

Cancer

A seventy-year-old veteran mountaineer developed widespread bone metastases from multiple myeloma. Powerful treatments relieved his pain somewhat and apparently arrested further spread. A few months after finishing his treatment, he climbed a 14,000-foot mountain faster and more easily than his partner.

There is no evidence that going to high altitude has a bad effect on cancer. In fact, many years ago Al Barach, a visionary physician, proposed treating certain cancers by having the patient breathe oxygen at half sea-level partial pressure, which is equivalent to going to 18,000 feet. The justification was that fast-growing cancer cells require more oxygen than do normal cells, and their growth might be slowed. Only a few limited studies were done, but the concept was revisited in the 1990s when a promising new treatment for cancer was studied based on depriving the tumor of oxygen and also of food by decreasing its blood supply. Because cancers grow more rapidly than normal tissue, they are more susceptible to oxygen lack and "starvation." Unless anemia or some other impediment decreases oxygen delivery to cells, someone with a disease likely soon to be terminal should grasp every pleasure he or she can.

Advanced Age

Chapter 17, "Limits to Work at Altitude," discussed the many things that age does to slow us down. In deciding whether an elderly person can or should go to altitude, the doctor should pay extra attention to several of these. Vital capacity—the largest breath we can take—decreases slightly but steadily with age, thus decreasing one of the best ways of dealing with hypoxia. The maximum achievable heart rate (MAHR) decreases with age, so the older we get, the less increase we can expect in the rate and output of the heart when pushed. We may, hopefully, grow wiser, but memory, along with reflexes, work capacity, and strength, all worsen. On the other hand, the older one is, the less likely one is to develop AMS, at least up to 10,000 feet, which is about as high as most older persons want to go. Still, many men and women over seventy have climbed to 18,000 feet and higher, and several who were over ninety have walked up Mount Fuji (12,395 feet). A very few over seventy have summited even higher peaks. Age by itself is not a deterrent—if you think you can, and if you long to climb or just visit the mountains, age alone should not stop you.

High Blood Pressure

Systemic blood pressure usually increases slightly with altitude, but over time it tends to level off or return to sea-level values. People with hypertension are likely to increase their blood pressure more than others do, even at moderate altitude. High blood pressure alone is not a contraindication to a visit to the mountains, although the individual had better not try one of the major summits. It is important to remember that a single blood pressure reading in any setting is often misleading because blood pressure is so labile and changes so much and so quickly in different circumstances.

Pulmonary artery pressure (PAP) also increases with age and increases further with cold and altitude, but this does not seem to increase the risk of HAPE in the elderly. Increased PAP may cause more breathlessness than expected, which suggests that some fluid is collecting in the lung interstitial space, but this happens in many people without progressing to HAPE. Unless one's activity at sea level is limited due to lung disease, this is not a reason to avoid altitude—where the air is fresher, and actually easier to breathe because it is thinner. This is good news for people with asthma, most of whom tolerate altitude well unless they have badly hurt their lungs over the years.

Heart Disease

Many people with known heart disease, or those who might be at risk for various reasons, ask about going to the mountains. Herb Hultgren, a distinguished cardiologist who studied high altitude for forty years, is conservative in his recommendations. In his published articles and book *High Altitude Medicine* he describes several cases, paraphrased as follows:

> A seventy-year-old physician with stable angina required several nitroglycerine tablets daily, plus several cardiac drugs. He flew to 8,000 feet, where he had repeated episodes of angina for thirty-six hours, but these decreased, and by the end of a week he was having no more episodes than at sea level. On return home his former condition was unchanged.
>
> An elderly businessman had slowly worsening angina for twenty-two years after a heart attack; this limited his activity. He flew to Denver (5,280 feet), and drove over a 12,000-foot pass and down to a resort at 8,200 feet. His angina was very severe on the pass and continued at the resort, forcing him to return home. He did not show evidence of further heart damage.

The first patient tolerated the altitude reasonably well despite his coronary artery disease. This is not unusual, and in fact some patients actually have less angina at moderate altitude. In the second individual, the coronary disease was more serious and he was fortunate not to have precipitated another heart attack.

In fact, myocardial infarcts are uncommon at altitude, some believe less frequent than in a comparable population at sea level. David Shlim reported that of 148,000 trekkers in Nepal who went to 9,000 to 17,000 feet, about 10 percent were over fifty; six left a trek early because of "heart symptoms" but there were no deaths due to heart disease. Maggiorini's large survey of climbers and hikers in the Alps showed no evidence of increased heart disease. (See Table 2.) However, despite these encouraging studies, the belief that moderate hypoxia actually dilates coronary arteries and improves angina is, unfortunately, a myth.

Ben Levine, a practicing cardiologist and active researcher in high-altitude physiology, reported a well-controlled study of fifteen men and five women visiting a resort at 8,200 feet for five days. Of the twenty subjects, who averaged sixty-eight years of age, 35 percent had known coronary heart disease and an additional 50 percent were considered at high risk of undetected underlying heart disease. They tolerated the altitude and daily treadmill exercise well. One man had a myocardial infarct after exercise on the fifth day, but the night before he had experienced severe angina, which he did not mention before the test. Forty-five percent of the group had symptoms of mild AMS. A battery of heart studies led the researchers to conclude:

> Patients with coronary artery disease who are well compensated at sea level are likely to do well at moderate altitude, although with acute exposure ischemia may be provoked at...lower work rates.

What should an older person with heart symptoms do if he or she wants to go the mountains? Everything depends on the individual's condition, and an evaluation should be performed by a cardiologist who understands more than a little about high altitude. A careful history and physical examination, plus a few of the more appropriate tests, are necessary. In general, recognizing that individuals differ and that the differences may be crucial, a person with angina due to mild coronary artery disease who is active at sea level can probably go safely to moderate altitude and do somewhat less than his or her usual sea-level activities.

Congestive heart failure, whether compensated or not, is evidence that the heart has been damaged or is an inadequate pump. The additional load of moderate hypoxia may not be well tolerated even with medication, and it is advised, again considering the individual, not to take the risk.

Congenital heart disease, valvular disease, valve replacements, enlargement of the heart, and frequent rhythm disturbances may be added risks and require careful evaluation. When feasible, marginal cases can be evaluated by exposing the patient to at least six hours of mild hypoxia, but this is hard to arrange.

Older and recent exercise protocols for testing at sea level are unreliable predictors of altitude tolerance.

What about cardiac bypass? After a patient has had a successful bypass, heart function generally improves greatly and surgeons like to consider the heart to be, if not "as good as new," at least nearly so. Although some disagree, many believe that a fully recovered bypass patient can safely go to altitude. In fact, several have gone very high in the Himalayas soon after bypass, without difficulty. The outlook after dilation of a plugged coronary artery by balloon angioplasty has not been evaluated fully. In any case, each person must be individually evaluated.

Blood Problems

Anemia exaggerates the impact of altitude because there is less hemoglobin to transport oxygen, and the heart tries to make up for this by faster, more forceful beats. One can tolerate mild anemia at altitude, but not if hemoglobin is less than about 8 grams. Leukemia might pose a problem, as would any illness that interferes with oxygen transport.

Two uncommon red cell problems are sickle cell anemia and sickle cell trait, also discussed in Chapter 4, "Moving Blood: Circulation." Persons with sickle cell trait or thalassemia (a similar mutant hemoglobin) are likely to have problems if they go to altitude.

Pulmonary Disease

Chapter 12, "Hypoxia in Everyday Life," discussed how individuals with lung problems like chronic obstructive pulmonary disease (COPD) adjust to hypoxia. Of the 30 million people with COPD in the United States, one group tolerates moderate altitude quite well—notably the "pink puffers," who often have a nearly normal arterial oxygen pressure and saturation, although their carbon dioxide is low and their pH is on the alkaline side. They are able to maintain good oxygenation at sea level by automatically overbreathing all the time. If blood studies and the usual pulmonary function studies and chest X rays confirm this diagnosis, many can go safely to 8,000 to 9,000 feet. In fact, many veteran miners have COPD from years of dust inhalation—yet are able to live and work even higher than this.

By contrast, "blue bloaters" breathe less than a healthy person, but rely on increased hemoglobin to sustain oxygen delivery. These people do not adjust to altitude, and if they go much higher than 5,000 feet without supplemental oxygen, they will be at risk for HAPE and perhaps even right heart failure. Those with advanced COPD do not tolerate air travel well. However, breathing oxygen helps the patient considerably and enables him or her to fly in commercial aircraft and even to visit altitude, provided that additional oxygen is breathed at all times. "Blue bloaters" usually have a high pulmonary artery pressure, and HAPE could be a significant risk without the extra oxygen.

Other Illnesses

As climbing and skiing became more popular, many people with chronic illnesses began to go to mountain resorts and then to higher and higher mountains. A good deal of reliable information has come from experience and from a few careful studies, but we need more—and no two individuals are quite the same.

Epilepsy is not a contraindication if it is well controlled, and hypoxia does not seem to increase the frequency or severity of attacks. Obviously, someone who is taking medicine should be careful to not stop taking it.

There is little or no evidence that *mental illness* is worsened by altitude, and in fact the calm beauty of mountains has soothed many disturbed persons.

Diabetes is not a contraindication to sojourning at high altitude, but may be more difficult to control during a climb. Exertion will use up blood and liver sugars and thus decrease the need for insulin, and may even cause insulin shock. At altitude, however, some people show an increase in blood sugar during or after exertion, indicating that the insulin dose might need to be increased for some people. Individuals with severe or "brittle" diabetes planning to exercise in the mountains might be wise to take frequent fingertip blood samples and adjust insulin accordingly. Insulin is not damaged by freezing.

Taking Medications

There is little authoritative information about the use of medications at altitude. We are a pill-taking culture, and although the chemistries and the actions and interactions of many drugs are well documented, we do not know much about how hypoxia affects them.

Diamox and *dexamethasone* are discussed in Chapter 15, "Prevention and Treatment." Several of the people on Everest in 1996 carried syringes loaded with dexamethasone and some were given the injection in the belief it would quickly give them a little extra strength in the crisis.

Progesterone has been used to increase ventilation and prevent AMS, with little benefit or adverse effect for short-term use. *Nifedipine*, like other cardiac calcium channel blockers, lowers both systemic and pulmonary blood pressure, and is good treatment for HAPE. For those who have had HAPE or are considered HAPE-susceptible, a small dose of nifedipine before (and perhaps during) a trip above 10,000 feet is a good preventive measure; it is not advisable for non-susceptibles.

The use of *birth control pills* (BCPs) at altitude is controversial: Some believe they may increase the risk of thrombosis and embolism, already increased by the thickened blood and by the release of biologically active substances by hypoxia. Those BCPs that contain progesterone may help slightly.

Aspirin and other *nonsteroidal anti-inflammatory drugs* (NSAIDs) may cause stomach irritation and even a little bleeding, but they are less irritating when taken with food. At one time it was thought that by preventing platelet clumping, aspirin might alleviate some altitude illness, but this has not proven to be the case. NSAIDs are of some help in relieving altitude headache but have no other effect on hypoxia.

A few stories have surfaced reporting that *tricyclic antidepressants* have caused a severe reaction to hypoxia, and in fact one patient with severe COPD died from respiratory arrest in the hospital allegedly because he was given an antidepressant. *Barbiturates* and *tranquilizers* have a greater and more prolonged effect when taken at altitude than they do at sea level, and are unwise, certainly above 18,000 feet, because the small, persistent effect may further blur judgment. One of the very short-acting sedatives is thought to have precipitated hallucinations and brief mild mental changes on a few occasions. Most climbers believe—some with firsthand experience—that *alcohol* is more powerful on a mountain where "one drink does the work of two."

Stimulants like tea and coffee are part of contemporary life at any altitude; high on a mountain, disrupted sleep may be further disrupted by caffeine. In place of boiling, water is often sterilized by adding *iodine*, which will not affect altitude tolerance. *Amphetamines* have been used for extra energy in a crisis: In 1950 Maurice Herzog was said to have taken dexedrine on top of Annapurna, the first 8,000-meter peak to be climbed. The resulting euphoria may have caused the careless loss of his gloves and severe frostbite, but it may also have saved his life. Just how much extra energy amphetamines provide during a crisis such as the one on Everest in 1996 is hard to determine. Certainly amphetamines, like other stimulants, are not to be taken casually anywhere.

Medicines prescribed for high blood pressure are likely to need dose adjustment at altitude, and other *cardiac drugs* may also need to be changed. It would be prudent to consult a local doctor at altitude if possible. These are individual issues that should be addressed by your own doctor before a trip—though he or she may not have guidelines any more definite than these!

The bottom line is that although we know a great deal about the chemistry of medications and their metabolic and degradation pathways, we have very little good information about their effects and effectiveness at altitude. Many drugs are broken down and eliminated by the liver, which has a high demand for oxygen, and some laboratory studies indicate that these, and perhaps others, are not well handled at altitude or during chronic hypoxia.

Using Illegal Drugs

Many climbers have used *marijuana* on mountains and, depending on whom you ask and how candid the responses, the effects may be called great, indifferent, or bad. Marijuana does blur awareness, especially of unpleasant stimuli, which is one reason it is taken. If it disturbs reaction times or judgment, that would not be helpful on a difficult climb. *Morphine* and other opiates blunt the respiratory drive and can be expected to increase the likelihood of HAPE and AMS/HACE. Nevertheless, morphine is valuable as a last resort for treating HAPE.

In general it is probably safe to assume that any medication will be more potent at altitude—which may be good news or bad.

EARLY WARNING SIGNS
The Brain and Central Nervous System

Although cognitive thought and mental processes are the most dangerously effected by altitude, they are by far the most difficult to study. Nevertheless, the more primitive functions of the brain can be studied. In Chapter 8, "The Spectrum of High-Altitude Illness: AMS/HACE," ataxia and clumsiness of the fine motions of the fingers were discussed as early symptoms, or rather as an early sign. Attempts to quantify these changes have been difficult until recently, when a rather complex technique called *posturography* has been tried at moderate altitude. The subject stands on a slightly moveable platform and is positioned, both with the eyes opened and the eyes closed, and photographed with a special high-speed camera. Even small motions are easily detected in the subject's balance. Not surprisingly, these small motions are an early indication of HACE, but what is surprising is that ataxia is also seen before any other evidence of HACE appears. The difficulty disappears with oxygen or descent. The technique is impractical except in a laboratory environment, such as a decompression chamber, but it does provide evidence of the early effect of hypoxia: subtle changes in the brain.

Another sophisticated technique very precisely measures the time intervals in pronouncing simple words in response to various questions. There are many other pencil-and-paper, electrical, electronic, or mechanical devices, but they all have the common drawback of the subject being slightly affected by the fact that he or she is being observed.

The Eye and Vision

The eye, being easily accessible, has been extensively studied at high altitude. Among the very early studies were those done by Ross McFarland prior to World War II. In a meticulously crafted series of studies, he showed that night vision (vision in dim light) decreases with increasing altitude, so that at 10,000 feet it is approximately half of what it is at sea level. This is because in dim light the rods in the retina are used rather than the cones, and because the rods are situated around the periphery of the retina, one can see at night much better in the peripheral vision than in the central! Color vision did not seem to be affected.

Beginning in World War II, aircraft could fly much higher than it was safe for pilots to go, unless they breathed extra oxygen. Training for night flying became particularly important, as did the early detection of hypoxia. The dimming of vision was an early warning of hypoxia but, unfortunately, this warning often came too late for many of the pilots who might have lost their oxygen supply.

At extreme altitude, climbers have experienced a variety of visual changes, all the way from dimmed vision to total blindness. (See Chapter 9, "Vision and the Eye at Altitude.")

To say that the mountain environment is different is to state the obvious! Below 10,000 feet the difference may be noticeable but not dangerous. The higher one goes, the more powerful is the combined impact of cold, exhaustion, and lack of oxygen, food, water, and sleep. Each of these may be moderated but not eliminated. Together they make very high mountains potentially lethal. Terrible in beauty, awesome, fickle in weather, the mountain environment truly can be a death zone.

But approached with experience, educated caution, humility, and reverence, mountains have been and always will be a reservoir of beauty and inspiration.

As for the mountaineers, Walter Lippman, philosopher-cum-journalist, wrote in the *New York Times* many decades ago:

The world is a better place...because it contains human beings who do...the useless, brave, noble, divinely foolish, and the very wisest things that are done by man. And what they prove...is that man is no mere creature of his habits, no automaton in his routine, but that in the dust of which he is made there is also fire, lighted now and then by great winds from the sky.

GLOSSARY

Acapnia: Literally, no carbon dioxide. Often used to describe a condition in which the partial pressure of carbon dioxide in the blood is lower than normal. See also **Hypocapnea**.

Acclimatization: Changes in response to altitude that develop over weeks or months.

Accommodations: Changes in response to altitude that occur within minutes.

Acephalgic migraine: Migraine without headache, commonly vision related.

Acetazolamide: A carbonic anhydrase inhibiting drug—known by its brand name, Diamox—that promotes diuresis (production of urine) and may reduce the symptoms of mild acute mountain sickness (AMS).

Acetylcholine: A neurotransmitter that stimulates skeletal muscle.

Acidosis: A metabolic condition in which the body can no longer buffer hydrogen ions in the blood, causing blood pH to drop (become acidic). It may be caused by inadequate respiration or metabolic disturbance.

Active transport: The process by which cells "pump" a substance across the cell membrane against a higher concentration, requiring energy expenditure through metabolism.

Adaptation: Changes responsive to altitude that take generations.

Adenosine diphosphate (ADP): A molecule composed of an adenine, a ribose, and two phosphates. ADP is formed when ATP (see **Adenosine triphosphate**) gives up energy to power a cellular process.

Adenosine monophosphate (AMP): A molecule composed of an adenine, a ribose, and one phosphate.

Adenosine triphosphate (ATP): A molecule composed of an adenine, a ribose and three phosphates. ATP can be formed from ADP (see **Adenosine diphosphate**) by the addition of energy or can give up energy to power cellular processes and become ADP.

Adipose: Fat-containing cells or tissue.

Adrenergic: Activated by or able to release epinephrine or related substances; related to the sympathetic nervous system, or having physiologic effects similar to epinephrine. See also **Epinephrine**, **Sympathetic nervous system**.

Adult respiratory distress syndrome (ARDS): A type of pulmonary edema that results from severe trauma or toxic shock.

Aldosterone: A steroid hormone that controls salt and water balance.

Allele: One of multiple forms of any gene.

Alpha-1-protease inhibitor (AAT): Also known as alpha-1-antitrypsin, this protein inhibits the enzyme neutrophil elastase. Severe AAT deficiency leads to pulmonary disease.

Altitude: Geographers and cartographers use feet or meters to define height above sea level. Physiologists prefer to express altitude in terms of barometric pressure, using torr or millimeters of mercury (mm Hg).

Alveolar: Pertaining to the air sacs in the lung.

Alveolar–arterial (A–a) gradient: The difference in the partial pressure of oxygen between alveolar air and arterial blood in the lungs.

Alveolar proteinosis: A rare lung disease in which phospholipid accumulates in the alveoli.

Alveolus (plural alveoli): The tiny air spaces in the lung where oxygen and carbon dioxide pass between air and blood.

Amaurosis fugax: A temporary interference of vision ("a shade coming down over the eyes"), related to constricting of the blood vessels that supply the eye.

Ambient: Relating to the environment surrounding us. Customarily refers to air, temperature, or humidity.

Amenorrhea: Abnormal absence of menses.

Anaerobic: Occurring in the absence of oxygen.

Anastomosis (plural anastomoses): An opening between two normally separated spaces, such as a communication or convergence between blood vessels.

Angiogenesis: The process in which new capillary blood vessels are formed.

Angiotensin II: The active form of angiotensin, which acts as a strong vasoconstrictor that causes a rise in blood pressure. See also **Renin.**

Angiotensin-converting enzyme (ACE): An enzyme responsible for producing the active form of angiotensin. ACE inhibitors are drugs used to lower high blood pressure. See also **Angiotensin II, Renin.**

Anoxemia: Literally means no oxygen in blood. See also **Hypoxia.**

Anoxia: Literally means no oxygen. See also **Hypoxia.**

Antidiuretic hormone (ADH): A hormone produced in the hypothalamus and released from the posterior pituitary gland that suppresses urine formation and stimulates contraction of blood vessel endothelial muscle.

Antioxidant: A substance (for example, vitamin E) that slows or prevents the reaction of oxygen with other chemicals (oxidation).

Arcuate nucleus: A part of the brain that senses oxygen and carbon dioxide levels and controls breathing and waking during sleep.

Arteriole: A small artery, usually one that leads to a capillary. See also **Capillaries.**

Arteriosclerosis: Formation of lipid-filled plaques in the arteries.

Ataxia: Customarily refers to staggering gait, but also applies to clumsiness with arms, hands, or fingers.

Atmospheric: Pertaining to the air that envelops the earth.

Atrial natriuretic peptide (ANP): A hormone secreted by small granules in the muscle fibers of the atria of the heart. Causes salt and water loss in the urine.

Atrium (plural **atria**): A heart chamber; there are two atria, the left and the right.

Autonomic nervous system: The part of the brain and peripheral nerves that automatically controls the functions we cannot willfully control, among them the heart and blood pressure and movement of the muscles that control breathing.

Axon: The long portion of the nerve cell that usually conducts impulses away from the cell body.

Barometer: A device developed by Evangelista Torricelli, from Gaspar Berti, to measure the weight of the atmosphere that envelops the earth, commonly expressed as torr, or millimeters of mercury (mm Hg) barometric pressure.

Basal metabolic rate (BMR): The amount of energy used at rest to maintain basic life functions. See also **Total metabolic rate.**

Basement membrane: The layer of protein fibers that separates epithelial tissues (tissues that cover open body surfaces such as the alveoli and blood vessels) from deeper tissues.

Beta-agonists: Also called beta-adrenergic agonists, drugs that activate adrenergic receptors. They stimulate the heart and cause bronchodilation.

Beta blockers: Drugs that block the activity of adrenergic receptors. They slow the heart and lower blood pressure.

Bronchus (plural **bronchi, bronchioles**): Branch of the trachea or windpipe; bronchioles lead from the trachea, subdivide into progressively smaller tubes, and end at the alveoli.

Buffer: A salt formed by the combination of a weak acid with a strong base (or vice versa) that absorbs hydrogen ions under acid conditions but gives them up under alkaline conditions, thus resisting a change in pH.

Calorie: A unit of measurement of energy; the amount of energy required to raise one gram of 15° C water one degree centigrade.

Cannula: A tube for insertion in a cavity, duct, or vessel.

Capillaries: Tiny, thin-walled vessels that form a network that carries blood from the smallest arterioles to the smallest venules.

Carbohydrate: A class of compounds composed of of carbon, hydrogen, and oxygen—sugars, starches, and celluloses—a major food class.

Carbonate–bicarbonate buffer system: Carbonic acid (H_2CO_3) is formed in the blood from the combination of carbon dioxide (CO_2) and water

(H_2O). Carbonic acid then breaks down to bicarbonate ($H_2CO_3^-$) and hydrogen ions (H^+). These chemicals act as a buffer system because they resist changes in pH. When acid is added to the blood, some of the hydrogen ions combine with bicarbonate minimizing the change in pH. When acid is removed from the blood, more carbonic acid breaks down, replacing some of the lost hydrogen ions. This also minimizes the change in pH.

Carbonic anhydrase: An enzyme that facilitates conversion of carbon dioxide to carbonic acid in red blood cells and to bicarbonate in the kidneys.

Carboxy–hemoglobin: The compound formed when carbon monoxide attaches to hemoglobin, displacing oxygen.

Cardiac output: The measure of the blood flow through the heart to the systemic circulation in one minute; a product of the heart rate and the stroke volume. See also **Heart rate**, **Stroke volume**.

Carotid: Large artery on each side of the neck, supplying the head with blood. Each has a smaller bulge called the carotid sinus, which monitors blood pressure. A collection of specialized cells adjacent to each artery (carotid bodies, or glomus) monitors oxygen in blood.

Carrying capacity: The amount of oxygen that the blood can carry when fully saturated. Usually described in volumes percent, i.e., the number of milliliters of gas in 100 milliliters of blood.

Catheter: A tubular device for insertion into canals, passages, vessels, or cavities for medical purposes.

Cell membrane: A semipermeable barrier surrounding the cell made up of a double layer (bilayer) of fat (lipid) molecules. Also called **plasma membrane** or plasmalemma.

Cerebellum: The part of the brain primarily responsible for controlling muscle tone and balance.

Cerebrospinal fluid (CSF): The fluid that bathes the brain and spinal cord. In patients with HACE, the worse the symptoms, the higher the CSF pressure is likely to be.

Cerebrovascular accident (CVA): See **Stroke**.

Cholecystokinin (CCK): A protein secreted in the upper intestine that causes gall bladder contraction and has other effects on the gastric system. CCK may mediate satiety.

Computerized tomography (CT): A scanning x-ray procedure used for diagnosis.

Coronary arteries: The two arteries, right and left, that stem from the aorta and supply oxygen to the tissues of the heart.

Corpus callosum: The band of fibers connecting the cerebral hemispheres.

Corpus cavernosum: Erectile tissue that can be distended by filling with blood; found in the penis and clitoris.

Cotton wool spots: Whitish areas seen in the retina of the eye, indicating swelling or edema, without bleeding.

Cyanosis, cyanotic: A bluish color of lips and nail beds (and, in extreme cases, of skin) due to lack of oxygen in the blood, which leaves some of the hemoglobin in the unsaturated form.

Cyclic guanosine monophosphate (cGMP): A messenger molecule that has the effect of reducing the calcium level in the arterial smooth muscle.

Cystic fibrosis (CF): A recessive genetic defect that results in abnormality of the glands that produce sweat or mucus and also causes severe lung damage.

Cytoplasm: The contents of the cell exterior to the nuclear membrane. See also **Nucleus**.

Cytosol: The fluid portion of the cell, exclusive of organelles and membranes. See also **Organelle**.

Dendrite: A branching portion of the nerve cell that usually conducts impulses toward the cell body.

Deoxyribonucleic acid (DNA): The double helix of two nucleic acid chains that make up the chromosomes and form the molecular basis of heredity.

Dexamethasone: A steroid medication that acts to control inflammation and may be useful in the treatment of severe acute mountain sickness (AMS).

Diabetes mellitus: A disorder of carbohydrate metabolism characterized by insufficient production or utilization of insulin. See also **Insulin**.

Diaphragm: The muscular partition separating the chest and abdominal cavity that can expand the thoracic cavity to cause inspiration of air into the lungs.

Diffusion: The movement of one substance through another, for example, of a gas through a barrier such as a cell wall, or of a gas or a dissolved substance throughout the gas or liquid in which it is dissolved.

Diuretic: A substance, either natural or synthetic, that increases the formation of urine.

Dopamine: A neurotransmitter that acts in the brain.

Doubleproduct: The product of the heart rate and blood pressure, a rough measure of fitness.

Dyspnea: Shortness of breath; difficulty breathing.

Edema: Fluid that accumulates in the loose tissue between the cells, or within cells, or within the alveoli or interstitial space of the lungs.

Elastase: An enzyme that breaks down elastin and collagen. See also **Elastin**.

Elastin: A glycoprotein that forms the fibers found in connective tissue.

Electron transport system (ETS): The mitochondrial electron transport chain involved in the process of energy conversion.

Embolus (plural emboli): An abnormal particle (as an air bubble or blood clot) circulating in the blood.

Endothelins: A family of substances, released by endothelial cells; one of the endothelins constricts blood vessels in direct opposition to nitric oxide. See also **Nitric oxide**.

Endothelium: The lining of blood vessels.

Endothelium-derived relaxing factor (EDRF): A powerful vasodilator that has been identified as a simple chemical substance, nitric oxide (NO).

Enzyme: A protein that speeds chemical reactions and determines which reactions occur in living organisms.

Epinephrine: A sympathetic hormone secreted by the adrenal medulla that acts as a potent vasoconstrictor (raising blood pressure), heart stimulant, and bronchial dilator. Also known as adrenaline.

Epithelium: Cells that line all free body surfaces including the alveoli, blood vessels, and skin.

Erythrocyte: Red blood cell.

Erythropoietin (EPO): A hormone produced in the kidney that promotes the production of red blood cells.

Estradiol: A female sex hormone produced by the ovaries.

Fibrosis: Formation of fibrous tissue.

Frontal lobes: The portion of the brain responsible for higher cognitive thought.

Furosemide: A potent diuretic medication, known by the brand name Lasix.

Gamow bag: A bag large enough to accept a person and which can be pressurized by pumping. Useful as an emergency treatment of acute mountain sickness (AMS) when descent is not immediately possible.

Gene: The molecular unit of inheritance that occupies a specific part of the chromosome and determines the structure of a particular protein or the function of other genetic material.

Glia: Supportive cells that surround and protect brain cells. Special glial cells protect the brain capillaries from overdistension.

Glomerulus (plural **glomeruli**): A part of the kidney where filtration of the blood takes place.

Glucose: A six-carbon sugar found in many foods, and the major source of energy for many organisms.

Glucose transporter: A membrane protein that binds one molecule of glucose in the interstitial fluid outside the cell and deposits it into the cytoplasm inside the cell. See also **Glucose**.

Glycogen: A long chain of glucose molecules found mainly in liver and muscle tissue as an energy store. Also called animal starch.

Glycolysis: The conversion of a sugar, usually glucose, to pyruvate to generate ATP without using oxygen. See also **Adenosine triphosphate**, **Anaerobic**.

Glycoprotein: Proteins with attached sugar units, commonly found on the cell's plasma membrane.

Gray matter: Neural tissue of the brain and spinal cord that contains cells, blood vessels, and nerve fibers. See also **White matter**.

Heart rate: The number of beats of the heart per minute, determined by taking the pulse. Varies with age, size, and cardiovascular health.

Hematocrit (HCT): The percentage of whole blood occupied by cells (mostly red blood cells). Describes the red cell mass.

Hemoglobin (Hb): A complex substance containing four iron atoms (which combine loosely with oxygen) and a protein (a species-specific globin) that determines the type of hemoglobin. Different animals have a metallic ion other than iron and different proteins.

Heterozygous: Having two different alleles of the same gene. See also **Allele**.

Hilum: The part of the lung through which the bronchus passes.

Homozygous: Having two copies of the same allele. See also **Allele**.

Hormone: Proteins produced by one tissue that reach distant tissues by way of the bloodstream and impact the function of the cells in those tissues.

Human leukocyte antigen (HLA): Proteins on the surface of cells that are important in activating immune system response.

Hypercapnia: Excessive carbon dioxide in blood.

Hypocapnea: Insufficient carbon dioxide in blood. This term is more precise, though less often used, than acapnia. See also **Acapnia**.

Hypoglycemia: Abnormally low blood concentration of glucose (sugar).

Hyponatremia: Abnormally low blood concentration of sodium.

Hypothalamus: A portion of the brain situated below the thalamus that secretes substances that influence pituitary function and metabolism.

Hypothermia: A condition of abnormally low body temperature.

Hypoxemia: A condition of below-normal oxygen content in arterial blood.

Hypoxia: Lack of oxygen. This has largely replaced the older, less accurate term **anoxia** (literally, "no oxygen"). **Anoxemia** refers to inadequate oxygen in the blood and is used instead of the more precise but clumsy word **hypoxemia**.

Hypoxia inducible factor (HIF): A protein that is produced in the presence of hypoxia and, in turn, stimulates the production of many substances that are important in acclimatization.

Hypoxic pulmonary vasoconstriction (HPV): A condition in which certain branches of the pulmonary arteries feeding poorly oxygenated lung areas are constricted, resulting in blood being shunted toward areas of the lung where the alveolar oxygen level is higher and the blood can more readily pick up oxygen.

Hypoxic ventilatory response (HVR): The change in rate and/or depth of breathing dictated by a decrease in the partial pressure of oxygen in the inspired air. It is an index of the sensitivity of the respiratory center to oxygen lack.

Insulin: A pancreatic hormone essential for the metabolism of carbohydrates. See also **Diabetes mellitus**.

Intercellular: Literally, between cells.

Intercostal muscle: Skeletal muscle between the ribs.

Interferon: A family of glycoproteins that play a role in fighting viral infection and cancer. See also **Glycoprotein**.

Interleukin: One of a variety of polypeptides that play a role in regulating the immune system and fighting infection.

Intermittent hypoxia: The situation in which tissues are alternately deprived of oxygen and then resupplied with it.

Intermittent upper airway obstruction (IUAO): A big name for simple snoring.

Interstitial: Pertaining to loose tissue (less accurately "interstitial space") between cells, the interstitium.

Intracellular: Literally, within cells.

Krebs cycle: See **Tricarboxylic acid cycle**.

Leptin: A hormone released from fat cells when energy stores are high that reduces appetite and increases energy expenditure.

Leukocytes: White blood cells that fight infection.

Lipid: A fat or fat-like substance.

Luteinizing hormone (LH): A female sex hormone produced in the pituitary that is involved in ovulation.

Lymph: Fluid that bathes the tissues, passes into lymphatic ducts, and is discharged into the blood through the thoracic duct.

Lymphatic system: Tissues that produce and store infection-fighting cells along with the network of vessels that carry lymph. See also **Lymph**.

Macula: The area of the retina responsible for central vision.

Magnetic resonance imaging (MRI): A scanning x-ray procedure used for diagnosis.

Maximal breathing capacity: The largest volume of air one can breathe in one minute.

Maximal oxygen uptake: The amount of oxygen one can acquire while working at peak capacity. It indicates the volume of air one can move, as well as the volume of oxygen passing from lungs to blood, and is the standard measurement of fitness and work capacity. Often abbreviated as VO_2 **max**.

Maximum achievable heart rate (MAHR): Roughly defined as "200 minus half one's age," MAHR is the fastest rate (in beats per minute) at which the heart can beat with normal electrical conduction.

Membrane: A thin, single-cell-thick covering for cells or organs. The characteristics of each membrane have developed to match its function. See also **Basement membrane**.

Membrane potential: Each living cell membrane carries a minute electric charge (bioelectric potential) that maintains the cell's integrity and enables it to fulfill its particular function. Cell death occurs when the membrane potential falls to zero.

Metabolic rate: The amount of oxygen consumed per minute. Usually measured under basal (resting, fasting) conditions, corrected for body surface area, called **basal metabolic rate (BMR).**

Metabolism: The chemical changes in living cells that produce energy needed for vital activities, assimilate new materials, and maintain the organism.

Mitochondria: Small cellular organelles in which energy production (production of **adenosine triphosphate**, or ATP) and cellular respiration (use of oxygen) take place.

Monge's disease: An alternative name for chronic mountain sickness (CMS), after Carlos Monge, who first described the condition in 1925 as a pathological loss of adaptation to high altitude characterized by severe polycythemia.

Mutation: A change in the genetic material, usually a single gene, that can be passed on hereditarily.

Myoglobin: An iron-containing pigment, similar to hemoglobin but with a higher affinity for oxygen, found in skeletal muscle where it acts as an oxygen storage protein.

Myosin: The contractile protein of muscle.

Neurotransmitter: A chemical that transmits a nerve impulse across a synapse. See also **Synapse.**

Nifedipine: A calcium channel-blocking drug used to treat angina that works by dilating the coronary arteries, reducing arterial pressure, and decreasing the oxygen utilization of the heart.

Nitric oxide (NO): An endogenous compound, produced by the enzyme nitric oxide synthase, that acts as a potent vasodilator.

Nitric oxide synthase (NOS): An enzyme that catalyzes the formation of nitric oxide. Two forms of NOS are inducible NOS (iNOS) and endothelial NOS (eNOS). When the production of iNOS is stimulated, it produces a large amount of NO quickly and locally. By contrast, eNOS produces a constant, low-level concentration of NO throughout the circulation.

Nonsteroidal anti-inflammatories (NSAIDs): A class of drugs that reduce inflammation, ease pain, and lower fever.

Norepinephrine: The neurotransmitter of the sympathetic nervous system. Known also as noradrenaline. Norepinephrine is most commonly released from a sympathetic nervous system nerve to stimulate an organ (such as the heart), while epinephrine is the major product released by the adrenal medulla. It too can stimulate the heart but must reach it via the blood. See also **Epinephrine, Sympathetic nervous system.**

Nucleus: The cellular organelle, essential to cellular reproduction and protein synthesis, that contains the chromosomes and is surrounded by a membrane.

Occipital: Pertaining to the back part of the head.

Oligomenorrhea: Abnormally infrequent or scanty menstrual flow.

Organelle: A specialized part of the cell, akin to a "little organ."

Osmotic pressure: Pressure in a fluid that depends on the number of particles dissolved in that fluid.

Oxygen-carrying capacity: See **Carrying capacity**.

Oxygen cascade: Shorthand description of the progressive decreases in partial pressure of oxygen as that gas moves from outside (ambient) air into lungs (alveoli), into blood, and finally into the cells, where it is used by the mitochondria.

Oxygen content: The amount of oxygen in blood, usually defined as milliliters of oxygen in 100 milliliters of blood. When hemoglobin is fully saturated, oxygen content equals carrying capacity. But when less saturated, capacity is greater than content.

Oxygen transport system: Rather loosely used phrase that describes the process of acquisition of oxygen by breathing in, the passage of oxygen from lungs into blood, carriage of oxygen throughout the body by hemoglobin, and, finally, passage of oxygen from blood into the cells.

Oxy–hemoglobin (Hb–O_2): The combination of oxygen and hemoglobin, used to define the dissociation curve relating partial pressure of oxygen to percentage of hemoglobin saturated with oxygen.

Papilledema: Edema of the optic disc of the retina, commonly caused by increased intracranial pressure.

Parasympathetic nervous system: Part of the autonomic nervous system that slows the heart and enhances digestion.

Partial pressure: The pressure that one gas in a mixture of gases would exert if it were the only gas present. The number of molecules of a particular gas present, divided by the total number of molecules in the mixture, gives the percentage of that particular gas in the mixture. This percentage multiplied by the total pressure of the gas mixture gives the partial pressure of that particular gas. Because we know the percentage of oxygen in air (20.93 percent), if we know the barometric pressure, we can easily determine the partial pressure of oxygen at that pressure and thus at that altitude.

Passive transport: The diffusion of a substance across a cell membrane without the input of metabolic energy. See also **Active transport**.

Perfusion: Flow of blood through tissues or organs, such as the lungs.

pH: A logarithmic term used to define degree of acidity or alkalinity.

Phlebotomy: A puncture of a vein for the withdrawal of blood.

Phosphodiesterase (PDE): An enzyme that breaks down cyclic AMP (see **Adenosine monophosphate**, an important intracellular messenger).

Some vasoactive substances such as NO (see **Nitric oxide**) work by modifying PDE function.

Phosphorylation: The addition of a phosphate group to a molecule, usually supplied by ATP, to another molecule. See also **Adenosine triphosphate**.

Phrenic nerve: The motor nerve of the diaphragm. See also **Diaphragm**.

Physical activity level (PAL): The total metabolic rate divided by the basal metabolic rate; a measure of how much physical activity a person can perform without losing weight.

Plasma: Liquid portion of blood.

Plasma membrane: See **Cell membrane**.

Polycythemia: An overabundance of red blood cells.

Progesterone: A pregestational hormone that promotes the buildup of the glandular uterine lining.

Protease: An enzyme that breaks down proteins.

Pulmonary artery pressure (PAP): Blood pressure in the pulmonary arteries. Increased PAP is a hallmark of high altitude pulmonary edema (HAPE).

Pulmonary function tests (PFT): A battery of tests used to measure the physical characteristics of the lungs, the efficacy of respiratory muscles, and the physiology of air exchange. Especially useful in detecting and defining the causes of many breathing problems. See also **Vital capacity**.

Pyruvic acid: An intermediate compound in the metabolism of carbohydrate, fat, and protein.

Reactive oxygen species (ROS): Chemicals such as hydrogen peroxide, free oxygen radicals, and superoxide that are formed in cells in the process by which cells use oxygen to extract energy from nutrients in the mitochondria.

Receptor: A molecular structure on the surface of a cell that selectively binds a specific substance such as a hormone or neurotransmitter. This binding produces a particular physiological effect.

Renin: An enzyme responsible for the production of angiotensin I, the precursor of the active form, angiotensin II. See also **Angiotensin II**.

Respiration: Term commonly used to describe the process of breathing (inspiration and expiration). Sometimes used to define the entire process of getting and using oxygen. Or, more narrowly, used to refer to the consumption of oxygen and formation of carbon dioxide by cells or tissues.

Respiratory center: A collection of highly specialized cells located in the lower part of the brain (the midbrain) that controls the rate and depth of breathing in response to blood carbon dioxide and/or pH. Primarily controlled by carbon dioxide.

Respiratory equivalent, respiratory quotient (RQ), respiratory exchange ratio (RER): Carbon dioxide output divided by oxygen input.

Retina: The layers of nerve tissue, blood vessels, and receptor organs in the back of the eye.

Retinopathy, retinal hemorrhages: Abnormalities in the retina; at high altitude due to increased blood flow and high altitude retinal hemorrhages (HARH).

Ribonucleic acid (RNA): A single-stranded nucleic acid that transfers information from DNA to the protein-building system of the cell. See also **Deoxyribonucleic acid, Ribosome.**

Ribosome: A granular organelle that is the cellular site of protein synthesis.

Secretion: Formation of a substance by specialized glands. Also used to describe active transport across cell membranes.

Signs and symptoms: Signs are indications that can be seen or heard by an observer; symptoms are sensations perceived only by the affected individual. The former are objective; the latter are subjective.

Sildenafil citrate: A drug, sold as Viagra, taken orally in the treatment of erectile dysfunction. It enhances the effects of nitric oxide (NO).

Sino–atrial node (S–A node): Located in the wall of the right atrium of the heart; stimulates the heart to beat at its own intrinsic rate.

Sodium–potassium pump: A cell membrane protein that constantly pushes sodium ions out of the cell while pulling potassium ions into the cell. It is one of many "pumps" that maintain proper concentrations of ions within cells by active transport across the membrane.

Steroid hormone: Any of the various hormones with a characteristic ring structure, such as the sex hormones and cortisone, which have anti-inflammatory properties.

Stroke: Blockage of a blood vessel that supplies brain tissue, caused either by blood clot or cerebral hemorrhage; also called **cerebrovascular accident (CVA).**

Stroke volume: The amount of blood pumped out of the heart by one ventricle during one contraction. See also **Cardiac output.**

Superoxide dismutase (SOD): An enzyme that catalyzes the breakdown of superoxide and thus protects cells against oxidative damage. See also **Antioxidant.**

Sympathetic nervous system: Part of the autonomic nervous system that speeds the heart and dilates the bronchi.

Synapse: The gap across which a nerve impulse passes from one neuron (nerve cell) to another. See also **Neurotransmitter.**

Thorax: The chest wall.

Thrombosis: The formation or presence of a blood clot within a blood vessel.

Thrombus (plural thrombi): A blood clot formed within a blood vessel.

Torr: Unit of pressure. (One torr is the pressure necessary to support a column of mercury one meter high at 0° C.) See **Barometer.**

Total metabolic rate: The basal metabolic rate plus the additional energy used to power any additional physical activity. See also **Basal metabolic rate.**

Trachea: The windpipe.

Transcranial Doppler ultrasound: Use of the Doppler effect in ultrasound to study the flow of blood in the brain.

Transcription: The construction of a messenger RNA molecule from the DNA template. See also **Deoxyribonucleic acid, Ribonucleic acid.**

Transient ischemic attack (TIA): A small, "silent" stroke. See also **Stroke.**

Tricarboxylic acid cycle (TCA): The sequence of reactions in a living organism that require oxygen and store energy in phosphate bonds. Also known as **Kreb's cycle** and citric acid cycle. See also **Adenosine triphosphate.**

Tyrosine hydroxylase (TH): An enzyme involved in the production of the neurotransmitter dopamine. See also **Dopamine.**

Vascular endothelial growth factor (VEGF): A protein that promotes the growth of blood vessels.

Ventilation: Movement of air in and out of the lungs.

Ventilation–perfusion mismatch: Imbalance or inequality between alveolar ventilation and perfusion (blood flow) in areas of the lung; also called V/Q inequity.

Ventricle: A heart chamber; there are two ventricles, left and right.

Vital capacity: Volume of air breathed out in a maximal exhalation after the fullest inspiration. Timed vital capacity refers to the volume that can be exhaled in a specific time, usually thirty seconds or one minute. See also **Pulmonary function tests.**

Vitreous: Glasslike; commonly refers to the clear, colorless jelly that fills the eye. Also called vitreous humor.

VO_2 max: See **Maximal oxygen uptake.**

White matter: Brain tissue, comprising the inner portion of the cerebrum, that carries information between the nerve cells of the brain and the spinal cord. See also **Corpus callosum, Gray matter.**

SELECTED BIBLIOGRAPHY

Abelson, A. E. "Altitude and Fertility." *Human Biology* 48 (1976): 83–91.

Acosta, I. "Of some mervellous effects of the windes, which are in some partes of the Indies." In *High Altitude Physiology,* edited by J. B. West, pp. 10–15. Stroudsberg, Pa.: Hutchinson Ross, 1981.

Adnot, S., B. Raffestin, and S. Eddahibi. "NO in the Lung." *Respiration Physiology* 101 (1995): 109–20.

Alexander, J. K. "Coronary Heart Disease at Altitude." *Texas Heart Institute Journal* 21 (1994): 261–66.

———. "Coronary Problems Associated with Altitude and Air Travel." *Cardiology Clinic* 13 (1995): 271–78.

Alvarez, A. "Sleep." *The New Yorker* (1992): 85–94.

Alvarez, W. C. "The Migrainous Scotomata as Studied in 618 Persons." *American Journal of Ophthalmology* 49 (1960): 489–504.

Anand, I. S., and Y. Chandrashekhar. "Subacute Mountain Sickness Syndromes: Role of Pulmonary Hypertension." In *Hypoxia and Mountain Medicine,* edited by J. R. Sutton, G. Coates, and C. S. Houston, pp. 241–51. Burlington, Vt.: Queen City Press, 1992.

Anand, I. S., R. M. Malhotra, Y. Chandrashekhar, H. K. Bali, S. S. Chauhan, S. K. Jindal, R. K. Bhandari, and P. L. Wahi. "Adult Subacute Mountain Sickness: A Syndrome of Congestive Heart Failure in Man at Very High Altitude." *Lancet* 335, no. 8689 (1990): 561–65.

Anonymous. "La Grotte du Chien." *Bulletin dela Société Méridionale de Spéléologie et de Préhistoire* 22, nos. 93–95 (1982).

Anonymous. "The Lake Louise Consensus on the Definition and Quantification of Altitude Illness." In *Hypoxia and Mountain Medicine,* edited by J. R. Sutton, G. Coates, and C. S. Houston, pp. 327–30. Burlington, Vt.: Queen City Press, 1992.

Appenzeller, O. "Altitude Headache." *Headache* 12 (1972): 126–29.

Arias-Stella, J., and H. Kryger. "Pathology of High Altitude Pulmonary Edema." *Archives of Pathology* 76 (1963): 43–53.

Arregui, A., J. Cabrera, F. Leon-Velarde, S. Paredes, D. Viscarra, and D. Arbaiza. "High Prevalence of Migraine in a High-Altitude Population." *Neurology* 41 (1991): 1668–69.

Asahina, K., M. Ikai, Y. Ogawa, and Y. Kuorda. "A Study of Acclimatization at Altitude in Japanese Athletes." *Schweiz Z Sportsmed* 14 (1967): 240–47.

Asmussen, E., and H. Chiodi. "The Effect of Hypoxemia on Ventilation and Circulation in Man." *American Journal of Physiology* 132 (1941): 426–36.

Aste-Salazar, H., and A. Hurtado. "The Affinity of Hemoglobin for Oxygen at Sea Level and at High Altitudes." *American Journal of Physiology* 142 (1944): 733–43.

Astrand, P. O. "The Respiratory Activity in Man Exposed to Prolonged Hypoxia." *Acta Physiologica Skandinavica* 30 (1954): 343–68.

Astrup, P. "Some Physiological and Pathological Effects of Moderate Carbon Monoxide Exposure." *British Medical Journal* 4 (1972): 447–52.

Atkins, J., B. Honigman, C. S. Houston, and R. C. Roach. "Elderly Population Has Decreased AMS Incidence at Moderate Altitude (Abstract)." In *Hypoxia and Molecular Medicine,* edited by J. R. Sutton, G. Coates, and C. S. Houston, p. 293. Burlington, Vt.: Queen City Press, 1993.

Baker, P. T. "Human Adaptation to High Altitude." *Science* 163, no. 3872 (1969): 1149–56.

Balke, B., J. T. Daniels, and J. A. Faulkner. "Training for Maximum Performance at Altitude." In *Exercise at High Altitude,* edited by R. Margaria, pp. 179–86. New York: Excerpta Medica, 1967.

Balke, B., and J. G. Wells. "Ceiling Altitude Tolerance Following Physical Training and Acclimatization." *Journal of Aviation Medicine* 29 (1958): 40–47.

Banchero, N., R. F. Grover, and J. A. Will. "Oxygen Transport in the Llama (Lama Glama)." *Respiration Physiology* 13 (1971): 102–15.

Barach, A. L., R. A. McFarland, and C. P. Seitz. "The Effects of Oxygen Deprivation on Complex Mental Functions." *Journal of Aviation Space Environmental Medicine* 8 (1937): 197–207.

Barbashova, Z. I. "Studies on the Mechanisms of Resistance to Hypoxia: A Review." *International Journal of Biometeorology* 11, no. 3 (1967): 243–54.

Barcroft, J. "Mountain Sickness." *Nature* 2855, no. 114 (1924): 90–92.

———. *Respiratory Function of the Blood. Part I: Lessons from High Altitude.* New York: Cambridge University Press, 1925.

Barcroft, J., M. Camis, and C. G. Mathison. "Report of the Monte Rosa Expedition of 1911." *Philosophical Transcripts of the Royal Society of London (Series B)* 206 (1914): 49–102.

Barcroft, J., A. Cooke, H. Hartridge, T. R. Parsons, and W. Parsons. "The Flow of Oxygen through the Pulmonary Epithelium." *Journal of Physiology* 53 (1920): 450–72.

Bärtsch, P., B. Merki, B. Kayser, M. Maggiorini, and O. Oelz. "Controlled Trial of the Treatment of Acute Mountain Sickness (AMS) with a Portable Hyperbaric Chamber (Abstract)." In *Hypoxia and Mountain Medicine,* edited by J. R. Sutton, G. Coates, and C. S. Houston, pp. 73–81. Burlington, Vt.: Queen City Press, 1992.

Bärtsch, P., S. Shaw, M. Francioli, M. P. Gnadinger, and P. Weidmann. "Atrial Natriuretic Peptide in Acute Mountain Sickness." *Journal of Applied Physiology* 65 (1988): 1929–37.

Baume, Louis. *Sivalaya.* Seattle: The Mountaineers Books, 1980.

Basnyat, B., J. H. Gertsch, E. W. Johnson, F. Castro-Marin, Y. Inoue, and

C. Yeh. "Efficacy of Low-Dose Acetazolamide (125 mg BID) for the Prophylaxis of Acute Mountain Sickness: A Prospective, Double-Blind, Randomized, Placebo-Controlled Trial. *High Altitude Medicine & Biology* 4, no. 1 (2003): 45–52.

Beall, C. M., K. P. Strohl, B. Gothe, G. M. Brittenham, M. Barragan, and E. Vargas. "Respiratory and Hematological Adaptations of Young and Older Aymara Men Native to 3600 m." *American Journal of Human Biology* 4 (1992): 17–26.

Bean, W. B. "Physical and Toxic Agents." In *Pathologic Physiology,* edited by W. A. Sodeman, p. 291. Philadelphia: Saunders, 1961.

Benoit, H., M. Germain, J. C. Barthelemy, C. Denis, J. Castells, D. Dormois, J. R. Lacour, and A. Geyssant. "Pre-Acclimatization to High Altitude Using Exercise with Normobaric Hypoxic Gas Mixtures." *International Journal of Sports Medicine* 13 (1992): S213–15.

Bernardi, L. "Interval Hypoxic Training." *Advances in Experimental Medicine and Biology,* 502 (2001): 377–99.

Bernier, Francis. *Travels in the Mogul Empire.* London: Pickering, 1826.

Bernstein, M. H. "Avian Respiratory Physiology and High Altitude Performance." In *Hypoxia: The Adaptations,* edited by J. R. Sutton, G. Coates, and J. E. Remmers, pp. 30–40. Philadelphia: BC Dekker, 1990.

Bert, P. *Barometric Pressure.* Bethesda, Md.: Undersea Medical Society, 1978.

Billings, C. E., R. E. Brashears, R. Bason, and D. K. Mathews. "Medical Observations During 20 Days at 3,800 Meters." *Archives of Environmental Health* 18 (1969): 987–95.

Blaschko, H. *Mountain Sickness, Handbuch des Offentlicher Gesundheitswesens.* Berlin: Herman Eulenberg, 1882.

Bligh, J., and D. Chauca. "The Effect of Cold and Hypoxia on the Pulmonary Arterial Pressure and Its Possible Significance in the Occurrence of High Mountain Sickness." Unpublished paper, 1982.

Block, A. J., P. G. Boysen, J. W. Wynne, and L. A. Hunt. "Sleep Apnea, Hypocapnea and Oxygen Desaturation in Normal Subjects." *New England Journal of Medicine* 300, no. 10 (1979): 513–17.

Bohr, C. "The Influence of Section of the Vagus Nerve on the Disengagement of Gases in the Air Bladder of Fishes." *Journal of Physiology* 15 (1894): 494–500.

Bortz, W. M. "Disuse and Aging." *Journal of the American Medical Association* 248, no. 10 (1982): 1203–08.

Boukreev, A. *The Climb.* New York: St. Martin's Press, 1997.

Boycott, A. E., and J. S. Haldane. "The Effects of Low Atmospheric Pressures on Respiration." *Journal of Physiology* 37 (1908): 355–77.

Boyle, R. "Two New Experiments Touching the Measure of the Force of the Spring of Air Compress'd and Dilated." In *High Altitude Physiology,* edited by J. B. West, pp. 70–75. Stroudsberg, Pa.: Hutchinson Ross, 1981.

Bradwell, A. R., A. D. Wright, C. Imray, and R. Fletcher. "Progesterone in Acute Mountain Sickness." In *Hypoxia and the Brain,* edited by J. R. Sutton, C. S. Houston, and G. Coates. Burlington, Vt.: Queen City

Press, 1995.

Bradwell, A. R., A. D. Wright, M. Winterborn, and C. Imray. "Acetazol-amide and High Altitude Diseases." *International Journal of Sports Medicine* 13 (1992): S63–64.

Brendel, W., J. R. Weingart, and L. R. Haas. "Medical Statement Analysis of 3200 High-Altitude Climbers." *Medical Science and Sports Medicine* 19 (1985): 180–91.

Brooks, M. M. "Effect of Methylene Blue on Performance Efficiency at High Altitudes." *Aviation Space and Environmental Medicine* 16 (1945): 251–62.

———. "Methylene Blue, An Antidote to Altitude Sickness." *Journal of Aviation Space and Environmental Medicine* 18, no. 3 (1948): 298–99.

Broome, J. R., M. A. Stoneham, J. M. Beeley, J. S. Milledge, and A. S. Hughes. "High Altitude Headache: Treatment with Ibuprophen." *Journal of Aviation Space and Environmental Medicine* 65 (1994): 19–20.

Brown, P. "Cheyne–Stokes Respiration." *Journal of Medicine* 30 (1961): 849–60.

Campbell, E. J. "The Evolution of Oxygen." In *Hypoxia: Man at Altitude,* edited by J. R. Sutton, N. L. Jones, and C. S. Houston, pp. 2–7. New York: Thieme-Stratton, 1982.

Chang, K. C., C. G. Morrill, and H. Chai. "Impaired Response to Hypoxia After Bilateral Carotid Body Resection for Treatment of Bronchial Asthma." *Chest* 73 (1978): 667–69.

Cournand, A. "The Historical Development of the Concepts of Pulmonary Circulation." In *Pulmonary Circulation,* edited by W. R. Adams and I. Veith. New York: Grune and Stratton, 1959.

Coward, F. A. "Mountain Sickness as Observed in the Andes." *Journal of the South Carolina Medical Association* 2 (1906): 123–25.

Creel, D. J., A. S. Crandall, and M. Swartz. "Hyperopic Shift Induced By High Altitude After Radial Keratotomy." *Journal of Refractive Surgery* 13 (1997): 398–400.

Curran, Jim. *K2: The Story of the Savage Mountain.* London: Hodder and Stoughton, 1995.

———. *K2: Triumph and Tragedy.* London: Hodder and Stoughton, 1987.

Curran, W. S., and W. G. B. Graham. "Long-Term Effects of Glomectomy." *Annual Review of Respiratory Diseases* 103 (1970): 566–8.

Dent, C. T. "Can Mount Everest Be Ascended?" *The Nineteenth Century* (1892): 604–13.

Dill, David B. *Life Heat and Altitude.* Cambridge: Harvard University Press, 1938.

Dill, D. B., H. T. Edwards, A. Folling, S. A. Oberg, A. M. Pappenheimer, and J. H. Talbott. "Adaptations of the Organism to Changes in Oxygen Pressure." *Journal of Physiology* 71 (1931): 47–83.

Dobell, C. *Antony van Leeuwenhoek and His Little Animals.* New York: Harcourt Brace, 1932.

Douglas, C. G., J. S. Haldane, Y. Henderson, and E. C. Schneider. "The Physiological Effects of Low Atmospheric Pressure as Observed on

Pikes Peak, Colorado." *Proceedings of the Royal Society of London (Series B)* 85 (1912): 65–67.

Druml, W., H. Steltzer, W. Waldhausl, K. Lenz, A. Hammerle, H. Vierhapper, S. Gasic, and O. F. Wagner. "Endothelin-1 in Adult Respiratory Distress Syndrome." *Annual Review of Respiratory Diseases* 148 (1993): 1169–73.

Fagan, K. A., and J. V. Weil. "Potential Genetic Contributions to Control of the Pulmonary Circulation and Ventilation at High Altitude." *High Altitude Medicine & Biology* 2, no. 2 (2001): 165–71.

Fa-Hsien. *The Travels of Fa-Hsien (399–414 AD).* Cambridge: Cambridge University Press, 1923.

Fishman, A. P. "Pulmonary Hypertension—Beyond Vasodilator Therapy." *New England Journal of Medicine* 338, no. 5 (1998): 321–22.

Fitzgerald, M. P. "Further Observations on the Changes in the Breathing and the Blood at Various High Altitudes." *Proceedings from the Royal Society of London (Series B)* 88 (1914): 248–58.

Fitzgerald, W. G. "How High Can We Climb?" *Technical World Magazine* (December 1907): 383–91.

Fleming, D. "Galen on the Motions of the Blood in the Heart and Lungs." *Isis* 46 (1955): 13–21.

Freshfield, D. W. "The Conquest of Mount Everest." *Alpine Journal* 1 (1924): 1–11.

Fulco, C. S., P. B. Rock, S. R. Muza, E. Lammi, B. Braun, A. Cymerman, L. G. Moore, and S. F. Lewis. "Gender Alters Impact of Hypobaric Hypoxia on Adductor Pollicis Muscle Performance." *Journal of Applied Physiology* 91 (2001): 100–108.

Fulton, J. F., and L. G. Wilson. *Selected Readings in the History of Physiology,* 2d. ed. Springfield, Ill.: Charles C. Thomas, 1966.

Ge, R. L., and G. Helun. "Current Concept of Chronic Mountain Sickness: Pulmonary Hypertension–Related High-Altitude Heart Disease." *Wilderness and Environmental Medicine* 12, no. 3 (2001): 190–94.

Giaid, A., and D. Saleh. "Reduced Production of Endothelial Nitric Oxide Synthase in the Lungs of Patients with Pulmonary Hypertension." *New England Journal of Medicine* 333, no. 4 (1995): 214–21.

Gibbs-Smith, C. H. A. *A History of Flying.* New York: Praeger, 1953.

Gilbert, D. L. "The First Documented Description of Mountain Sickness: The Andean or Pariacaca Story." *Respiration Physiology* 52 (1983): 327–47.

———. "The First Documented Report of Mountain Sickness: The China or Headache Story." *Respiration Physiology* 52 (1983): 315–26.

———. *Oxygen and Living Processes.* New York: Springer-Verlag, 1981.

Gilbert, R. D., W. J. Pearce, and L. D. Longo. "Fetal Cardiac and Cerebrovascular Acclimatization Responses to High-Altitude, Long-Term Hypoxia." *High Altitude Medicine & Biology* 4, no. 2 (2003): 203-13.

Gillespie, C. *Dictionary of Scientific Biography.* 16 vols. New York: Scribners, 1980.

Gippenreiter, E. G., and J. B. West. "High Altitude Medicine and Physiology in the Former Soviet Union." *Journal of Aviation Space and Environmental Medicine* 67 (1996): 576–84.

Gordon, B. L. *Medicine Throughout Antiquity.* Philadelphia: F. A. Davis, 1949.

Gribble, Francis. *The Early Mountaineers.* London: T. Fisher Unwin, 1899.

Hackett, P. H. "Medical Research on Mt. McKinley." *Annual of Sports Medicine* 4, no. 4 (1989): 232–44.

Hackett, P. H., and D. Rennie. "High-Altitude Pulmonary Edema." *Journal of the American Medical Association* 287, no. 17 (2002): 2275–78.

Hackett, P. H., R. C. Roach, R. B. Schoene, F. Hollingshead, and W. J. Mills. "The Denali Medical Research Project, 1982–85." *American Alpine Journal* 28, no. 2 (1986): 129–37.

Hackett, P. H., R. C. Roach, R. A. Wood, R. G. Foutch, R. T. Meehan, D. Rennie, and W. J. Mills, Jr. "Dexamethasone for Prevention and Treatment of Acute Mountain Sickness." *Journal of Aviation Space and Environmental Medicine* 59 (1988): 950–54.

Hackett, P. H., P. R. Yarnell, R. Hill, K. Reynard, J. Heit, and J. McCormick. "High Altitude Cerebral Edema and MR Imaging: Clinical Correlation and Pathophysiology." *Journal of the American Medical Association* 280, no. 22 (1998): 1920–25.

Haider, M. "A History of the Moguls of Central Asia." In *The Tarikh-I-Rashida,* edited by N. Elias. Lahore, Pakistan: Book Traders, 1896.

Haldane, J. S. "Acclimatisation to High Altitudes." *Physiological Review* 7, no. 3 (1927): 363–83.

———. *Respiration.* Oxford: Clarendon Press, 1935.

Haldane, J. S., A. M. Kellas, and E. L. Kennaway. "Experiments on Acclimatisation to Reduced Atmospheric Pressure." *Journal of Physiology* 53 (1919): 181–206.

Hannon, J. P. "High Altitude Acclimatization in Women." In *The Effects of Altitude on Physical Performance,* edited by R. F. Goddard, pp. 37–44. Chicago: Athletic Institute, 1966.

Harvey, W. *De Motu Cordis.* Springfield, Ill.: Thomas, 1957.

Heath, D. *Man at High Altitude.* Edinburgh: Churchill Livingstone, 1989.

Hebbel, R. P., J. W. Eaton, R. S. Kronenberg, E. D. Zanjani, L. G. Moore, and E. M. Berger. "Human Llamas: Adaptation to Altitude in Subjects with High Hemoglobin Oxygen Affinity." *Journal of Clinical Investigation* 62 (1978): 593–600.

Hecht, H. H. "A Sea Level View of Altitude Problems." *American Journal of Medicine* 50 (1971): 703–708.

Hecht, H. H., H. Kuida, R. L. Lange, J. L. Thorne, A. M. Brown, R. Carlisle, A. Ruby, and F. Ukradyha. "Brisket Disease, II. Clinical Features and Hemodynamic Observations in Altitude-Dependent Right Heart Failure of Cattle." *American Journal of Medicine* 32 (1962): 171–83.

Henderson, Yandell. *Adventures in Respiration.* Baltimore, Md.: Williams and Wilkins, 1939.

———. "Life at Great Altitudes." *Yale Review* 3NS (1914): 759–73.

Honigman, B., M. K. Theis, J. Koziol-McLain, R. C. Roach, R. Yip, C. S. Houston, and L. G. Moore. "Acute Mountain Sickness in a General Tourist Population at Moderate Altitude." *Annals of Internal Medicine* 118, no. 8 (1993): 587–92.

Hornbein, T. F. and R. B. Schoene. "High Altitude: An Exploration of Human Adaptation." *Lung Biology in Health and Disease* 161 (2000).

Houston, C. S., and Bengt Kayser. *Proceedings of the Hypoxia Symposia 1977–1997.* Burlington, Vt: Queen City Press, 1998.

Hultgren, H. *High Altitude Medicine.* Stanford, Calif.: Hultgren, 1996.

———. "High Altitude Pulmonary Edema at a Ski Resort." *West Journal of Medicine* 164 (1996): 222–27.

———. "High Altitude Pulmonary Edema: Current Concepts." *Annual Review of Medicine* 47 (1986): 267–84.

Hultgren, H. N., and W. Spickard. "Medical Experiences in Peru." *Stanford Medical Bulletin* 18, no. 2 (1960): 76–95.

Hurtado, A. "Chronic Mountain Sickness." *Journal of the American Medical Association* 120 (1942): 1278–82.

———. *Life at High Altitudes.* Washington, D.C.: Pan American Health Organization, 1966.

———. "Studies at High Altitude. Blood Observations on the Indian Natives of the Peruvian Andes." *American Journal of Physiology* 100 (1932): 487–505.

Kamio, S., and S. Ohmori. "Hematological, Biochemical, and Immunological Study During 24 Hour Japan Mountaineering Stamina Race." *Japanese Journal of Mountain Medicine* 17 (1997): 77–82.

Karpouzis, K. M., and E. L. Spierings. "Circumstances of Onset of Chronic Headache in Patients Attending a Specialty Practice." *Headache* 39 (1999): 317-20.

Kayser, B. "Acute Mountain Sickness in Western Tourists Around the Thorong Pass (5400 m) in Nepal." *Journal of Wilderness Medicine* 2 (1991): 110–17.

Kellogg, R. H. "La Pression Barométrique: Paul Bert's Hypoxia Theory and Its Critics." *Respiration Physiology* 34 (1978): 1–28.

———. "Some High Points in Altitude Physiology." In *Environmental Stress: Individual Human Adaptations,* edited by L. J. Folinsbee, J. A. Wagner, J. F. Borgia, B. L. Drinkwater, J. A. Gliner, and J. F. Bedi, pp. 317–24. New York: Academic Press, 1978.

Keys, A. "The Physiology of Life at High Altitudes; The International High Altitude Expedition to Chile, 1935." *Scientific Monthly* 43 (1936): 289–312.

Khan, D. A., M. Aslam, and Z. U. Khan. "Changes in Plasma Electrolytes During Acclimatization at High Altitude." *Journal of the Pakistani Medical Association* 46, no. 6 (1996): 128–31.

Khoo, M. C. K., J. D. Anholm, Song-wan Ko, R. Downey, A. C. Powles, J. R. Sutton, and C. S. Houston. "Dynamics of Periodic Breathing and Arousal During Sleep at Extreme Altitude." *Respiration Physiology* 103 (1996): 33–43.

Kimmelberg, H. K. "Current Concepts of Brain Edema." *Neurosurgery Journal* 83 (1995): 1051–59.

Klausen, T., H. Christensen, J. M. Hansen, O. J. Nielsen, N. Fogh-Andersen, and N. V. Olsen. "Human Eythropoietin Response to Hypocapnic Hypoxia, Normocapnic Hypoxia and Hypocapnic Normoxia." *European Journal of Applied Physiology* 74, no. 5 (1996): 475–80.

Klausen, T., T. D. Poulsen, N. Fogh-Anderson, J. P. Richalet, and O. J. Nielsen. "Diurnal Variations of Serum Erythropoietin at Sea Level and Altitude." *European Journal of Applied Physiology and Occupational Medicine* 72, no. 4 (1996): 297–302.

Kleger, G. R., P. Bärtsch, P. Vock, L. J. Roberts, and P. E. Ballmer. "Evidence Against an Increase in Capillary Permeability in Subjects Exposed to High Altitude." *Journal of Applied Physiology* 81, no. 5 (1996): 1917–23.

Krakauer, Jon. *Into Thin Air.* New York: Villard, 1997.

Krogh, A. "The Supply of Oxygen to Tissues and the Control of Capillary Circulation." *Journal of Physiology* 52 (1919): 457–74.

Kronecker, H. "Mountain Sickness." *The Medical Magazine* 4, no. 7 (1895): 651–66.

Lafflen, D., D. Poquin, G. Savourey, P. A. Barraud, C. Raphel, and J. Bittel. "Cognitive Performance During Short Acclimation to Severe Hypoxia." *Journal of Aviation Space and Environmental Medicine* 68 (1997): 993–97.

Landon, P. *The Opening of Tibet.* New York: Doubleday, Page, 1905.

Last, H. "Empedocles and His Klepsydra Again." *Classics Quarterly* XVIII (1924): 169–73.

Lavoisier, A. *Elements of Chemistry, Book 1, Great Books Foundation.* Chicago: Henry Regnery, 1949.

Levine, B. D. "Intermittent Hypoxic Training: Fact and Fancy." *High Altitude Medicine & Biology* 3, no. 2 (2002): 177–93.

Lieberman, P., A. Protopapas, and B. G. Kanki. "Speech Production and Cognitive Deficits on Mt. Everest." *Journal of Aviation Space and Environmental Medicine* 66 (1995): 857–64.

Longstaff, T. G. "Mountain Sickness and Its Probable Causes." Doctoral thesis, Edinburgh, 1906.

Lowenstein, C. J., J. L. Dinerman, and S. H. Snyder. "Nitric Oxide, a Physiologic Messenger." *Annals of Internal Medicine* 120 (1994): 227–37.

Marx, J. L. "Neurobiology: Researchers High on Endogenous Opiates." *Science* (1976): 1227–29.

Mayow, J. "Medico–Physical Works." In *Alembic Club Reprints*, no. 17. Edinburgh: E&S Livingston, 1957.

Menon, N. D. "High Altitude Pulmonary Edema." *New England Journal of Medicine* 273, no. 2 (1965): 66–73.

Middleton, D. *Victorian Lady Travellers.* Chicago: University of Chicago Press, 1982.

Middleton, W. E. K. *The History of the Barometer.* Baltimore, Md.: Johns Hopkins University Press, 1964.

Monge, C. *Acclimatization in the Andes.* Baltimore, Md.: Johns Hopkins University Press, 1948.

Mooney, B. *Altitude-Rated Places: A Medical Atlas.* New Orleans, La.: McNaughton and Gunn, 1993.

Moore, L. G. "Fetal Growth Restriction and Maternal Oxygen Transport during High Altitude Pregnancy." *High Altitude Medicine and Biology* 4, no. 2 (2003): 141-56.

Morse, W. K. *Chinese Medicine.* New York: Hoeber, 1934.

Mosso, A. *Life of Man on the High Alps.* London: T. Fisher Unwin, 1898.

Mummery, A. *My Climbs in the Alps and Caucasus.* London: T. Fisher Unwin, 1894.

Murray, H. *Historical Account of Discoveries and Travels in Asia from the Earliest Times to the Present.* Edinburgh: Constable, 1820.

Naeje, R. "Pulmonary Circulation at High Altitude." *Respiration* 64 (1997): 429–34.

Needham, J. *Science and Civlization in China, Vol. 2: History of Scientific Thought.* New York: Cambridge University Press, 1969.

Noakes, T. D. "Hyponatremia during Endurance Running." *Medicine and Science in Sports and Exercise* 24, no. 4 (1992): 403–405.

Pearce, W. J. "Mechanisms of Hypoxic Cerebral Vasodilation." *Pharmacologic Therapeutics* 65, no. 1 (1995): 75–91.

Perkins, J. F. "Historical Development of Respiratory Physiology." In *Handbook of Physiology, Section 3, Vol. 1: Respiration,* edited by W. O. Fenn and H. Rahn, pp. 1–62. Washington, D.C.: American Physiological Society, 1964.

Pinker, S. *How the Mind Works.* New York: Norton, 1997.

Pinkerton, J. *A General Collection of the Best and Most Interesting Voyages and Travels in All Parts of the World.* London: Longman, 1808.

Poirier, J. P. *Lavoisier: Chemist, Biologist, Economist.* Philadelphia: University of Pennsylvania Press, 1996.

Pollard, A. J., S. Niermeyer, P. Barry, P. Bärtsch, F. Berghold, R. A. Bishop, C. Clarke, S. Dhillon, T. E. Dietz, A. Durmowicz, B. Durrer, M. Eldridge, P. Hackett, D. Jean, S. Kriemler, J. A. Litch, D. Murdoch, A. Nickol, J. P. Richalet, R. Roach, D. R. Shlim, U. Wiget, M. Yaron, G. Zubieta-Castillo, Sr., and G. R. Zubieta-Calleja, Jr. "Children at High Altitude: An International Consensus Statement by an Ad Hoc Committee of the International Society for Mountain Medicine, March 12, 2001." *High Altitude Medicine and Biology* 2, no. 3 (2001) 389–403.

Priestley, J. *The Discovery of Oxygen, Alembic Club Reprints No.7.* Edinburgh: E&S Livingston, 1961.

Prioreschi, P. *A History of Medicine, Vol. 3: Roman Medicine.* 1st ed. Omaha, Neb.: Horatius, 1998.

———. *A History of Medicine, Vol. 2: Greek Medicine.* 2nd ed. Omaha, Neb.: Horatius, 1996.

Pugh, G. "Cardiac Output in Muscular Exercise at 5800 m (19,000 ft)." *Journal of Applied Physiology* 19, no. 3 (1964): 441–47.

Ravenhill, T. H. "Some Experiences of Mountain Sickness in the Andes."

Journal of Tropical Medicine and Hygiene 16, no. 20 (1913): 313–20.

Reeves, J. T., and R. F. Grover. *Attitudes on Altitude: Pioneers in Medical Research on Colorado's High Mountains.* Boulder, Colo.: University Press of Colorado, 2001.

Renniek, I. D. B. "See Nuptse and Die." *Lancet* II (1976): 1177–79.

Richalet, J.P. "High Altitude Pulmonary Edema: Still a Place For Controversy?" *Thorax* 50 (1995): 923–29.

Roach, R.C., and P. H. Hackett. "Frontiers of Hypoxia Research: Acute Mountain Sickness." *The Journal of Experimental Biology* 204 (2001): 3161–70.

Roach, R. C., C. S. Houston, B. Honigman, R. A. Nicholas, M. Yaron, C. K. Grissom, J. K. Alexander, and H. N. Hultgren. "How Well Do Older Persons Tolerate Moderate Altitude?" *Western Journal of Medicine* 162 (1995): 32–36.

Samaja, M. "Blood Gas Transport at High Altitude." *Respiration* 64 (1997): 895–99.

Sandoval, D. A., and K. S. Matt. "Effects of the Oral Contraceptive Pill Cycle on Physiological Responses to Hypoxic Exercise." *High Altitude Medicine & Biology* 4, no. 1 (2003): 61–72.

Sartori C., Y. Allemann, H. Duplain, M. Lepori, M. Egli, E. Lipp, D. Huter, P. Turini, O. Hugli, S. Cook, P. Nicod, and U. Scherer. "Salmeterol for the Prevention of High-Altitude Pulmonary Edema." *New England Journal of Medicine* 346 (2002): 1631–36.

Saussure, H.-B. de. In *A General Collection of the Best and Most Interesting Voyages and Discoveries in All Parts of the World,* edited by J. Pinkerton. London: Longman, 1813.

Scherrer, U., L. Vollenweider, A. Delabays, M. Savcic, U. Eichenberger, C. R. Kleger, A. Fikrle, P. E. Ballmer, and P. Bärtsch. "Inhaled Nitric Oxide for High-Altitude Pulmonary Edema." *New England Journal of Medicine* 334, no. 10 (1996): 624–29.

Schirlo, C., V. Pavlicek, A. Jacomet, J. S. R. Gibbs, E. Koller, O. Oelz, M. Seebauer, and J. Kohl. "Characteristics of the Ventilatory Response in Subjects Susceptible to High Altitude Pulmonary Edema During Acute and Prolonged Hypoxia." *High Altitude Medicine and Biology 3,* no. 3 (2002): 267–76.

Schoene, R. B. "Control of Breathing at High Altitude." *Respiration* 64 (1997): 407–15.

Serebrovskaya, T. V. "Intermittent Hypoxia Research in the Former Soviet Union and the Commonwealth of Independent States: History and Review of the Concept and Selected Applications." *High Altitude Medicine & Biology* 3, no. 2 (2002): 205–21.

Severinghaus, J. W. "Sightings." *High Altitude Medicine & Biology* 2, no. 2 (2001): 135–140.

———. "Sightings." *High Altitude Medicine & Biology* 3, no. 2 (2002): 149–55.

———. "Sightings." *High Altitude Medicine & Biology* 3, no. 3 (2002): 257–63.

Shlim, D. R., and J. Gallie. "The Causes of Death Among Trekkers in Nepal." *International Journal of Sports Medicine* no. 13, suppl. 1 (1992): S74–S75.

Singh, I. "High Altitude Pulmonary Edema." *Lancet* 1 (1965): 229–232.

Singh, I., P. K. Khana, M. C. Srivistava, M. Lal, S. B. Roy, and C. S. Subramanyam. "Acute Mountain Sickness." *New England Journal of Medicine* 280 (1969): 175–184.

Soutiere, S. E., and C. G. Tankersley. "Challenges Implicit to Gene Discovery Research in the Control of Ventilation during Hypoxia." *High Altitude Medicine and Biology* 2, no. 2 (2001): 191–200.

Speer, S. T. *On the Physiological Phenomena of Mountain Sickness.* London: T. Richards, 1853.

Spierings E. L. "Mechanism of Migraine and Action of Antimigraine Medications." *Medical Clinics of North America* 85 (2001): 943–58.

Stager, C. "Killer Lake." *National Geographic* (September 1987): 404–20.

Stamler, J. S., L. Jia, J. P. Eu, T. J. McMahon, I. T. Demchenko, J. Bonaventura, K. Gernert, and C. A. Piantadosi. "Blood Flow Regulation by S-Nitrosohemoglobin in the Physiological Oxygen Gradient." *Science* 276 (1997): 2034–36.

Stickney, E. J., and J. C. Van Liere. *Anoxia: Its Effects on the Body.* Chicago: University of Chicago Press, 1962.

Stray-Gundersen, J., R. F. Chapman, and B. D. Levine. "'Living High— Training Low': Altitude Training Improves Sea Level Performance in Male and Female Elite Runners." *Journal of Applied Physiology* 91 (2001): 1113–20.

Swenson, E. R., M. Maggiorini, S. Mongovin, J. S. R. Gibbs, I. Greve, H. Mairbäurl, and P. Bärtsch. "Pathogenesis of High-Altitude Pulmonary Edema: Inflammation Is Not an Etiologic Factor." *Journal of the American Medical Association* 287, no. 4 (2002): 2228–36.

Tate, R. M., and T. L. Petty. "Primary Pulmonary Edema (ARDS)." *Annual Review of Medicine* (1984): 471–93.

Torricelli, E. "Torricelli's Letters on the Pressure of the Atmosphere." In *High Altitude Physiology,* edited by J. B. West, pp. 60–63. Stroudsberg, Pa.: Hutchinson Ross, 1981.

Torrington, K. G. "Recurrent High Altitude Illness Associated with Right Pulmonary Artery Occlusion from Granulomatous Mediastinitis." *Chest* 96, no. 6 (1989): 1422–24.

Tschop, M., C. J. Strasburger, G. Hartmann, J. Biollaz, and P. Bärtsch. "Raised Leptin Concentrations at High Altitude Associated with Loss of Appetite." *Lancet* 352 (1998): 1119–20.

Tschudi, J. J. *Travels in Peru.* London: David Bogue, 1847.

Utiger, D., U. Eichenberger, D. Bernasch, R. W. Baumgartner, and P. Bärtsch. "Transient Minor Improvement of High Altitude Headache by Sumatriptan." *High Altitude Medicine and Biology* 3, no. 4 (2002): 387–93.

Vitzthum, V. J., and A. S. Wiley. "The Proximate Determinants of Fertility in Populations Exposed to Chronic Hypoxia." *High Altitude Medicine and Biology* 4, no. 2 (2003): 125–39.

Voelkel, N. "Appetite Suppressants and Pulmonary Hypertension." *Thorax* no. 52, suppl. 3 (1997): S63–S67.

Walsh, M. N., and W. M. Boothby. "The Demonstration of Air Bubbles in the Spinal Fluid under Atmospheric Pressures Produced in a Low Pressure Chamber Simulating Those Obtaining During Rapid Ascents in Airplanes." *Proceedings of the Staff Meetings of the Mayo Clinic* 16, no. 15 (1941): 225–28.

Ward, M. P., J. S. Milledge, and J. B. West. *High Altitude Medicine and Physiology.* London: Chapman and Hall, 1995.

West, J. B. "Alexander M. Kellas and the Physiological Challenge of Mt. Everest." *Journal of Applied Physiology* 63, no. 1 (1987): 3–11.

———. "Book Review." *High Altitude Medicine and Biology* 3, no. 2 (2002): 243–44.

———. "Commuting to High Altitude: Value of Oxygen Enrichment of Room Air." *High Altitude Medicine & Biology* 3, no. 2 (2002): 223–35.

———. *Everest: The Testing Place.* New York: McGraw Hill, 1985.

———. *High Altitude Physiology.* Stroudsburg, Pa.: Hutchinson Ross, 1981.

———. *High Life: A History of High-Altitude Physiology and Medicine.* New York: Oxford University Press, 1998.

———. "Oxygen Enrichment of Room Air to Relieve Hypoxia of High Altitude." *Respiration Physiology* 99 (1995): 225–32.

Wilson, L. G. "Erasistratus, Galen, and the Pneuma." *Bulletin of the History of Medicine* 33, no. 4 (1959): 295–314.

———. "The Transformation of Ancient Concepts of Respiration in the Seventeenth Century." *Isis* 51, no. 3 (1960): 161–72.

Woods, D. R., and H. E. Montgomery. "Angiotensin-Converting Enzyme and Genetics at High Altitude." *High Altitude Medicine and Biology* 2, no. 2 (2001): 201–10.

Woodworth, J. A. "Brief Notes and Bibliography of History of Mountain Medicine." *Appalachia* (1976): 81–93.

Workman, W. H. "Some Altitude Effects at Camps Above 20,000 feet." *Appalachia* 13 (1908): 350–59.

Yaron M., S. Niermeyer, K. N. Lindgren, B. Honigman, J. D. Strain, and C. B. Cairns. "Physiologic Response to Moderate Altitude Exposure among Infants and Young Children." *High Altitude Medicine and Biology* 4, no. 1 (2003): 53–59.

Zanger, T. "The Danger of Railway Trips to High Altitudes for Elderly People." *Lancet* (June 20, 1903): 1730–35.

Zuntz, N., A. Loewy, F. Muller, and W. Caspari. *High Altitude Climates and Walking in the Mountains.* Berlin: Bong, 1906.

APPENDIX: HISTORICAL FIGURES IN ALTITUDE PHYSIOLOGY

Trying to discover who did what, and when, is one of the most fascinating aspects of research. The deeper you dig, the further you look, the more likely you are to find unsung heroes—people whose work precedes, often by many years, that of those now better known. Fame often seems to be capricious in its choice of whom to anoint. Often those whose names have endured are those who have sifted the work of others and put together many pieces to make something new and important. Most of us are able to reach however high we do because we stand on the shoulders of those who have gone before.

Here are noted the names and brief biographies of some well-known and some obscure persons whose intuition, labor, courage, genius, or ability to bring together the observations of others enabled them to expand our knowledge and our skills. Only a few are here: Most of those in our century have been omitted, and regretfully many others have been left out. Certainly there are many others who are no longer remembered at all.

Fabricius ab Aquapendente (1537–1619). This Italian surgeon (usually called Hieronymus) is best known for his outstanding studies of anatomy and embryology. He succeeded his teacher Gabriel Fallopius as professor of surgery at the University of Padua, and his fame spread throughout Europe. Among his many works is a description of the valves in veins, which permit blood to flow in only one direction. This observation, along with a beautiful engraved illustration, was picked up by William Harvey as an essential part of his description of the circulation of the blood twenty years after he had studied under Fabricius ab Aquapendente.

Anaxagoras (500–428 B.C.). One of the philosophers during the Golden Age of Pericles in Athens, Anaxagoras built on the principles advanced by Empedocles, holding that matter was infinitely divisible, and that all things were held together in an apparently uniform and motionless form. He wrote only one important paper and has not had much permanent impact.

Aristotle (384–322 B.C.). Of all the great philosopher–scientists in the Golden Age of Greece, Aristotle is one of the best known. His scientific concepts were based on logic: He believed the universe to be finite and centered around Earth. Outside of his universe there could be nothing; inside of it there could be no emptiness, i.e., no vacuum. He believed in the four basic elements of fire, air, water, and earth as defined by Empedocles, but rejected the latter's atomic theory. Some consider Aristotle the founder of anatomy because of his studies of the heart and circulatory system. He believed that the pulsation of the heart was due to "boiling" of the blood, which then flowed to the lungs to be cooled. Because of the way he prepared his animals for study, he did not recognize that there were four rather than three chambers in the heart, nor did he distinguish between arteries and veins or recognize the existence of the heart valves. His influence on all of the sciences endured for a thousand years, being challenged successfully only during the Renaissance.

Baliani, Giovanni Batista (1582–1666). Although trained in the law and following the career of a public servant, the Italian Baliani was a gifted and imaginative amateur in physics, whose correspondence with Galileo in 1630 explained why lift pumps and siphons were limited in the height at which they could function. Baliani's concept of atmospheric pressure was correct but rejected by Galileo, but not by Evangelista Torricelli, after Gaspar Berti described his first barometer.

Barcroft, Joseph (1872–1947). Together with Paul Bert, Bruce Dill, and John S. Haldane, Barcroft is one of the figures most closely associated with studies of high altitude. Born in England, he graduated with a doctorate in physiology from Kings College, Cambridge, and remained there as professor of physiology until his death. For some years he studied glands of internal secretion with Ernest Starling, and for a time with Haldane, soon developing better techniques for measuring gas exchanges. After several discouraging years studying the oxy–hemoglobin dissociation curve (the relationship between oxygen partial pressure and the fraction of hemoglobin that has bound oxygen), Barcroft was the first to show how the concentration of different salts, temperature, and acidity affected the shape of the curve. Brought up as a Quaker, he disagreed with the pacifist stand the group took during World War I, and served with distinction in the medical corps. Experience with troops gassed with chlorine led him to study respiratory physiology, revisiting the question of oxygen secretion in the lungs, about which he disagreed with Haldane. He soon became interested in altitude sickness and made several mountain expeditions, for which he is best known among altitude specialists today. He also showed that the spleen serves as a reservoir for blood, releasing a significant amount when needed (such as following bleeding) to restore circulating volume.

Beeckman, Isaac (1588–1637). Primarily interested in physics, mechanics, and meteorology, Beeckman was a progressive and influential Dutch thinker much concerned with teaching physics and mathematics to the common man. He believed that the universe was infinite, he subscribed to the atomic theory, and he came close to understanding the circulation of the blood. He challenged convention by proclaiming that air had weight, and seems to have understood how pumps worked, and perhaps accepted the possibility that a vacuum could exist.

Bernard, Claude (1813–1878). Although Bernard became one of the best-known French physiologists, he was an average student, passing examinations only with difficulty. Fortunately, he came under the influence of some of the great physicians of his time, fell in love with physiological experimentation rather than medical practice, and received many honors for his studies of digestive enzymes, liver function, and the autonomic nervous system. He was a great experimenter, and as his studies advanced, his horizons widened and the concept of the constancy of the internal environment became central to most of his experiments and writing. Apparently he was the first to recognize that carbon monoxide kills by replacing oxygen on hemoglobin in red blood cells, and he was a pioneer in the study of both toxic and beneficial medications. His great contribution was the principle of homeostasis—the tendency of organisms to maintain their internal stability.

Bert, Paul (1833–1886). Truly the father of altitude physiology, Bert was also a zoologist, physiologist, and pioneer in transplant surgery, and his textbooks on natural history, zoology, and the physical sciences were widely printed and translated. His countryman Claude Bernard had the greatest influence on Bert's career, and was largely responsible for his major work on barometric pressure. Although less well known than his work at high altitude, his studies of hemoglobin and how it combines with oxygen were even more important, as they explained how oxygen is carried to the tissues from the lungs. Deeply saddened by the death from acute hypoxia of two of his young colleagues during the flight of the balloon *Zenith,* he gave up research. He then became more active and prominent in French politics, and was appointed governor general of Indo-China, where he died soon after.

Berti, Gaspar (1600–1643). Although this Italian professor of mathematics was primarily interested in astronomy and physics, his major contribution to science was construction of the apparatus that led to the modern barometer, which he built sometime between 1640 and his death in 1643. None of Berti's own writing has survived, and what we know of his work comes from secondary sources. At first he could not believe that a vacuum existed above the water column in his crude barometer because the sound of a bell could be heard ringing in the space, but his friend and biographer Emmanuel Maignan showed him that the sound was transmitted by a metal arm holding the bell! Berti described the device to Evangelista Torricelli, who made it practical.

Black, Joseph (1728–1799). In addition to having a busy and distinguished medical practice in Edinburgh, Black was a brilliant and popular chemistry teacher, lecturing without notes, demonstrating his experiments with unfailing success, and attracting students from all over the world. His experimental methods were very precise, and he was the first to describe the qualities of carbon dioxide, which he called "fixed air" and recognized as a product of animal metabolism. His experiments with heat were even more important. Black recognized that air was necessary for all forms of combustion, was quite ambiguous in his treatment of the phlogiston theory, and, after Antoine-Laurent Lavoisier's work was known, gradually abandoned the phlogiston theory.

Boerhaave, Hermann (1668–1738). Holding three of the five professorships in the medical school at Leiden in the Netherlands, Boerhaave was one of the great teachers of his time, attracting students from all over Europe. He not only lectured for four or five hours a day, he was also a brilliant bedside teacher and established the modern system of history, physical examination, diagnosis, course of illness, and outcome. He did not have a clear concept of red blood cells, and his somewhat ambivalent interest in alchemy is indicative of the confusion that still existed in science in Europe during that time. With extraordinary patience, he studied the possibility of transmutation of elements; for example, distilling a portion of mercury 500 times, shaking a sample of mercury continuously for eight and a half months and then distilling it repeatedly, and even boiling one sample of mercury for fifteen and a half years.

Borrichius (Borch), Olaus (1626–1690). Ole Borch, a Dane, studied medicine first but became better known as a professor of botany and chemistry. He had a large and busy medical practice and wrote extensively about a wide variety of subjects. In one of his many experiments, in 1678 he decomposed potassium nitrate to generate oxygen, but, like many others before him, did not realize the importance of what he had done.

Boyle, Robert (1627–1691). Born in Ireland, Boyle achieved major influence through his extraordinary work in philosophy, chemistry, and physics and as a founder of and principal influence in the Royal Society of London. Of his wide interests, his best-known work concerned the physics of air. By 1650 he had heard of Otto von Guericke's air pump, adopted an improved design by Robert Hooke, and confirmed the observations of Evangelista Torricelli and Gaspar Berti. He demonstrated that sound could not be transmitted in a vacuum. Throughout his life, Boyle studied the behavior of gases, the vacuum, and the properties of matter. He supported the concept of atomic structure of all matter, although he used the less specific term "corpuscle." He was a great experimenter, and described all of his experiments in immense detail so that others might repeat them.

Cesalpino, Andrea (1519–1603). Cesalpino was an Italian philosopher and physician, a follower of Aristotle, and a pioneer in the study of circulation. He realized that the heart pumped blood throughout the body through the arteries, and received blood from the veins. He described the valves of the heart and pulmonary vessels, although he failed to put together a coherent picture of circulation as William Harvey later did.

Dalton, John (1766–1844). Son of an English Quaker weaver, Dalton was entirely self-educated in physics and chemistry. After several stints of teaching in small schools and giving private lessons, he was drawn to examine the properties of gases and liquids, specifically of atmospheric humidity and rain. He kept meticulous daily meteorological records, and after five years published his first description of the individual properties of each gas in a mixture of several gases. After some controversy, this was formulated as Dalton's law of partial pressures and became fundamental to all studies of atmosphere and physiology.

Empedocles (490–430 B.C.). This early Greek philosopher originated the four-element theory of matter, believing that earth, water, air, and fire were the "roots of all things" and that there were two forces—love and hate—that moved humankind. He believed that animals developed both by chance and by natural selection, and Darwin quoted his work as cited by Aristotle. Only a few of his writings have survived, and most are overlaid with legend. He is said to have stopped an epidemic by diverting two rivers, to have changed the climate in a valley by building a wall across a gorge, and to have revived a woman who had been without pulse or respiration for thirty days. His alleged fatal leap into the volcanic crater of Etna may be myth, or—impelled by belief in his immortality—a fatal prank!

Galen (129–199). Few physicians have more profoundly influenced medicine than did this Roman who served as physician to the gladiators after completing twelve years of medical studies. He believed in a "fourfold scheme" that included the four humors of the body, the four elements, the four seasons, the ages of man, and other factors in a harmonious whole. His greatest work was titled *Anatomical Procedures* but was based on observation rather than dissection. He accepted the view of Erasistratus that blood entered the right ventricle from the right atrium (which received blood from the veins) and was prevented from returning by the tricuspid valve. From the right ventricle it went to the lungs by the pulmonary artery and nourished the lungs. He felt that the heart worked like a bellows, actively dilating and passively contracting. He showed that the heart and vessels always contained blood, while Erasistratus had thought that sometimes they could contain air. Galen is best known for his immense pharmacopeia, which dictated medical treatment for many centuries.

Galilei, Galileo (1564–1642). His is one of the most famous names in mathematics, physics, and astronomy. This Italian was a firm supporter of Copernicus, and for this he was examined by the Inquisition and condemned to prison, but the sentence was commuted to house arrest for life. His most famous studies were made possible by the thirty-power telescope he developed in 1609, and he is best known for his work in astronomy and in the motions of falling bodies. Galileo treated the existence of a vacuum in a curious way. Having been told that suction pumps and siphons could not lift water beyond a certain height, he explained this with the theory that water had its own inner limited tensile strength, just as a rope or wire will break of its own weight if it's long enough. He failed to understand that the weight of the atmosphere was the cause of the siphon phenomenon, and rejected it even after Giovanni Baliani had clearly explained it to him.

Guericke, Otto von (1602–1686). Born in Hamburg, he was destined for politics and studied law, but was attracted by the concept of space and soon became a convert of Copernicus. He wondered about the possibility of a vacuum, how heavenly bodies might affect each other across the emptiness of space, and whether space was indeed bounded or limitless. In 1647 he made the first functioning suction pump and ten years later constructed the famous Magdeburg Sphere, which consisted of two hemispheres made of heavy copper, fitted tightly together with a gasket, and then evacuated. Teams of horses could not pull the hemispheres apart until a valve was opened, which convincingly demonstrated the pressure of the atmosphere.

Hales, Stephen (1677–1761). Born to an old and distinguished English family, Hales took a general education at Cambridge, where he was strongly influenced by Issac Newton's heritage and by the distinguished scholar William Stukeley. Throughout his life he was a clergyman. Although he had no formal medical training, his curiosity and ingenuity led him into pioneering studies of blood pressure and circulation, for which he was made a member of the Royal Society. At the time, the magnitude of the arterial blood pressure was unknown, with some contending that it was very large and might actually power muscle contraction. Hales's simple measurement of the arterial blood pressure in a mare ensured him permanent fame, and led him to further studies of the heart, the veins and capillaries, and the mechanics of blood flow. He was very versatile, and his most original—though less known—work involved the force that could raise the sap in plants and trees, often to great heights. He demonstrated transpiration, showing that leaves give off not only moisture but also tiny bubbles of gas. This led him to study the gas laws and the composition of air as defined by Robert Hooke, John Mayow, and Robert Boyle. He repeated Mayow's experiments, placing either a candle or a small animal under a bell jar and demonstrating that some element in air was consumed before the candle was extinguished or the animal died. Taking this a bit further in a series of rebreathing experiments on himself, he showed that some element of air was consumed and another gas produced by the body, which would not support life. This convinced him that "fresh air" was essential to health and led him to invent ventilators for purifying the air in hospitals and on shipboard, a major advance in public health.

Harvey, William (1578–1657). After undergraduate studies at Cambridge, Harvey left England to complete his medical degree under some of the great anatomists in Italy. Upon returning to London, he became a distinguished physician and an important influence in the Royal College of Physicians, doing his historic work on circulation in his free time. He had broad interests and a wide circle of friends outside of the sciences, and was untiring in his studies of the entire animal world, though he is best known for his "discovery" of the action of the heart and circulation. Most of his papers on other areas of natural history were lost in the Great Fire of London. Though Harvey followed Aristotle rather than Galen, his unique contribution came from his ability to put together many theories and observations of others and his own dissections and calculations to produce the first complete and accurate explanation of the coursing of blood through arteries, veins, and capillaries, impelled by the heart as a pump. Many others had accurately described parts of the system—Galen's concept of the greater circulation was one bit, and Renaldo Colombo's description of the circulation through the lungs another, but Harvey was the first to make a coherent description of the whole. The logical steps through which he reached his conclusions are fascinatingly detailed in his great book *De Motu Cordis,* a first edition of which is said to be the most expensive book in the world!

Hooke, Robert (1635–1702). Although described as sickly all of his life, Hooke was a precocious genius whose talents included mathematics, mechanics, and physiology. Before he was eighteen he had mastered geometry and playing the organ, and described thirty ways of flying; he then entered Oxford, where he was befriended by some of the most brilliant men of his time. As assistant to Robert Boyle, he built an improved version of Otto von Guericke's air pump, and undoubtedly contributed importantly to formulating Boyle's famous gas laws. By 1660 he had invented a method for using a spring instead of a pendulum to drive a clock, and actually drew up a patent for this, although Christian Huygens built the first spring watch in 1674. He was made a member of the Royal Society, becoming curator responsible for several new scientific demonstrations for each weekly meeting. He published his most important book, *Micrographia,* in 1665, containing hundreds of observations made through a beautiful microscope that he had specially made to his specifications. Less well known are Hooke's studies of air, combustion, and respiration. He showed that the function of breathing was to supply fresh air to the lungs rather than to cool or to pump blood and, along with John Mayow, Robert Boyle, and Richard Lower, came close to isolating oxygen. He was a tireless inventor, producing brilliant and innovative ideas and a variety of scientific instruments. He was described by his contemporaries as a difficult man in an age of difficult men whose life was punctuated by bitter quarrels that refused to be settled.

Ibn-al-Nafis (circa 1208–1288). Only in the last thirty-five years has the work of this great Egyptian physician been rediscovered, and even today his contributions to medicine are inadequately recognized. In his early thirties he planned a comprehensive 300-volume medical text of which 80 volumes were published. Primarily a surgeon, he defined three stages for each operation: diagnosis, during which a patient entrusts the surgeon with his life; the operation; and, finally, postoperative care. His most extraordinary contribution was his description of the pulmonary circulation in 1242, centuries before Michael Servetus, Renaldo Colombo, and William Harvey. He wrote:

> This is the right cavity of the two cavities of the heart. When the blood in this cavity has become thin, it must be transferred into the left cavity, where the pneuma is generated. But there is no passage between these two cavities, the substance of the heart there being impermeable. It neither contains a visible passage, as some people have thought, nor does it contain an invisible passage which would permit the passage of blood, as Galen thought. The pores of the heart there are compact and the substance of the heart is thick. It must, therefore, be that when the blood has become thin, it is passed into the arterial vein (pulmonary artery) to the lung, in order to be dispersed inside the substance of the lung, and to mix with the air. The finest parts of the blood are then strained, passing into the venous artery (pulmonary vein) reaching the left of the two cavities of the heart, after mixing with the air and becoming fit for the generation of pneuma....

It is said that his religion and compassion prevented him from dissection, which might have led him to an accurate definition of the total circulation. Whether or not reports of his work reached and influenced his successors is hotly debated today.

Lavoisier, Antoine-Laurent (1743–1794). Although best known for his studies of oxygen (and he is sometimes credited with having been the first to make it), this Parisian was a distinguished chemist, geologist, and social reformer as well, and it was indeed his activity as a humanitarian and reformer that led to his execution during the Reign of Terror in the French Revolution. In his mid-twenties he first became interested in the properties of air, which led in 1775 to his "discovery" of oxygen, some two years after he had received a letter from Carl Wilhelm Scheele describing how to make that gas. Stephen Hales, Joseph Black, Joseph Priestley, and others were also studying the atmosphere, and although Lavoisier at first knew little of their work, he recognized the significance of Priestley's work as soon as he learned of it. His own description of oxygen, its preparation, and its properties was published in 1775, a few weeks after Priestley's.

In 1782–83, following some leads from Henry Cavendish and Priestley, Lavoisier showed that water was not a simple material but a combination of "inflammable air" (hydrogen) and "dephlogistigated air" (oxygen). He immediately understood the importance of the Montgolfier balloon ascents in 1783, and during the next two years made a number of hydrogen balloons that rose even better, but his interest in balloons was soon displaced by work on his monumental chemistry textbook, completed only shortly before his death on the guillotine.

Lower, Richard (1631–1691). Lower became one of the most distinguished practitioners of medicine in London and was also recognized as among the finest English physiologists after William Harvey. He became interested in the attempts by Christopher Wren to infuse blood and medication directly into veins, and performed the first successful blood transfusion between dogs in 1665, and between humans in 1667. These studies led to extensive work in cardiopulmonary physiology, and in 1669 he published definitive experiments showing that dark red venous blood became bright red during its passage through the lungs. Thus he rounded out Harvey's work and laid the basis for much of what would follow.

Malpighi, Marcello (1628–1694). Italian-born Malpighi received his doctorates in medicine and philosophy at the age of twenty-five, and has since been known as the father of microscopic anatomy, although he also practiced medicine throughout his life. Giovanni Borelli, a distinguished naturalist, was his lifelong friend, and stimulated his interest in the physiology of plants and animals. He was the first Italian to be elected to the Royal Society of London, and in 1669 was made an honorary member. Malpighi acquired one of the new microscopes made by Robert Hooke, with which he examined capillary blood flow. This enabled him to show the connections between arteries and veins in the lung, providing the linkage that William Harvey had not been able to make decades before. He founded the study of histology.

Mayow, John (1643–1679). Born in London and educated at Oxford, Mayow accomplished a great deal in his short life. By the age of twenty-seven he had published two important books on respiration. His studies of the "nitro-aerial spirit" did more than those by others to show that something in air was necessary for, and consumed by, both living animals and a burning candle. He perceived too that a gas (which, a century later, was identified as oxygen) entered the blood through the lungs. Some consider Mayow the most important investigator in the distinguished English group that made such advances in the seventeenth century.

Mosso, Angelo (1846–1910). At twenty-four Mosso graduated summa cum laude from the University of Turin medical school in Italy and studied physiology under several distinguished scientists, becoming professor of physiology in 1879 at Turin. His Institute of Physiology established a station in the Alps to study human physiology at high altitude in 1895. Some of his most important work was the invention of scientific instruments, notably a plethysmograph for measuring blood flow and pressure, and an ergograph for measuring muscle activity and fatigue. In 1904 he developed locomotor ataxia and was forced to give up his physiological and political activities, but turned to archaeology, where he made equally noteworthy contributions.

Paracelsus, Theophrastus (1493–1541). The real name of this extraordinary Swiss was von Hohenheim. Where or even whether he took formal medical training is unknown, but he did serve as a military surgeon, and he understood that most diseases were of external origin, describing silicosis and tuberculosis as occupational diseases, and recognizing for the first time that syphilis could be congenital. He understood and used the anesthetic and sedative qualities of certain volatile liquids similar to ether, and used mercury and other chemicals as medications. He was a great and pioneering physician, an able chemist, and uncompromisingly destructive toward tradition.

Pascal, Blaise (1623–1662). Born in France and brought up and educated by his father, a widower, young Pascal became interested in mathematics and physics, and before he was twenty published several new mathematical concepts. He invented and built a mechanical device to do simple addition and subtraction, which enjoyed limited success. By 1646 he had repeated Gaspar Berti's experiment and was corresponding with Torricelli about barometers, and expanded the study to prove that a vacuum was possible. After being caught up in the controversy over his alleged role in Florin Perier's demonstration that barometric pressure decreases as altitude increases, he returned to mathematics and published more books and papers, for which he is best known.

Priestley, Joseph (1733–1804). Because he was born in England and educated for the ministry, it is not surprising that Priestley's initial writings were theological discussions of the nature of matter. They aroused great controversy, but throughout all of his work runs a vein of religious conviction that occasionally confuses or obscures his great original contributions.

He began to study gases at the age of thirty-seven and became one of the outstanding gas chemists of the world, making many new gases, such as ammonia and sulfur and nitrogen, and of course working on oxygen. He seems to have cultivated the role of poor scientist, in contrast to Antoine-Laurent Lavoisier, with whom his competitive rivalry sharpened with time. In 1770 he began publication of a series of six important books on gases that were widely studied and influential, and showed the strong influence of Stephen Hales. Priestley's major clash with Lavoisier came over the latter's demonstration of the composition of water and his claim for priority in discovering oxygen. Priestley clung to the phlogiston theory even after his voluntary exile to Pennsylvania because of his support of the French Revolution. His demonstration that green plants can convert carbon dioxide to oxygen was beautifully designed and explained why atmospheric oxygen was not wholly consumed by combustion and life on earth.

Ravenhill, Thomas (1882–1952). This Englishman is best known for his work as physician to a mining company in the Andes, where he saw and described three forms of mountain sickness. He served as surgeon in some of the worst action of World War I and was so physically and mentally broken by his experiences that he never returned to medicine. His single publication (1908) is comprehensive and accurate, and after long obscurity has become widely known and cited. Ravenhill became a well-known artist after that war.

Saussure, Horace-Benedict de (1740–1799). Although de Saussure is best known for his interest in Mont Blanc, his degree in philosophy from Geneva was in physics, and he was a distinguished mathematician, botanist, and geologist as well. This Frenchman made studies of the transmission of heat and cold, electricity, and magnetism on Mont Blanc, and observed his own pulse and respiration on all his mountain ascents. His extensive studies of geology, meteorology, and physiology were published in his four-volume work *Voyages dans les Alpes,* a collector's item until reprinted recently. In 1760 he made his first visit to Chamonix and became passionately interested in Mont Blanc, and the reward that he offered to the person who would reach the summit first undoubtedly hastened the ascent.

Scheele, Carl Wilhelm (1742–1786). Born, educated, and living his entire life in Sweden, Scheele was primarily a pharmacist and chemist whose ingenuity, curiosity, and persistence made him one of the most distinguished scientists of his time. Before he was twenty years old, he challenged the phlogiston theory and undertook a series of experiments on plants and animals that convinced him that life was supported by some element in air that was converted in the animal to a gas that would not support life. Although he took voluminous notes, he was slow to publish, and his notebooks have only recently been deciphered. On September 30, 1774, he wrote to thank Antoine-Laurent Lavoisier for one of the latter's books and in his letter gave detailed instructions on how to prepare oxygen, together with basic information on its chemical and physiological properties—the earliest-known written description of oxygen. Scheele knew that some English scientist was following similar studies, and sent to the printer in December 1775 a manuscript in which he described the preparation of oxygen, which would support combustion, and of nitrogen, which would not. Publication was delayed for various reasons, and by the time his book appeared, in July 1777, others had published, and credit for Scheele's discoveries went to them. He did important work in both organic and inorganic chemistry, but is almost unknown for his most important contribution.

Servetus, Michael (1511–1553). Servetus was born and first educated in philosophy in Spain, where his religious studies raised in him doubts about the Holy Trinity that made him a fugitive and later led to his execution. He went to France and studied law, where he published his most heretical work, for which he was most criticized. He became a proofreader for a publisher, and this aroused his interest in medicine, which he studied in Paris and later practiced. His most important book was a theological text, important mainly because in one section of it he describes the circulation of the blood from the heart through the pulmonary artery to the lungs and back to the heart. Servetus understood that some "vital spirit" entered the lungs, passed into the blood, and was carried back to the heart and throughout the body. He was on the threshold of comprehending the circulation of the blood, but his text was primarily a religious one, and all but three copies were destroyed when he was burned at the stake for heresy, seventy-five years before Harvey's announcement.

Stahl, Georg Ernst (1660–1734). Allegedly intolerant and narrow-minded, and undoubtedly controversial, Stahl was an outstanding and active German physician and academician, a chemist, and a natural philosopher. He devoted much of his attention to distinguishing between the living and the nonliving and the anima that separates them. He preached preventive medicine and felt that doctors had to deal with the entire body and mind rather than individual organs. Strongly influenced by the chemist J. I. Becher, Stahl apparently originated the name "phlogiston" to define combustibility. Although he recognized that phlogiston and air were related, he believed that phlogiston was an element rather than a quality, and considered carbon as almost pure phlogiston. Although the phlogiston theory was wrong, it stimulated much of the essential study that was to follow in the next century.

Starling, Ernest (1866–1927). Born in Jamaica, part of the British Commonwealth, Starling made major contributions to human physiology. He pioneered modern understanding of fluid balance between the blood and interstitial (tissue) fluids, and factors that impact the contractile force of the heart. His hypotheses are the basis of what we understand about edema. He coined the word "hormone" for substances that are secreted by what we know as glands of internal secretion and carried throughout the body to affect functions. During his studies of poison gas in World War I, he prepared functioning heart-lung organs, and from these derived his "Law of the Heart" describing how the amount of blood that the heart pumps is determined by the amount of blood that flows into it.

Sylvius, aka Franciscus de la Boe (1614–1672). Born in the Netherlands, this physician–anatomist's work helped to change the reliance of medicine from mystical speculation to a rational application of basic chemical and physical laws. Sylvius believed that the important processes of life and of illness occur in the blood, and therefore diseases could be treated chemically. He was a distinguished influential professor and was ahead of his time in understanding the process of respiration.

Torricelli, Evangelista (1608–1647). This Italian physicist and mathematician is memorialized in the term "torr," which is commonly used as a measure of barometric pressure. Whether he influenced Gaspar Berti's great experiment is unclear, but once he learned of it, he had the wit to see its importance and to use mercury in place of water, thereby making the first true barometer.

Vesalius, Andreas (1514–1564). Born in Brussels, Vesalius revolutionized medicine by the dissections he made on hundreds of human cadavers and by publishing the first textbook of anatomy. These studies and his public lectures led him to challenge many of Galen's conclusions as based on animal rather than human observations. These, plus beautiful engravings of parts of the human anatomy in his textbook, make him the father of human anatomy. Vesalius's demonstration of the valves in human veins predated Harvey by twenty years, and Harvey may have studied under him in Padua. His textbook was so well done and became so influential that Vesalius was appointed to the court of Philip II, King of Spain.

INDEX

ABOUT THE AUTHORS

An M.D., scientist, mountaineer, and teacher, **Charles S. Houston** is one of the leading authorities on high-altitude medicine. He began climbing in 1925, organized a British–American expedition to Nanda Devi in 1936, and led expeditions that almost climbed K2 in 1938 and 1953. He began his study of the effects of high altitude as a naval flight surgeon during World War II, and in the mid-1940s directed Operation Everest—an acclimatization study that used a decompression chamber to simulate an altitude of 29,000 feet. From 1967 to 1975 he directed high-altitude studies in the Canadian Yukon, and in 1985 was the principal investigator for Operation Everest II.

As an internist, he practiced general medicine and later taught medicine at the University of Vermont (until 1979). Dr. Houston believes strongly that medical knowledge can be made accessible and interesting to the general public. He has written almost a hundred scientific papers, coauthored four books, and written extensively for mountaineering journals. He lives in Burlington, Vermont, and has three children and six grandchildren. His wife of fifty-eight years died recently.

David E. Harris developed an interest in pulmonary and cardiovascular physiology while working as a nurse anesthetist at Johns Hopkins Hospital in the 1980s. He received his doctorate in physiology from the University of Vermont College of Medicine in 1990 and is currently an associate professor at Lewiston-Auburn College, University of Southern Maine, where he teaches anatomy and physiology and researches the impact of heart disease prevention programs. Dr. Harris has published articles in peer-reviewed journals on a wide range of topics, including physiology, disease prevention, education, and natural history. A climber of no renown, little ability, but boundless enthusiasm, David currently lives in Maine with his wife Barbara, an avid sea kayaker, and a menagerie of animals too numerous to mention.

A science writer and editor, **Ellen J. Zeman** received her doctorate in chemistry from Northwestern University in 1987. Dr. Zeman has written for and edited scientific and medical journals, magazines, encyclopedias, and reference books covering many fields—from solid-state electronics to cardiology—and especially enjoys bringing complex or obscure subjects to life for a general audience. She has served on the staff of several peer-reviewed journals and was technical editor of the *Encyclopedia of Sports Science* and the *Macmillan Encyclopedia of Energy*. Ellen lives with her family in Burlington, Vermont, and enjoys hiking and skiing the gentle Green Mountains.

Contact Information:
Charles S. Houston
77 Ledge Road
Burlington, VT 05401
(802) 863-6441

David E. Harris
24 Woodline Ave.
Lisbon Falls, ME 04252

Ellen J. Zeman
111 Rivermount Terrace
Burlington, VT 05401
ezeman@adelphia.net

OTHER TITLES YOU MIGHT ENJOY FROM
THE MOUNTAINEERS BOOKS

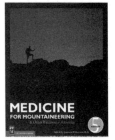
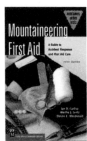
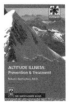
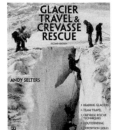
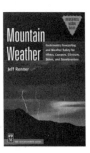